# HESI A2
# Full Study Guide

Smart Edition Media
36 Gorham Street
Suite 1
Cambridge, MA 02138
800-496-5994

Email: info@smarteditionmedia.com

Library of Congress Cataloging-in-Publication Data
Smart Edition Media.
HESI: Full Study Guide, Test Strategies and Secrets/Smart Edition Media.

ISBN: 978-1-949147-09-4, 1st edition

1. HESI.
2. Study Guides.
3. Health Education Systems Incorporated
4. Nursing
5. Careers

**Disclaimer:**

The opinions expressed in this publication are the sole works of Smart Edition Media and were created independently from any National Evaluation Systems or other testing affiliates. Between the time of publication and printing, specific standards as well as testing formats and website information may change that are not included in part or in whole within this product. Smart Edition Media develops sample test questions, and they reflect similar content as on real tests; however, they are not former tests. Smart Edition Media assembles content that aligns with exam standards but makes no claims nor guarantees candidates a passing score.

**Printed in the United States of America**

HESI: Full Study Guide, Test Strategies and Secrets/Smart Edition Media. ISBN: 978-1-949147-09-4

# HESI A2 PRACTICE ONLINE

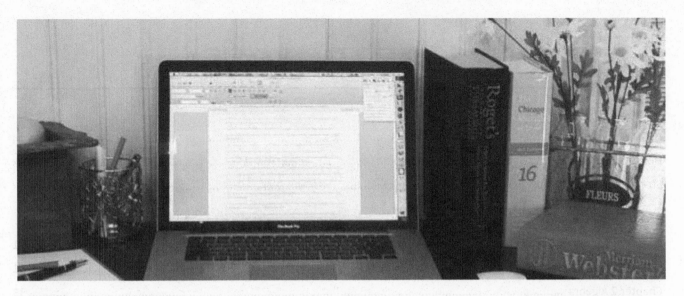

Smart Edition Media's Online Learning Resources allow you the flexibility to study for your exam on your own schedule and are the perfect companion to help you reach your goals! You can access online content with an Internet connection from any computer, laptop, or mobile device.

## Online Learning Resources

Designed to enable you to master the content in quick bursts of focused learning, these tools cover a complete range of subjects, including:

- English Language Arts
- Reading
- Math
- Science
- Writing

Our online resources are filled with test-taking tips and strategies, important facts, and practice problems that mirror questions on the exam.

## Online Sample Tests & Flashcards

Access additional full-length practice tests online!

Use these tests as a diagnostic tool to determine areas of strength and weakness before embarking on your study program or to assess mastery of skills once you have completed your studies.

**FLASHCARDS**  **GAMES**  **QUIZZES**  **TESTS**

Go to the URL: **https://smarteditionmedia.com/pages/hesi-online-resources** and follow the password/login instructions.

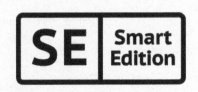

# TABLE OF CONTENTS

# INTRODUCTION

## HESI OVERVIEW

The HESI Admissions Assessment Exam or HESI A2, is an exam that is often selected by nursing schools and programs during the application process as a requirement for admission. The test is taken by prospective students in order to assess their skills and abilities in areas such as English, Math, and Science.

There are other tests that are similar to the HESI exam, some of which may be required by your nursing program of choice. In addition, there are a total of 10 sections of the HESI exam that can be taken. Since every school utilizes the HESI differently, score requirements will also vary. Be sure to contact your school for their exact exam requirements before you begin the admissions process.

Entrance exams, like the HESI, help school administrators determine how a student is likely to perform in nursing school based on how well they perform on the test. Studies have also shown that entrance exam results are linked to how well students perform during their first year in nursing school, as well as measure their outcome for success and completion of the nursing program. These tests also act as a preparation for the Registered Nurse licensure exam, the NCLEX, after graduation. The HESI specifically aims to prepare students for taking the NCLEX exam.

## ABOUT THIS BOOK

This book provides you with an accurate and complete representation of The HESI Admissions Assessment Exam (HESI) and includes the core sections found on the exam: Math, Vocabulary and general knowledge, Reading Comprehension, Grammar, Chemistry, Biology, Physics, Anatomy & Physiology.

The reviews in this book are designed to provide the information and strategies you need to do well on all of these sections of the exam. The two full-length practice tests in the book are based on the HESI and contain questions similar to those you can expect to encounter on the official test. A detailed answer key follows each practice quiz and test. These answer keys provide explanations designed to help you completely understand the test material. Each explanation references the book chapter to allow you to go back to that section for additional review, if necessary.

## ONLINE SAMPLE TESTS

The purchase of this book grants you access to three additional full-length practice tests online. You can locate these exams on the Smart Edition Media website.

Go to the URL: **https://smarteditionmedia.com/pages/hesi-online-resources** and follow the password/login instructions.

# HESI Basics

## Test dates

- The test may be offered every few weeks.

- Check with you nursing school/program on when/if they administer the test

## How to register for the HESI exam

- Go to the EVOLVE main website and choose *I'm a Student*

- Choose *Register for Distance Testing* → *Register* → *Redeem/Checkout*

- You will then make an Evolve account, read registered user agreement, Choose *Yes, I accept, SUBMIT*

- Once you have registered, you will be able to access *My Content* under the *HESI Assessment Student Access* link

- Select *Payments:* Here you will be able to choose test date and location

- Follow the prompts and *Proceed to Checkout*

**Price:** $35-70. The cost will vary among the school/testing center administering the test

## Where do I take the test?

- The test is administered by many nursing schools or community colleges.

- May be able to take it at a testing center

- Check with your school/program of choice for available dates and locations

- Many schools/programs will offer the test in accordance to the application due dates.

## How long is the test?

- The time of the test will vary based on how many sections you are required to take.

- 4 hours is the allotted time for the entire test

- Must be completed in one testing session

- Arrive 30 minutes early to allow for check-in

## What subjects are on the test?

- Test subjects and admission criteria will vary amongst programs. Check with your nursing school/program about which section they require.

- *Test subjects may include: Math, Vocabulary and general knowledge, Reading Comprehension, Grammar, Chemistry, Biology, Physics, Anatomy & Physiology*

- Your school may also require a *Learning Style/Personality Profile* exam

**How many questions are on the test?** This will vary according to test subjects required

**How long does it take to get the test score?** You will receive your score immediately once you have completed the exam

**What if I fail the test?** You may be able to retake the test; however, the test is only offered.

- Check with your program/school for their requirements on retesting

- There may be a waiting period for retaking the test

## How long are scores valid?

- Check with your nursing program for this information

**What to bring/not bring to the test?**

Bring:

- Government Issued Photo ID (Driver's license, Passport, Green card)

- Receipt of payment of the test OR payment for test (if not paid for in advance)

- Login information (Username and Password)

    - You will need to create an account when registering for the test.

Do not bring

- Books or study material

- Calculator (one will be provided to you)

- Electronics of any kind (cell/smart phone, digital/smart watches, beepers/pagers, tablet)

- Food or Drink

# HESI VS NCLEX…WHAT'S THE DIFFERENCE?

Upon finishing nursing school, all students must sit for the nursing licensure exam, NCLEX, in order to become a registered nurse (RN) and to become licensed to practice nursing in your state.

The HESI is known to be a predictor or practice exam to prepare students for the NCLEX. Schools may require HESI for entrance into the nursing program but may also be used as a mid-curricular exam (to see how well a student is being prepared), or an exit exam (at the end of nursing school, to identify their preparedness to take the NCLEX).

Some schools may require the HESI exit exam in order to graduate. Just remember, all school are different and have different requirements when it comes to the HESI. But, if you do have to take it, consider yourself lucky as you will be adequately prepared when you sit for the NCLEX.

In conclusion, in order to become a licensed RN, everyone MUST take the NCLEX. The HESI is generally only required as either an entrance exam into nursing school or an exit exam.

Schools that require the HESI will vary.

# HOW TO USE THIS BOOK

Studies show that most people begin preparing for college-entry exams approximately 8 weeks before their test date. If you are scheduled to take your test in sooner than 8 weeks, do not despair! Smart Edition Media has designed this study guide to be flexible to allow you to concentrate on areas where you need the most support.

Whether you have 8 weeks to study—or much less than that—we urge you to take advantage of our online diagnostic tests to determine areas of strength and weakness, if you have not done so already. The diagnostic tests are arranged by subject area and can be found online at **www.smarteditionmedia.com**.

Once you have completed the online diagnostic tests, use this information to help you create a study plan that suits your individual study habits and time frame. If you are short on time, look at your diagnostic test results to determine which subject matter could use the most attention and focus the majority of your efforts on those areas. While this study guide is organized to follow the order of the actual test, you are not required to complete the book from beginning to end, in that exact order.

# HOW THIS BOOK IS ORGANIZED

Take a look at the Table of Contents. Notice that each **Section** in the study guide corresponds to a subtest of the exam. These sections are broken into **Chapters** that identify the major content categories of the exam.

Each chapter is further divided into individual **Lessons** that address the specific content and objectives required to pass the exam. Some lessons contain embedded example questions to assess your comprehension of the content "in the moment." All lessons contain a bulleted list called **"Let's Review."** Use this list to refresh your memory before taking a practice quiz, test, or the actual exam. A **Practice Quiz**, designed to check your progress as you move through the content, follows each chapter.

Whether you plan on working through the study guide from cover to cover, or selecting specific sections to review, each chapter of this book can be completed in one sitting. If you must end your study session before finishing a chapter, try to complete your current lesson in order to maximize comprehension and retention of the material.

# STUDY STRATEGIES AND TIPS

## MAKE STUDY SESSIONS A PRIORITY.

- Use a calendar to schedule your study sessions. Set aside a dedicated amount of time each day/week for studying. While it may seem difficult to manage, given your other responsibilities, remember that in order to reach your goals, it is crucial to dedicate the time now to prepare for this test. A satisfactory score on your exam is the key to unlocking a multitude of opportunities for your future success.

- Do you work? Have children? Other obligations? Be sure to take these into account when creating your schedule. Work around them to ensure that your scheduled study sessions can be free of distractions.

---

**TIPS FOR FINDING TIME TO STUDY.**

Wake up 1-2 hours before your family for some quiet time

Study 1-2 hours before bedtime and after everything has quieted down

Utilize weekends for longer study periods

Hire a babysitter to watch children

---

## TAKE PRACTICE TESTS

- Smart Edition Media offers practice tests, both online and in print. Take as many as you can to help be prepared. This will eliminate any surprises you may encounter during the exam.

## KNOW YOUR LEARNING STYLE

- Identify your strengths and weaknesses as a student. All students are different and everyone has a different learning style. Do not compare yourself to others.

- Howard Gardner, a developmental psychologist at Harvard University, has studied the ways in which people learn new information. He has identified seven distinct intelligences. According to his theory:

"we are all able to know the world through language, logical-mathematical analysis, spatial representation, musical thinking, the use of the body to solve problems or to make things, an understanding of other individuals, and an understanding of ourselves. Where individuals differ is in the strength of these intelligences—the so-called profile of intelligences—and in the ways in which such intelligences are invoked and combined to carry out different tasks, solve diverse problems, and progress in various domains."

- Knowing your learning style can help you to tailor your studying efforts to suit your natural strengths.

- What ways help you learn best? Videos? Reading textbooks? Find the best way for you to study and learn/review the material

---

**WHAT IS YOUR LEARNING STYLE?**

**Visual-Spatial** – Do you like to draw, do jigsaw puzzles, read maps, daydream? Creating drawings, graphic organizers, or watching videos might be useful for you.

**Bodily-Kinesthetic** – Do you like movement, making things, physical activity? Do you communicate well through body language, or like to be taught through physical activity? Hands-on learning, acting out, role playing are tools you might try.

**Musical** – Do you show sensitivity to rhythm and sound? If you love music, and are also sensitive to sounds in your environments, it might be beneficial to study with music in the background. You can turn lessons into lyrics or speak rhythmically to aid in content retention.

**Interpersonal** – Do you have many friends, empathy for others, street smarts, and interact well with others? You might learn best in a group setting. Form a study group with other students who are preparing for the same exam. Technology makes it easy to connect, if you are unable to meet in person, teleconferencing or video chats are useful tools to aid interpersonal learners in connecting with others.

**Intrapersonal** – Do you prefer to work alone rather than in a group? Are you in tune with your inner feelings, follow your intuition and possess a strong will, confidence and opinions? Independent study and introspection will be ideal for you. Reading books, using creative materials, keeping a diary of your progress will be helpful. Intrapersonal learners are the most independent of the learners.

**Linguistic** – Do you use words effectively, have highly developed auditory skills and often think in words? Do you like reading, playing word games, making up poetry or stories? Learning tools such as computers, games, multimedia will be beneficial to your studies.

**Logical-Mathematical** – Do you think conceptually, abstractly, and are able to see and explore patterns and relationships? Try exploring subject matter through logic games, experiments and puzzles.

---

### CREATE THE OPTIMAL STUDY ENVIRONMENT

- Some people enjoy listening to soft background music when they study. (Instrumental music is a good choice.) Others need to have a silent space in order to concentrate. Which do you prefer? Either way, it is best to create an environment that is free of distractions for your study sessions.

- Have study guide – Will travel! Leave your house: Daily routines and chores can be distractions. Check out your local library, a coffee shop, or other quiet space to remove yourself from distractions and daunting household tasks will compete for your attention.

- Create a Technology Free Zone. Silence the ringer on your cell phone and place it out of reach to prevent surfing the Web, social media interactions, and email/texting exchanges. Turn off the television, radio, or other devices while you study.

- Are you comfy? Find a comfortable, but not *too* comfortable, place to study. Sit at a desk or table in a straight, upright chair. Avoid sitting on the couch, a bed, or in front of the TV. Wear clothing that is not binding and restricting.

- Keep your area organized. Have all the materials you need available and ready: Smart Edition study guide, computer, notebook, pen, calculator, and pencil/eraser. Use a desk lamp or overhead light that provides ample lighting to prevent eye-strain and fatigue.

### HEALTHY BODY, HEALTHY MIND

- Consider these words of wisdom from Buddha, "To keep the body in good health is a duty—otherwise we shall not be able to keep our mind strong and clear."

> **KEYS TO CREATING A HEALTHY BODY AND MIND:**
>
> Drink water – Stay hydrated! Limit drinks with excessive sugar or caffeine.
>
> Eat natural foods – Make smart food choices and avoid greasy, fatty, sugary foods.
>
> Think positively – You can do this! Do not doubt yourself, and trust in the process.
>
> Exercise daily – If you have a workout routine, stick to it! If you are more sedentary, now is a great time to begin! Try yoga or a low-impact sport. Simply walking at a brisk pace will help to get your heart rate going.
>
> Sleep well – Getting a good night's sleep is important, but too few of us actually make it a priority. Aim to get eight hours of uninterrupted sleep in order to maximize your mental focus, memory, learning, and physical wellbeing.

### FINAL THOUGHTS

- Remember to relax and take breaks during study sessions.

- Review the testing material. Go over topics you already know for a refresher.

- Focus more time on less familiar subjects.

# EXAM PREPARATION

In addition to studying for your upcoming exam, it is important to keep in mind that you need to prepare your mind and body as well. When preparing to take an exam as a whole, not just studying, taking practice exams, and reviewing math rules, it is critical to prepare your body in order to be mentally and physically ready. Often, your success rate will be much higher when you are *fully* ready.

Here are some tips to keep in mind when preparing for your exam:

### SEVERAL WEEKS/DAYS BEFORE THE EXAM

- Get a full night of sleep, approximately 8 hours

- Turn off electronics before bed

- Exercise regularly

- Eat a healthy balanced diet, include fruits and vegetable

- Drink water

## THE NIGHT BEFORE

- Eat a good dinner

- Pack materials/bag, healthy snacks, and water

- Gather materials needed for test: your ID and receipt of test. You do not want to be scrambling the morning of the exam. If you are unsure of what to bring with you, check with your testing center or test administrator.

- Map the location of test center, identify how you will be getting there (driving, public transportation, uber, etc.), when you need to leave, and parking options.

- Lay your clothes out. Wear comfortable clothes and shoes, do not wear items that are too hot/cold

- Allow minimum of ~8 hours of sleep

- Avoid coffee and alcohol

- Do not take any medications or drugs to help you sleep

- Set alarm

## THE DAY OF THE EXAM

- Wake up early, allow ample time to do all the things you need to do and for travel

- Eat a healthy, well-rounded breakfast

- Drink water

- Leave early and arrive early, leave time for any traffic or any other unforeseeable circumstances

- Arrive early and check in for exam. This will give you enough time to relax, take off coat, and become comfortable with your surroundings.

Take a deep breath, get ready, go! You got this!

# SECTION I
# MATHEMATICS

# Math: 50 questions, 50 minutes

**Areas assessed:** Numbers, Basic Operations, Measurement, and Algebra.

**MATH TIPS**

- Read the questions thoroughly and slowly. Reread if necessary. The order/value they are expecting may be different that you are anticipating.

- Brush up on decimals, ratios, fractions, PEMDAS, percentages.

- Know addition, subtraction, multiplication, division problems.

- Be sure to know how to add, subtract, multiply, and divide fractions.

- Brush up on common math rules. i.e. when adding a fraction, they must have same common denominator.

- You will be able to use a calculator. It will be provided by the testing center.

# Chapter 1 Numbers, Basic Operations, and Measurement

## Basic Addition and Subtraction

This lesson introduces the concept of numbers and their symbolic and graphical representations. It also describes how to add and subtract whole numbers.

## Numbers

A **number** is a way to quantify a set of entities that share some characteristic. For example, a fruit basket might contain nine pieces of fruit. More specifically, it might contain three apples, two oranges, and four bananas. Note that a number is a quantity, but a **numeral** is the symbol that represents the number: 8 means the number eight, for instance.

Although number representations vary, the most common is **base 10.** In base-10 format, each **digit** (or individual numeral) in a number is a quantity based on a multiple of 10. The base-10 system designates 0 through 9 as the numerals for zero through nine, respectively, and combines them to represent larger numbers. Thus, after counting from 1 to 9, the next number uses an additional digit: 10. That number means 1 group of 10 ones plus 0 additional ones. After 99, another digit is necessary, this time representing a hundred (10 sets of 10). This process of adding digits can go on indefinitely to express increasingly large numbers. For whole numbers, the rightmost digit is the

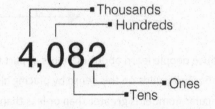

ones place, the next digit to its left is the tens place, the next is the hundreds place, then the thousands place, and so on.

Classifying numbers can be convenient. The chart below lists a few common number sets.

| Sets of Numbers | Members | Remarks |
| --- | --- | --- |
| **Natural numbers** | 1, 2, 3, 4, 5,... | The "counting" numbers |
| **Whole numbers** | 0, 1, 2, 3, 4,... | The natural numbers plus 0 |
| **Integers** | ..., −3, −2, −1, 0, 1, 2, 3,... | The whole numbers plus all negative whole numbers |
| **Real numbers** | All numbers | The integers plus all fraction/decimal numbers in between |
| **Rational numbers** | All real numbers that can be expressed as $p/q$, where $p$ and $q$ are integers and $q$ is nonzero | The natural numbers, whole numbers, and integers are all rational numbers |
| **Irrational numbers** | All real numbers that are not rational | The rational and irrational numbers together constitute the entire set of real numbers |

## Example

**Jane has 4 pennies, 3 dimes, and 7 dollars. How many cents does she have?**

A.  347

B.  437

C.  734

D.  743

The correct answer is **C.** The correct solution is 734. A penny is 1 cent. A dime (10 pennies) is 10 cents, and a dollar (100 pennies) is 100 cents. Place the digits in base-10 format: 7 hundreds, 3 tens, 4 ones, or 734. **See Lesson: Basic Addition and Subtraction.**

# The Number Line

The **number line** is a model that illustrates the relationships among numbers. The complete number line is infinite and includes every real number—both positive and negative. A ruler, for example, is a portion of a number line that assigns a **unit** (such as inches or centimeters) to each number. Typically, number lines depict smaller numbers to the left and larger numbers to the right. For example, a portion of the number line centered on 0 might look like the following:

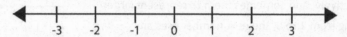

Because people learn about numbers in part through counting, they have a basic sense of how to order them. The number line builds on this sense by placing all the numbers (at least conceptually) from least to greatest. Whether a particular number is greater than or less than another is determined by comparing their relative positions. One number is greater than another if it is farther right on the number line. Likewise, a number is less than another if it is farther left on the number line. Symbolically, < means "is less than" and > means "is greater than." For example, 5 > 1 and 9 < 25.

## Example

**Place the following numbers in order from greatest to least: 5, –12, 0.**

A.  0, 5, –12

B.  –12, 5, 0

C.  5, 0, –12

D.  –12, 0, 5

**BE CAREFUL!**
When ordering negative numbers, think of the number line. Although –10 > –2 may seem correct, it is incorrect. Because –10 is to the left of –2 on the number line, –10 < –2.

The correct answer is **C.** The correct solution is 5, 0, –

12. Use the number line to order the numbers. Note that the question says *from greatest to least*. **See Lesson: Basic Addition and Subtraction.**

2

# Addition

**Addition** is the process of combining two or more numbers. For example, one set has 4 members and another set has 5 members. To combine the sets and find out how many members are in the new set, add 4 and 5 to get the **sum.** Symbolically, the expression is 4 + 5, where + is the **plus sign.** Pictorially, it might look like the following:

$$\begin{matrix} \circ\ \circ \\ \circ\ \circ \end{matrix} \quad + \quad \begin{matrix} \circ\ \circ \\ \circ\ \circ\ \circ \end{matrix} \quad = \quad \begin{matrix} \circ\ \circ\ \circ\ \circ \\ \circ\ \circ\ \circ\ \circ\ \circ \end{matrix}$$

To get the sum, combine the two sets of circles and then count them. The result is 9.

> **KEY POINT**
>
> The order of the numbers is irrelevant when adding.

Another way to look at addition involves the number line. When adding 4 + 5, for example, start at 4 on the number line and take 5 steps to the right. The stopping point will be 9, which is the sum.

Counting little pictures or using the number line works for small numbers, but it becomes unwieldy for large ones—even numbers such as 24 and 37 would be difficult to add quickly and accurately. A simple algorithm enables much faster addition of large numbers. It works with two or more numbers.

> **STEP BY STEP**
>
> **Step 1.** Stack the numbers, vertically aligning the digits for each place.
>
> **Step 2.** Draw a plus sign (+) to the left of the bottom number and draw a horizontal line below the last number.
>
> **Step 3.** Add the digits in the ones place.
>
> **Step 4.** If the sum from Step 3 is less than 10, write it in the same column below the horizontal line. Otherwise, write the first (ones) digit below the line, then **carry** the second (tens) digit to the top of the next column.
>
> **Step 5.** Going from right to left, repeat Steps 3–4 for the other places.
>
> **Step 6.** If applicable, write the remaining carry digit as the leftmost digit in the sum.

## Example

**Evaluate the expression 154 + 98.**

A. 250

B. 252

C. 352

D. 15,498

The correct answer is **B**. The correct solution is 252. Carefully follow the addition algorithm (see below). The process involves carrying a digit twice. **See Lesson: Basic Addition and Subtraction.**

$$
\begin{array}{r} 154 \\ + 98 \\ \hline \end{array}
\rightarrow
\begin{array}{r} \overset{1}{1}54 \\ + 98 \\ \hline 2 \end{array}
\rightarrow
\begin{array}{r} \overset{11}{1}54 \\ + 98 \\ \hline 52 \end{array}
\rightarrow
\begin{array}{r} \overset{11}{1}54 \\ + 98 \\ \hline 252 \end{array}
$$

# Subtraction

**Subtraction** is the inverse (opposite) of addition. Instead of representing the sum of numbers, it represents the difference between them. For example, given a set containing 15 members, subtracting 3 of those members yields a **difference** of 12. Using the **minus sign,** the expression for this operation is $15 - 3 = 12$. As with addition, two approaches are counting pictures and using the number line. The first case might involve drawing 15 circles and then crossing off 3 of them; the difference is the number of remaining circles (12). To use the number line, begin at 15 and move left 3 steps to reach 12.

Again, these approaches are unwieldy for large numbers, but the subtraction algorithm eases evaluation by hand. This algorithm is only practical for two numbers at a time.

---

**STEP BY STEP**

**Step 1.** Stack the numbers, vertically aligning the digits in each place. Put the number you are subtracting *from* on top.

**Step 2.** Draw a minus sign (–) to the left of the bottom number and draw a horizontal line below the stack of numbers.

**Step 3.** Start at the ones place. If the digit at the top is larger than the digit below it, write the difference under the line. Otherwise, **borrow** from the top digit in the next-higher place by crossing it off, subtracting 1 from it, and writing the difference above it. Then add 10 to the digit in the ones place and perform the subtraction as normal.

**Step 4.** Going from right to left, repeat Step 3 for the rest of the places. If borrowing was necessary, make sure to use the new digit in each place, not the original one.

---

When adding or subtracting with negative numbers, the following rules are helpful. Note that $x$ and $y$ are used as placeholders for any real number.

$$x + (-y) = x - y$$

$$-x - y = -(x + y)$$

$$(-x) + (-y) = -(x + y)$$

$$x - y = -(y - x)$$

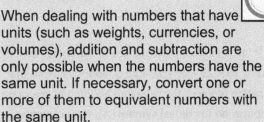

**BE CAREFUL!**

When dealing with numbers that have units (such as weights, currencies, or volumes), addition and subtraction are only possible when the numbers have the same unit. If necessary, convert one or more of them to equivalent numbers with the same unit.

## Example

**Kevin has 120 minutes to complete an exam. If he has already used 43, how many minutes does he have left?**

A. 43

B. 77

C. 87

D. 163

The correct answer is **B.** The correct solution is 77. The first step is to convert this problem to a math expression. The goal is to find the difference between how many minutes Kevin has for the exam and how many he has left after 43 minutes have elapsed. The expression would be 120 – 43. Carefully follow the subtraction algorithm (see below). The process will involve borrowing a digit twice. **See Lesson: Basic Addition and Subtraction.**

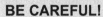

$$
\begin{array}{r} 120 \\ -\ 43 \\ \hline \end{array}
\longrightarrow
\begin{array}{r} {}^{1\,10}1\cancel{2}0 \\ -\ 43 \\ \hline 7 \end{array}
\longrightarrow
\begin{array}{r} {}^{0\ 1110}\cancel{1}\cancel{2}0 \\ -\ 43 \\ \hline 77 \end{array}
$$

## Let's Review!

- Numbers are positive and negative quantities and often appear in base-10 format.
- The number line illustrates the ordering of numbers.
- Addition is the combination of numbers. It can be performed by counting objects or pictures, moving on the number line, or using the addition algorithm.
- Subtraction is finding the difference between numbers. Like addition, it can be performed by counting, moving on the number line, or using the subtraction algorithm.

# MULTIPLICATION AND DIVISION

This lesson describes the process of multiplying and dividing numbers and introduces the order of operations, which governs how to evaluate expressions containing multiple arithmetic operations.

## Multiplication

Addition can be tedious if it involves multiple instances of the same numbers. For example, evaluating 29 + 29 is easy, but evaluating 29 + 29 + 29 + 29 + 29 is laborious. Note that this example contains five instances—or multiples—of 29. **Multiplication** replaces the repeated addition of the same number with a single, more concise operation. Using the **multiplication (or times) symbol** ($\times$), the expression is

$29 + 29 + 29 + 29 + 29 = 5 \times 29$

The expression contains 5 multiples of 29. These numbers are the **factors** of multiplication. The result is called the **product.** In this case, addition shows that the product is 145. As with the other arithmetic operations, multiplication is easy for small numbers. Below is the multiplication table for whole numbers up to 12.

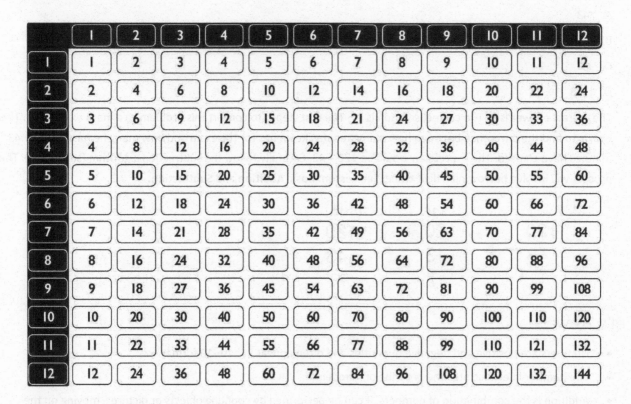

| | 1 | 2 | 3 | 4 | 5 | 6 | 7 | 8 | 9 | 10 | 11 | 12 |
|---|---|---|---|---|---|---|---|---|---|---|---|---|
| **1** | 1 | 2 | 3 | 4 | 5 | 6 | 7 | 8 | 9 | 10 | 11 | 12 |
| **2** | 2 | 4 | 6 | 8 | 10 | 12 | 14 | 16 | 18 | 20 | 22 | 24 |
| **3** | 3 | 6 | 9 | 12 | 15 | 18 | 21 | 24 | 27 | 30 | 33 | 36 |
| **4** | 4 | 8 | 12 | 16 | 20 | 24 | 28 | 32 | 36 | 40 | 44 | 48 |
| **5** | 5 | 10 | 15 | 20 | 25 | 30 | 35 | 40 | 45 | 50 | 55 | 60 |
| **6** | 6 | 12 | 18 | 24 | 30 | 36 | 42 | 48 | 54 | 60 | 66 | 72 |
| **7** | 7 | 14 | 21 | 28 | 35 | 42 | 49 | 56 | 63 | 70 | 77 | 84 |
| **8** | 8 | 16 | 24 | 32 | 40 | 48 | 56 | 64 | 72 | 80 | 88 | 96 |
| **9** | 9 | 18 | 27 | 36 | 45 | 54 | 63 | 72 | 81 | 90 | 99 | 108 |
| **10** | 10 | 20 | 30 | 40 | 50 | 60 | 70 | 80 | 90 | 100 | 110 | 120 |
| **11** | 11 | 22 | 33 | 44 | 55 | 66 | 77 | 88 | 99 | 110 | 121 | 132 |
| **12** | 12 | 24 | 36 | 48 | 60 | 72 | 84 | 96 | 108 | 120 | 132 | 144 |

When dealing with large numbers, the multiplication algorithm is more practical than memorization. The ability to quickly recall the products in the multiplication table is nevertheless crucial to using this algorithm.

> **STEP BY STEP**
>
> **Step 1.** Stack the two factors, vertically aligning the digits in each place.
>
> **Step 2.** Draw a multiplication symbol (×) to the left of the bottom number and draw a horizontal line below the stack.
>
> **Step 3.** Begin with the ones digit in the lower factor. Multiply it with the ones digit from the top factor.
>
> **Step 4.** If the product from Step 3 is less than 10, write it in the same column below the horizontal line. Otherwise, write the first (ones) digit below the line and carry the second (tens) digit to the top of the next column.
>
> **Step 5.** Perform Step 4 for each digit in the top factor, adding any carry digit to the result. If an extra carry digit appears at the end, write it as the leftmost digit in the product.
>
> **Step 6.** Going right to left, repeat Steps 3–4 for the other places in the bottom factor, starting a new line in each case.
>
> **Step 7.** Add the numbers below the line to get the product.

## Example

**A certain type of screw comes in packs of 35. If a contractor orders 52 packs, how many screws does he receive?**

A. 2

B. 57

C. 245

D. 1,820

The correct answer is **D.** The first step is to convert this problem to a math expression. The goal is to find how many screws the contractor receives if he orders 52 packs of 35 each. The expression would be 52 × 35 (or 35 × 52). Carefully follow the multiplication algorithm (see below).

**See Lesson: Basic Multiplication and Division.**

$$
\begin{array}{r} 52 \\ \times\,35 \\ \hline \end{array}
\rightarrow
\begin{array}{r} {}^{1} \\ 52 \\ \times\,35 \\ \hline 0 \end{array}
\rightarrow
\begin{array}{r} {}^{1} \\ 52 \\ \times\,35 \\ \hline 260 \end{array}
\rightarrow
\begin{array}{r} {}^{1} \\ 52 \\ \times\,35 \\ \hline 260 \\ 6 \end{array}
\rightarrow
\begin{array}{r} {}^{1}\;{}^{1} \\ 52 \\ \times\,35 \\ \hline 260 \\ 56 \end{array}
\rightarrow
\begin{array}{r} {}^{1}\;{}^{1} \\ 52 \\ \times\,35 \\ \hline 260 \\ 156 \end{array}
\rightarrow
\begin{array}{r} {}^{1}\;{}^{1} \\ 52 \\ \times\,35 \\ \hline 260 \\ +\,156 \\ \hline 1,820 \end{array}
$$

HESI

> **KEY POINT**
>
> As with addition, the order of numbers in a multiplication expression is irrelevant to the product. For example, $6 \times 9 = 9 \times 6$.

# Division

Division is the inverse of multiplication, like subtraction is the inverse of addition. Whereas multiplication asks how many individuals are in 8 groups of 9 ($8 \times 9 = 72$), for example, division asks how many groups of 8 (or 9) are in 72. Division expressions use either the / or ÷ symbol. Therefore, $72 \div 9$ means: How many groups of 9 are in 72, or how many times does 9 go into 72? Thinking about the meaning of multiplication shows that $72 \div 9 = 8$ and $72 \div 8 = 9$. In the expression $72 \div 8 = 9$, 72 is the **dividend,** 8 is the **divisor,** and 9 is the **quotient.**

When the dividend is unevenly divisible by the divisor (e.g., $5 \div 2$), calculating the quotient with a **remainder** can be convenient. The quotient in this case is the maximum number of times the divisor goes into the dividend plus how much of the dividend is left over. To express the remainder, use an R. For example, the quotient of $5 \div 2$ is 2R1 because 2 goes into 5 twice with 1 left over.

Knowing the multiplication table allows quick evaluation of simple whole-number division. For larger numbers, the division algorithm enables evaluation by hand.

Unlike multiplication—but like subtraction—the order of the numbers in a division expression is important. Generally, changing the order changes the quotient.

| **STEP BY STEP** | |
|---|---|
| **Step 1.** | Write the divisor and then the dividend on a single line. |
| **Step 2.** | Draw a vertical line between them, connecting to a horizontal line over the dividend. |
| **Step 3.** | If the divisor is smaller than the leftmost digit of the dividend, perform the remainder division and write the quotient (without the remainder) above that digit. If the divisor is larger than the leftmost digit, use the first two digits (or however many are necessary) until the number is greater than the divisor. Write the quotient over the rightmost digit in that number. |
| **Step 4.** | Multiply the quotient digit by the divisor and write it under the dividend, vertically aligning the ones digit of the product with the quotient digit. |
| **Step 5.** | Subtract the product from the digits above it. |
| **Step 6.** | Bring down the next digit from the quotient. |
| **Step 7.** | Perform Steps 3–6, using the most recent difference as the quotient. |
| **Step 8.** | Write the remainder next to the quotient. |

## Example

**Evaluate the expression 468 ÷ 26.**

A.  18                    B.  18R2                    C.  494                    D.  12,168

The correct answer is **A.** Carefully follow the division algorithm. In this case, the answer has no remainder. **See Lesson: Basic Multiplication and Division.**

$$26\overline{)468} \rightarrow \begin{array}{r} 1 \\ 26\overline{)468} \\ 26 \end{array} \rightarrow \begin{array}{r} 1 \\ 26\overline{)468} \\ -26 \\ \hline 20 \end{array} \rightarrow \begin{array}{r} 1 \\ 26\overline{)468} \\ -26\downarrow \\ \hline 208 \end{array} \rightarrow \begin{array}{r} 18 \\ 26\overline{)468} \\ -26\downarrow \\ \hline 208 \\ -208 \\ \hline 0 \end{array}$$

> **KEY POINT**
> Division by 0 is undefined. If it appears in an expression, something is wrong.

# Signed Multiplication and Division

Multiplying and dividing signed numbers is simpler than adding and subtracting them because it only requires remembering two simple rules. First, if the two numbers have the same sign, their product or quotient is positive. Second, if they have different signs, their product or quotient is negative.

As a result, negative numbers can be multiplied or divided as if they are positive. Just keep track of the sign separately for the product or quotient. Note that negative numbers are sometimes written in parentheses to avoid the appearance of subtraction.

## For Example:

$5 \times (-3) = -15$

$(-8) \times (-8) = 64$

$(-12) \div 3 = -4$

$(-100) \div (-25) = 4$

## Example

**Evaluate the expression $(-7) \times (-9)$.**

A.  −63                    B.  −16                    C.  16                    D.  63

The correct answer is **D.** Because both factors are negative, the product will be positive. Because the product of 7 and 9 is 63, the product of −7 and −9 is also 63. **See Lesson: Basic Multiplication and Division.**

# Order of Operations

By default, math expressions work like most Western languages: they should be read and evaluated from left to right. However, some operations take precedence over others, which can change this default evaluation. Following this **order of operations** is critical. The mnemonic **PEMDAS** (**P**lease **E**xcuse **M**y **D**ear **A**unt **S**ally) helps in remembering how to evaluate an expression with multiple operations.

---

**STEP BY STEP**

**P.**     Evaluate operations in parentheses (or braces/brackets). If the expression has parentheses within parentheses, begin with the innermost ones.

**E.**     Evaluate exponential operations. (For expressions without exponents, ignore this step.)

**MD.**   Perform all multiplication and division operations, going through the expression from left to right.

**AS.**    Perform all addition and subtraction operations, going through the expression from left to right.

---

Because the order of numbers in multiplication and addition does not affect the result, the PEMDAS procedure only requires going from left to right when dividing or subtracting. At those points, going in the correct direction is critical to getting the right answer.

Calculators that can handle a series of numbers at once automatically evaluate an expression according to the order of operations. When available, calculators are a good way to check the results.

**BE CAREFUL!**

When evaluating an expression like $4 - 3 + 2 \times 5$, remember to go from left to right when adding and subtracting or when multiplying and dividing. The first step in this case (MD) yields $4 - 3 + 10$. Avoid the temptation to add first in the next step; instead, go from left to right. The result is $1 + 10 = 11$, *not* $4 - 13 = -9$.

## Example

**Evaluate the expression 8 × (3 + 6) ÷ 3 − 2 + 5.**

A.  13            B.  17            C.  27            D.  77

The correct answer is **C.** Use the PEMDAS mnemonic. Start with parentheses. Then, do multiplication/division from left to right. Finally, do addition/subtraction from left to right.
**See Lesson: Basic Multiplication and Division.**

$8 \times (3 + 6) \div 3 - 2 + 5$

$8 \times 9 \div 3 - 2 + 5$

$72 \div 3 - 2 + 5$

$24 - 2 + 5$

$22 + 5$

$27$

## Let's Review!

- The multiplication table is important to memorize for both multiplying and dividing small whole numbers (up to about 12).
- Multiplication and division of large numbers by hand typically requires the multiplication and division algorithms.
- Multiplying and dividing signed numbers follows two simple rules: If the numbers have the same sign, the product or quotient is positive. If they have different signs, the product or quotient is negative.
- When evaluating expressions with several operations, carefully follow the order of operations; PEMDAS is a helpful mnemonic.

# DECIMAL AND FRACTIONS

This lesson introduces the basics of decimals and fractions. It also demonstrates changing decimals to fractions, changing fractions to decimals, and converting between fractions, decimals, and percentages.

## Introduction to Fractions

A fraction represents part of a whole number. The top number of a fraction is the **numerator,** and the bottom number of a fraction is the **denominator.** The numerator is smaller than the denominator for a **proper fraction.** The numerator is larger than the denominator for an **improper fraction.**

| Proper Fractions | Improper Fractions |
| --- | --- |
| $\frac{2}{5}$ | $\frac{5}{2}$ |
| $\frac{7}{12}$ | $\frac{12}{7}$ |
| $\frac{19}{20}$ | $\frac{20}{19}$ |

An improper fraction can be changed to **mixed number.** A mixed number is a whole number and a proper fraction. To write an improper fraction as a mixed number, divide the denominator into the numerator. The result is the whole number. The remainder is the numerator of the proper fraction, and the value of the denominator does not change. For example, $\frac{5}{2}$ is $2\frac{1}{2}$ because 2 goes into 5 twice with a remainder of 1. To write an improper fraction as a mixed number, multiply the whole number by the denominator and add the result to the numerator. The results become the new numerator. For example, $2\frac{1}{2}$ is $\frac{5}{2}$ because 2 times 2 plus 1 is 5 for the new numerator.

> **KEEP IN MIND**
> When comparing fractions, the denominators of the fractions must be the same.

When comparing fractions, the denominators must be the same. Then, look at the numerator to determine which fraction is larger. If the fractions have different denominators, then a **least common denominator** must be found. This number is the smallest number that can be divided evenly into the denominators of all fractions being compared.

To determine the largest fraction from the group $\frac{1}{3}, \frac{3}{5}, \frac{2}{3}, \frac{2}{5}$, the first step is to find a common denominator. In this case, the least common denominator is 15 because 3 times 5 and 5 times 3 is 15. The second step is to convert the fractions to a denominator of 15. The fractions with a denominator of 3 have the numerator and denominator multiplied by 5, and the fractions with a denominator of 5 have the numerator and denominator multiplied by 3, as shown below:

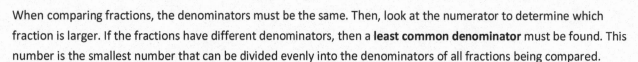

$$\frac{1}{3} \times \frac{5}{5} = \frac{5}{15}, \frac{3}{5} \times \frac{3}{3} = \frac{9}{15}, \frac{2}{3} \times \frac{5}{5} = \frac{10}{15}, \frac{2}{5} \times \frac{3}{3} = \frac{6}{15}$$

Now, the numerators can be compared. The largest fraction is $\frac{2}{3}$ because it has a numerator of 10 after finding the common denominator.

## Examples

1. **Which fraction is the least?**

   A. $\frac{3}{5}$       B. $\frac{3}{4}$       C. $\frac{1}{5}$       D. $\frac{1}{4}$

   The correct answer is **C.** The correct solution is $\frac{1}{5}$ because it has the smallest numerator compared to the other fractions with the same denominator. The fractions with a common denominator of 20 are $\frac{3}{5} = \frac{12}{20}, \frac{3}{4} = \frac{15}{20}, \frac{1}{5} = \frac{4}{20}, \frac{1}{4} = \frac{5}{20}$. **See Lesson: Decimals and Fractions.**

2. **Which fraction is the greatest?**

   A. $\frac{5}{6}$       B. $\frac{1}{2}$       C. $\frac{2}{3}$       D. $\frac{1}{6}$

   The correct answer is **A.** The correct solution is $\frac{5}{6}$ because it has the largest numerator compared to the other fractions with the same denominator. The fractions with a common denominator of 6 are $\frac{5}{6} = \frac{5}{6}, \frac{1}{2} = \frac{3}{6}, \frac{2}{3} = \frac{4}{6}, \frac{1}{6} = \frac{1}{6}$. **See Lesson: Decimals and Fractions.**

# Introduction to Decimals

A **decimal** is a number that expresses part of a whole. Decimals show a portion of a number after a decimal point. Each number to the left and right of the decimal point has a specific place value. Identify the place values for 645.3207.

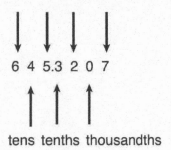

When comparing decimals, compare the numbers in the same place value. For example, determine the greatest decimal from the group 0.4, 0.41, 0.39, and 0.37. In these numbers, there is a value to the right of the decimal point. Comparing the tenths places, the numbers with 4 tenths (0.4 and 0.41) are greater than the numbers with three tenths (0.39 and 0.37).

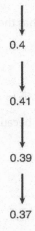

Then, compare the hundredths in the 4 tenths numbers. The value of 0.41 is greater because there is a 1 in the hundredths place versus a 0 in the hundredths place.

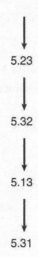

0.4

0.41

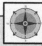

**KEEP IN MIND**

When comparing decimals, compare the place value where the numbers are different.

Here is another example: determine the least decimal of the group 5.23, 5.32, 5.13, and 5.31. In this group, the ones value is 5 for all numbers. Then, comparing the tenths values, 5.13 is the smallest number because it is the only value with 1 tenth.

5.23

5.32

5.13

5.31

## Examples

1. **Which decimal is the greatest?**

A.  0.07             B.  0.007             C.  0.7             D.  0.0007

The correct answer is **C.** The solution is 0.7 because it has the largest place value in the tenths.
**See Lesson: Decimals and Fractions.**

2. **Which decimal is the least?**

A.  0.0413           B.  0.0713           C.  0.0513           D.  0.0613

The correct answer is **A.** The correct solution is 0.0413 because it has the smallest place value in the hundredths place. **See Lesson: Decimals and Fractions.**

# Changing Decimals and Fractions

Three steps change a decimal to a fraction.

**STEP BY STEP**

**Step 1.** Write the decimal divided by 1 with the decimal as the numerator and 1 as the denominator.

**Step 2.** Multiply the numerator and denominator by 10 for every number after the decimal point. (For example, if there is 1 decimal place, multiply by 10. If there are 2 decimal places, multiply by 100).

**Step 3.** Reduce the fraction completely.

To change the decimal 0.37 to a fraction, start by writing the decimal as a fraction with a denominator of one, $\frac{0.37}{1}$.

Because there are two decimal places, multiply the numerator and denominator by 100, $\frac{0.37 \times 100}{1 \times 100} = \frac{37}{100}$. The fraction does not reduce, so $\frac{37}{100}$ is 0.37 in fraction form.

Similarly, to change the decimal 2.4 to a fraction start by writing the decimal as a fraction with a denominator of one, $\frac{0.4}{1}$, and ignore the whole number. Because there is one decimal place, multiply the numerator and denominator by 10, $\frac{0.4 \times 10}{1 \times 10} = \frac{4}{10}$. The fraction does reduce: $2\frac{4}{10} = 2\frac{2}{5}$ is 2.4 in fraction form.

The decimal $0.\overline{3}$ as a fraction is $\frac{0.\overline{3}}{1}$. In the case of a repeating decimal, let $n = 0.\overline{3}$ *and* $10 = 3.\overline{3}$. Then, $10n - n = 3.\overline{3} - 0.\overline{3}$, resulting in $9n = 3$ and solution of $n = \frac{3}{9} = \frac{1}{3}$. The decimal $0.\overline{3}$ is $\frac{1}{3}$ as a fraction.

## Examples

1. **Change 0.38 to a fraction. Simplify completely.**

   A. $\frac{3}{10}$ 　　　　　 B. $\frac{9}{25}$ 　　　　　 C. $\frac{19}{50}$ 　　　　　 D. $\frac{2}{5}$

   The correct answer is **C.** The correct solution is $\frac{19}{50}$ because $\frac{0.38}{1} = \frac{38}{100} = \frac{19}{50}$. **See Lesson: Decimals and Fractions.**

2. **Change $1.\overline{1}$ to a fraction. Simplify completely.**

   A. $1\frac{1}{11}$ 　　　　　 B. $1\frac{1}{9}$ 　　　　　 C. $1\frac{1}{6}$ 　　　　　 D. $1\frac{1}{3}$

   The correct answer is **B.** The correct solution is $1\frac{1}{9}$. Let n = $1.\overline{1}$ and 10n = $11.\overline{1}$. Then, $10n - n = 11.\overline{1} - 1.\overline{1}$, resulting in 9n = 10 and solution of n = $\frac{10}{9} = 1\frac{1}{9}$. **See Lesson: Decimals and Fractions.**

Two steps change a fraction to a decimal.

> **STEP BY STEP**
>
> **Step 1.** Divide the denominator by the numerator. Add zeros after the decimal point as needed.
>
> **Step 2.** Complete the process when there is no remainder or the decimal is repeating.

To convert $\frac{1}{5}$ to a decimal, rewrite $\frac{1}{5}$ as a long division problem and add zeros after the decimal point, $1.0 \div 5$. Complete the long division and $\frac{1}{5}$ as a decimal is 0.2. The division is complete because there is no remainder.

To convert $\frac{8}{9}$ to a decimal, rewrite $\frac{8}{9}$ as a long division problem and add zeros after the decimal point, $8.00 \div 9$. Complete the long division, and $\frac{8}{9}$ as a decimal is $0.\overline{8}$. The process is complete because the decimal is complete.

To rewrite the mixed number $2\frac{3}{4}$ as a decimal, the fraction needs changed to a decimal. Rewrite $\frac{3}{4}$ as a long division problem and add zeros after the decimal point, $3.00 \div 4$. The whole number is needed for the answer and is not included in the long division. Complete the long division, and $2\frac{3}{4}$ as a decimal is 2.75.

## Examples

1. **Change $\frac{9}{10}$ to a decimal. Simplify completely.**

   A. 0.75          B. 0.8          C. 0.85          D. 0.9

   The correct answer is **D.** The correct answer is 0.9 because $\frac{9}{10} = 9.0 \div 10 = 0.9$. **See Lesson: Decimals and Fractions.**

2. **Change $\frac{5}{6}$ to a decimal. Simplify completely.**

   A. 0.73          B. 0.7$\overline{6}$          C. 0.8$\overline{3}$          D. 0.86

   The correct answer is **C.** The correct answer is $0.8\overline{3}$ because $\frac{5}{6} = 5.000 \div 6 = 0.8\overline{3}$. **See Lesson: Decimals and Fractions.**

# Convert among Fractions, Decimals, and Percentages

Fractions, decimals, and percentages can change forms, but they are equivalent values.

There are two ways to change a decimal to a percent. One way is to multiply the decimal by 100 and add a percent sign. 0.24 as a percent is $0.24 \times 100 = 24\%$.

Another way is to move the decimal point two places to the right. The decimal 0.635 is 63.5% as a percent when moving the decimal point two places to the right.

Any decimal, including repeating decimals, can change to a percent. $0.\overline{3}$ as a percent is $0.\overline{3} \times 100 = 33.\overline{3}\%$.

# Example

**Write 0.345 as a percent.**

A.  3.45%

B.  34.5%

C.  345%

D.  3450%

The correct answer is **B.** The correct answer is 34.5% because 0.345 as a percent is $0.345 \times 100 = 34.5\%$. **See Lesson: Decimals and Fractions.**

There are two ways to change a percent to a decimal. One way is to remove the percent sign and divide the decimal by 100. For example, 73% as a decimal is $73 \div 100 = 0.73$.

Another way is to move the decimal point two places to the left. For example, 27.8% is 0.278 as a decimal when moving the decimal point two places to the left.

Any percent, including repeating percents, can change to a decimal. For example, $44.\overline{4}\%$ as a decimal is $44.\overline{4} \div 100 = 0.\overline{4}$.

# Example

**Write 131% as a decimal.**

A.  0.131        B.  1.31        C.  13.1        D.  131

The correct answer is **B.** The correct answer is 1.31 because 131% as a decimal is $131 \div 100 = 1.31$.

**See Lesson: Decimals and Fractions.**

Two steps change a fraction to a percent.

> **STEP BY STEP**
> **Step 1.**   Divide the numerator and denominator.
> **Step 2.**   Multiply by 100 and add a percent sign.

To change the fraction $\frac{3}{5}$ to a decimal, perform long division to get 0.6. Then, multiply 0.6 by 100 and $\frac{3}{5}$ is the same as 60%.

To change the fraction $\frac{7}{8}$ to a decimal, perform long division to get 0.875. Then, multiply 0.875 by 100 and $\frac{7}{8}$ is the same as 87.5%.

Fractions that are repeating decimals can also be converted to a percent. To change the fraction $\frac{2}{3}$ to a decimal, perform long division to get $0.\overline{6}$. Then, multiply $0.\overline{6}$ by 100 and the percent is $66.\overline{6}\%$.

## Example

**Write $2\frac{1}{8}$ as a percent.**

A.  21.2%          B.  21.25%          C.  212%          D.  212.5%

The correct answer is **D.** The correct answer is 212.5% because $2\frac{1}{8}$ as a percent is 2.125 x 100 = 212.5%. **See Lesson: Decimals and Fractions.**

Two steps change a percent to a fraction.

| STEP BY STEP |
| --- |
| **Step 1.**   Remove the percent sign and write the value as the numerator with a denominator of 100. |
| **Step 2.**   Simplify the fraction. |

Remove the percent sign from 45% and write as a fraction with a denominator of 100, $\frac{45}{100}$. The fraction reduces to $\frac{9}{20}$.

Remove the percent sign from 22.8% and write as a fraction with a denominator of 100, $\frac{22.8}{100}$. The fraction reduces to $\frac{228}{1000} = \frac{57}{250}$.

Repeating percentages can change to a fraction. Remove the percent sign from $16.\overline{6}$% and write as a fraction with a denominator of 100, $\frac{16.\overline{6}}{100}$. The fraction simplifies to $\frac{0.1\overline{6}}{1} = \frac{1}{6}$.

## Example

**Write 72% as a fraction.**

A.  $\frac{27}{50}$          B.  $\frac{7}{10}$          C.  $\frac{18}{25}$          D.  $\frac{3}{4}$

The correct answer is **C.** The correct answer is $\frac{18}{25}$ because 72% as a fraction is $\frac{72}{100} = \frac{18}{25}$.
**See Lesson: Decimals and Fractions.**

## Let's Review!

- A fraction is a number with a numerator and a denominator. A fraction can be written as a proper fraction, an improper fraction, or a mixed number. Changing fractions to a common denominator enables you to determine the least or greatest fraction in a group of fractions.

- A decimal is a number that expresses part of a whole. By comparing the same place values, you can find the least or greatest decimal in a group of decimals.

- A number can be written as a fraction, a decimal, and a percent. These are equivalent values. Numbers can be converted between fractions, decimals, and percents by following a series of steps.

# MULTIPLICATION AND DIVISION OF FRACTIONS

This lesson introduces how to multiply and divide fractions.

## Multiplying a Fraction by a Fraction

The multiplication of fractions does not require changing any denominators like adding and subtracting fractions do. To multiply a fraction by a fraction, multiply the numerators together and multiply the denominators together. For example, $\frac{2}{3} \times \frac{4}{5}$ is $\frac{2 \times 4}{3 \times 5}$, which is $\frac{8}{15}$.

Sometimes, the final solution reduces. For example, $\frac{3}{5} \times \frac{1}{9} = \frac{3 \times 1}{5 \times 9} = \frac{3}{45}$. The fraction $\frac{3}{45}$ reduces to $\frac{1}{15}$.

Simplifying fractions can occur before completing the multiplication. In the previous problem, the numerator of 3 can be simplified with the denominator of 9: $\frac{\cancel{3}^{1}}{5} \times \frac{1}{\cancel{9}_{3}} = \frac{1}{15}$. This method of simplifying only occurs with the multiplication of fractions.

**KEEP IN MIND**

The product of multiplying a fraction by a fraction is always less than 1.

### Examples

1. **Multiply $\frac{1}{2} \times \frac{3}{4}$.**

   A. $\frac{1}{4}$        B. $\frac{1}{2}$        C. $\frac{3}{8}$        D. $\frac{2}{3}$

   The correct answer is **C**. The correct solution is $\frac{3}{8}$ because $\frac{1}{2} \times \frac{3}{4} = \frac{3}{8}$.
   **See Lesson: Multiplication and Division of Fractions.**

2. **Multiply $\frac{2}{3} \times \frac{5}{6}$.**

   A. $\frac{1}{9}$        B. $\frac{5}{18}$        C. $\frac{5}{9}$        D. $\frac{7}{18}$

   The correct answer is **C**. The correct solution is $\frac{5}{9}$ because $\frac{2}{3} \times \frac{5}{6} = \frac{10}{18} = \frac{5}{9}$.
   **See Lesson: Multiplication and Division of Fractions.**

## Multiply a Fraction by a Whole or Mixed Number

Multiplying a fraction by a whole or mixed number is similar to multiplying two fractions. When multiplying by a whole number, change the whole number to a fraction with a denominator of 1. Next, multiply the numerators together and the denominators together. Rewrite the final answer as a mixed number. For example: $\frac{9}{10} \times 3 = \frac{9}{10} \times \frac{3}{1} = \frac{27}{10} = 2\frac{7}{10}$.

When multiplying a fraction by a mixed number or multiplying two mixed numbers, the process is similar.

For example, multiply $\frac{10}{11} \times 3\frac{1}{2}$. Change the mixed number to an improper fraction, $\frac{10}{11} \times \frac{7}{2}$. Multiply the numerators together and multiply the denominators together, $\frac{70}{22}$. Write the improper fraction as a mixed number, $3\frac{4}{22}$. Reduce if necessary, $3\frac{2}{11}$.

**KEEP IN MIND**

Always change a mixed number to an improper fraction when multiplying by a mixed number.

19

HESI

This process can also be used when multiplying a whole number by a mixed number or multiplying two mixed numbers.

## Examples

1. **Multiply** $4 \times \frac{5}{6}$.

   A. $\frac{5}{24}$      B. $2\frac{3}{4}$      C. $3\frac{1}{3}$      D. $4\frac{5}{6}$

   The correct answer is **C**. The correct solution is $3\frac{1}{3}$ because $\frac{4}{1} \times \frac{5}{6} = \frac{20}{6} = 3\frac{2}{6} = 3\frac{1}{3}$.

   **See Lesson: Multiplication and Division of Fractions.**

2. **Multiply** $1\frac{1}{2} \times 1\frac{1}{6}$.

   A. $1\frac{1}{12}$      B. $1\frac{1}{4}$      C. $1\frac{3}{8}$      D. $1\frac{3}{4}$

   The correct answer is **D**. The correct solution is $1\frac{3}{4}$ because $\frac{3}{2} \times \frac{7}{6} = \frac{21}{12} = 1\frac{9}{12} = 1\frac{3}{4}$.

   **See Lesson: Multiplication and Division of Fractions.**

# Dividing a Fraction by a Fraction

Some basic steps apply when dividing a fraction by a fraction. The information from the previous two sections is applicable to dividing fractions.

**STEP BY STEP**

**Step 1.** Leave the first fraction alone.

**Step 2.** Find the reciprocal of the second fraction.

**Step 3.** Multiply the first fraction by the reciprocal of the second fraction.

**Step 4.** Rewrite the fraction as a mixed number and reduce the fraction completely.

Divide, $\frac{3}{10} \div \frac{1}{2}$. Find the reciprocal of the second fraction, which is $\frac{2}{1}$.

Now, multiply the fractions, $\frac{3}{10} \times \frac{2}{1} = \frac{6}{10}$. Reduce $\frac{6}{10}$ to $\frac{3}{5}$.

Divide, $\frac{4}{5} \div \frac{3}{8}$. Find the reciprocal of the second fraction, which is $\frac{8}{3}$.

Now, multiply the fractions, $\frac{4}{5} \times \frac{8}{3} = \frac{32}{15}$. Rewrite the fraction as a mixed number, $\frac{32}{15} = 2\frac{2}{15}$.

## Examples

1. **Divide $\frac{1}{2} \div \frac{5}{6}$.**

   A. $\frac{5}{12}$        B. $\frac{3}{5}$        C. $\frac{5}{6}$        D. $1\frac{2}{3}$

   The correct answer is **B.** The correct solution is $\frac{3}{5}$ because $\frac{1}{2} \times \frac{6}{5} = \frac{6}{10} = \frac{3}{5}$. **See Lesson: Multiplication and Division of Fractions.**

2. **Divide $\frac{2}{3} \div \frac{3}{5}$.**

   A. $\frac{2}{15}$        B. $\frac{2}{5}$        C. $1\frac{1}{15}$        D. $1\frac{1}{9}$

   The correct answer is **D.** The correct solution is $1\frac{1}{9}$ because $\frac{2}{3} \times \frac{5}{3} = \frac{10}{9} = 1\frac{1}{9}$.
   **See Lesson: Multiplication and Division of Fractions.**

# Dividing a Fraction and a Whole or Mixed Number

Some basic steps apply when dividing a fraction by a whole number or a mixed number.

| | |
|---|---|
| **STEP BY STEP** | |
| **Step 1.** | Write any whole number as a fraction with a denominator of 1. Write any mixed numbers as improper fractions. |
| **Step 2.** | Leave the first fraction (improper fraction) alone. |
| **Step 3.** | Find the reciprocal of the second fraction. |
| **Step 4.** | Multiply the first fraction by the reciprocal of the second fraction. |
| **Step 5.** | Rewrite the fraction as a mixed number and reduce the fraction completely. |

Divide, $\frac{3}{10} \div 3$. Rewrite the expression as $\frac{3}{10} \div \frac{3}{1}$. Find the reciprocal of the second fraction, which is $\frac{1}{3}$. Multiply the fractions, $\frac{3}{10} \times \frac{1}{3} = \frac{3}{30} = \frac{1}{10}$. Reduce $\frac{3}{30}$ to $\frac{1}{10}$.

Divide, $2\frac{4}{5} \div 1\frac{3}{8}$. Rewrite the expression as $\frac{14}{5} \div \frac{11}{8}$. Find the reciprocal of the second fraction, which is $\frac{8}{11}$.

Multiply the fractions, $\frac{14}{5} \times \frac{8}{11} = \frac{112}{55} = 2\frac{2}{55}$. Reduce $\frac{112}{55}$ to $2\frac{2}{55}$.

# Examples

1. **Divide $\frac{2}{3} \div 4$.**

   A. $\frac{1}{12}$         B. $\frac{1}{10}$         C. $\frac{1}{8}$         D. $\frac{1}{6}$

   The correct answer is **D.** The correct answer is $\frac{1}{6}$ because $\frac{2}{3} \times \frac{1}{4} = \frac{2}{12} = \frac{1}{6}$.

   **See Lesson: Multiplication and Division of Fractions.**

2. **Divide $1\frac{5}{12} \div 1\frac{1}{2}$.**

   A. $\frac{17}{18}$         B. $1\frac{5}{24}$         C. $1\frac{5}{6}$         D. $2\frac{1}{8}$

   The correct answer is **A.** The correct answer is $\frac{17}{18}$ because $\frac{17}{12} \div \frac{3}{2} = \frac{17}{12} \times \frac{2}{3} = \frac{34}{36} = \frac{17}{18}$.

   **See Lesson: Multiplication and Division of Fractions.**

# Let's Review!

- The process to multiply fractions is to multiply the numerators together and multiply the denominators together. When there is a mixed number, change the mixed number to an improper fraction before multiplying.

- The process to divide fractions is to find the reciprocal of the second fraction and multiply the fractions. As with multiplying, change any mixed numbers to improper fractions before dividing.

# RATIOS, PROPORTIONS, AND PERCENTAGES

This lesson reviews percentages and ratios and their application to real-world problems. It also examines proportions and rates of change.

## Percentages

A **percent** or **percentage** represents a fraction of some quantity. It is an integer or decimal number followed by the symbol %. The word *percent* means "per hundred." For example, 50% means 50 per 100. This is equivalent to half, or 1 out of 2.

Converting between numbers and percents is easy. Given a number, multiply by 100 and add the % symbol to get the equivalent percent. For instance, 0.67 is equal to $0.67 \times 100 = 67\%$, meaning 67 out of 100. Given a percent, eliminate the % symbol and divide by 100. For instance, 23.5% is equal to $23.5 \div 100 = 0.235$.

Although percentages between 0% and 100% are the most obvious, a percent can be any real number, including a negative number. For example, $1.35 = 135\%$ and $-0.872 = -87.2\%$. An example is a gasoline tank that is one-quarter full: one-quarter is $\frac{1}{4}$ or 0.25, so the tank is 25% full. Another example is a medical diagnostic test that has a certain maximum normal result. If a patient's test exceeds that value, its representation can be a percent greater than 100%. For instance, a reading that is 1.22 times the maximum normal value is 122% of the maximum normal value. Likewise, when measuring increases in a company's profits as a percent from one year to the next, a negative percent can represent a decline. That is, if the company's profits fell by one-tenth, the change was –10%.

### Example

**If 15 out of every 250 contest entries are winners, what percentage of entries are winners?**

A.  0.06%          B.  6%          C.  15%          D.  17%

The correct answer is **B.** First, convert the fraction $\frac{15}{250}$ to a decimal: 0.06. To get the percent, multiply by 100% (that is, multiply by 100 and add the % symbol). Of all entries, 6% are winners. **See Lesson: Ratios, Proportions, and Percentages.**

## Ratios

A **ratio** expresses the relationship between two numbers and is expressed using a colon or fraction notation. For instance, if 135 runners finish a marathon but 22 drop out, the ratio of finishers to non-finishers is 135:22 or $\frac{135}{22}$. These expressions are equal.

Ratios also follow the rules of fractions. Performing arithmetic operations on ratios follows the same procedures as on fractions. Ratios should also generally appear in lowest terms. Therefore, the constituent numbers in a ratio represent the relative quantities of each side, not absolute quantities. For example, because the ratio 1:2 is equal to 2:4, 5:10, and 600:1,200, ratios are insufficient to determine the absolute number of entities in a problem.

> **BE CAREFUL!**
> Avoid confusing standard ratios with odds (such as "3:1 odds"). Both may use a colon, but their meanings differ. In general, a ratio is the same as a fraction containing the same numbers.

## Example

**If the ratio of women to men in a certain industry is 5:4, how many people are in that industry?**

A.  9                    B.  20                    C.  900                    D.   Not enough information

The correct answer is **D.** The ratio 5:4 is the industry's relative number of women to men. But the industry could have 10 women and 8 men, 100 women and 80 men, or any other breakdown whose ratio is 5:4. Therefore, the question provides too little information to answer. Had it provided the total number of people in the industry, it would have been possible to determine how many women and how many men are in the industry. **See Lesson: Ratios, Proportions, and Percentages.**

**KEY POINT**

Mathematically, ratios act just like fractions. For example, the ratio 8:13 is mathematically the same as the fraction $\frac{8}{13}$.

## Proportions

A **proportion** is an equation of two ratios. An illustrative case is two equivalent fractions:

$$\frac{21}{28} = \frac{3}{4}$$

This example of a proportion should be familiar: going left to right, it is the conversion of one fraction to an equivalent fraction in lowest terms by dividing the numerator and denominator by the same number (7, in this case).

Equating fractions in this way is correct, but it provides little information. Proportions are more informative when one of the numbers is unknown. Using a question mark (?) to represent an unknown number, setting up a proportion can aid in solving problems involving different scales. For instance, if the ratio of maple saplings to oak saplings in an acre of young forest is 7:5 and that acre contains 65 oaks, the number of maples in that acre can be determined using a proportion:

$$\frac{7}{5} = \frac{?}{65}$$

Note that to equate two ratios in this manner, the numerators must contain numbers that represent the same entity or type, and so must the denominators. In this example, the numerators represent maples and the denominators represent oaks.

$$\frac{7 \text{ maples}}{5 \text{ oaks}} = \frac{? \text{ maples}}{65 \text{ oaks}}$$

Recall from the properties of fractions that if you multiply the numerator and denominator by the same number, the result is an equivalent fraction. Therefore, to find the unknown in this proportion, first divide the denominator on the right by the denominator on the left. Then, multiply the quotient by the numerator on the left.

$$65 \div 5 = 13$$

$$\frac{7 \times 13}{5 \times 13} = \frac{?}{65}$$

The unknown (?) is $7 \times 13 = 91$. In the example, the acre of forest has 91 maple saplings.

**DID YOU KNOW?**

When taking the reciprocal of both sides of a proportion, the proportion still holds. When setting up a proportion, ensure that the numerators represent the same type and the denominators represent the same type.

## Example

**If a recipe calls for 3 parts flour to 2 parts sugar, how much sugar does a baker need if she uses 12 cups of flour?**

A.  2 cups

B.  3 cups

C.  6 cups

D.  8 cups

The correct answer is **D.** The baker needs 8 cups of sugar. First, note that "3 parts flour to 2 parts sugar" is the ratio 3:2. Set up the proportion using the given amount of flour (12 cups), putting the flour numbers in either the denominators or the numerators (either will yield the same answer):

$$\frac{3}{2} = \frac{12}{?}$$

Since $12 \div 3 = 4$, multiply $2 \times 4$ to get 8 cups of sugar. **See Lesson: Ratios, Proportions, and Percentages.**

# Rates of Change

Numbers that describe current quantities can be informative, but how they change over time can provide even greater insight into a problem. The rate of change for some quantity is the ratio of the quantity's difference over a specific time period to the length of that period. For example, if an automobile increases its speed from 50 mph to 100 mph in 10 seconds, the rate of change of its speed (its acceleration) is

$$\frac{100 \text{ mph} - 50 \text{ mph}}{10 \text{ s}} = \frac{50 \text{ mph}}{10 \text{ s}} = 5 \text{ mph per second} = 5 \text{ mph/s}$$

The basic formula for the rate of change of some quantity is

$$\frac{x_f - x_i}{t_f - t_i}$$

where $t_f$ is the "final" (or ending) time and $t_i$ is the "initial" (or starting) time. Also, $x_f$ is the (final) quantity at (final) time $t_f$, and $x_i$ is the (initial) quantity at (initial) time $t_i$. In the example above, the final time is 10 seconds and the initial time is 0 seconds—hence the omission of the initial time from the calculation.

According to the rules of fractions, multiplying the numerator and denominator by the same number yields an equivalent fraction, so you can reverse the order of the terms in the formula:

$$\frac{x_f - x_i}{t_f - t_i} = \frac{-1}{-1} \times \frac{x_f - x_i}{t_f - t_i} = \frac{x_i - x_f}{t_i - t_f}$$

The key to getting the correct rate of change is to ensure that the first number in the numerator and the first number in the denominator correspond to each other (that is, the quantity from the numerator corresponds to the time from the denominator). This must also be true for the second number.

## Example

**If the population of an endangered frog species fell from 2,250 individuals to 2,115 individuals in a year, what is that population's annual rate of increase?**

A.  –135%          B.  –6%          C.  6%          D.  135%

The correct answer is **B.** The population's rate of increase was –6%. The solution in this case involves two steps. First, calculate the population's annual rate of change using the formula. It will yield the change in the number of individuals.

$$\frac{2{,}115 - 2{,}250}{1 \text{ year} - 0 \text{ year}} = -135 \text{ per year}$$

Second, divide the result by the initial population. Finally, convert to a percent.

$$\frac{-135 \text{ per year}}{2{,}250} = -0.06 \text{ per year}$$

$$(-0.06 \text{ per year}) \times 100\% = -6\% \text{ per year}$$

Since the question asks for the *annual* rate of increase, the "per year" can be dropped. Also, note that the answer must be negative to represent the decreasing population. **See Lesson: Ratios, Proportions, and Percentages.**

## Let's Review!

- A percent—meaning "per hundred"—represents a relative quantity as a fraction or decimal. It is the absolute number multiplied by 100 and followed by the % symbol.

- A ratio is a relationship between two numbers expressed using fraction or colon notation (for example, $\frac{3}{2}$ or 3:2). Ratios behave mathematically just like fractions.

- An equation of two ratios is called a proportion. Proportions are used to solve problems involving scale.

- Rates of change are the speeds at which quantities increase or decrease. The formula $\frac{x_f - x_i}{t_f - t_i}$ provides the rate of change of quantity $x$ over the period between some initial (*i*) time and final (*f*) time.

# STANDARDS OF MEASURE

This lesson discusses the conversion within and between the standard system and the metric system and between 12-hour clock time and military time.

## Length Conversions

The basic units of measure of length in the standard measurement system are inches, feet, yards, and miles. There are 12 inches (in.) in 1 foot (ft.), 3 feet (ft.) in 1 yard (yd.), and 5,280 feet (ft.) in 1 mile (mi.).

The basic unit of measure of metric length is meters. There are 1,000 millimeters (mm), 100 centimeters (cm), and 10 decimeters (dm) in 1 meter (m). There are 10 meters (m) in 1 dekameter (dam), 100 meters (m) in 1 hectometer (hm), and 1,000 meters (m) in 1 kilometer (km).

> **BE CAREFUL!**
> There are some cases where multiple conversions must be performed to determine the correct units.

To convert from one unit to the other, multiply by the appropriate factor.

## Examples

1. **Convert 27 inches to feet.**

   A.   2 feet          B.   2.25 feet          C.   3 feet          D.   3.25 feet

   The correct answer is **B.** The correct solution is 2.25 feet. $27 \text{ in} \times \frac{1 \text{ ft}}{12 \text{ in}} = \frac{27}{12} = 2.25 \text{ ft}$.
   **See Lesson: Standards of Measure.**

2. **Convert 67 millimeters to centimeters.**

   A.   0.0067 centimeters                    B.   0.067 centimeters

   C.   0.67 centimeters                      D.   6.7 centimeters

   The correct answer is **D.** The correct solution is 6.7 centimeters. $67 \text{ mm} \times \frac{1 \text{ cm}}{10 \text{ mm}} = \frac{67}{10} = 6.7 \text{ cm}$.
   **See Lesson: Standards of Measure.**

## Volume and Weight Conversions

There are volume conversion factors for standard and metric volumes.

The volume conversions for standard volume are shown in the table.

| Measurement | Conversion |
|---|---|
| Pints (pt.) and fluid ounces (fl. oz.) | 1 pint equals 16 fluid ounces |
| Quarts (qt.) and pints (pt.) | 1 quart equals 2 pints |
| Quarts (qt.) and gallons (gal.) | 1 gallon equals 4 quarts |

The basic unit of volume for the metric system is liters. There are 1,000 milliliters (mL) in 1 liter (L) and 1,000 liters (L) in 1 kiloliter (kL).

There are weight conversion factors for standard and metric weights.

27

HESI

The basic unit of weight for the standard measurement system is pounds. There are

      16 ounces (oz.) in 1 pound (lb.) and

      2,000 pounds (lb.) in 1 ton (T).

The basic unit of weight for the metric system is grams.

**KEEP IN MIND**

The conversions within the metric system are multiples of 10.

| Measurement | Conversion |
| --- | --- |
| Milligrams (mg) and grams (g) | 1,000 milligrams equals 1 gram |
| Centigrams (cg) and grams (g) | 100 centigrams equals 1 gram |
| Kilograms (kg) and grams (g) | 1 kilogram equals 1,000 grams |
| Metric tons (t) and kilograms(kg) | 1 metric ton equals 1,000 kilograms |

## Examples

1. **Convert 8 gallons to pints.**

    A.  1 pint                      B.  4 pints

    C.  16 pints                D.  64 pints

    The correct answer is **D.** The correct solution is 64 pints. $8 \text{ gal} \times \frac{4 \text{ qt}}{1 \text{ gal}} \times \frac{2 \text{ pt}}{1 \text{ qt}} = 64$ pt.

    **See Lesson: Standards of Measure.**

2. **Convert 7.5 liters to milliliters.**

    A.  75 milliliters            B.  750 milliliters

    C.  7,500 milliliters        D.  75,000 milliliters

    The correct answer is **C.** The correct solution is 7,500 milliliters. $7.5 \text{ L} \times \frac{1,000 \text{ ml}}{1 \text{ L}} = 7,500$ mL.

    **See Lesson: Standards of Measure.**

3. **Convert 12.5 pounds to ounces.**

    A.  142 ounces              B.  150 ounces

    C.  192 ounces              D.  200 ounces

    The correct answer is **D.** The correct solution is 200 ounces. $12.5 \text{ lb} \times \frac{16 \text{ oz}}{1 \text{ lb}} = 200$ oz.

    **See Lesson: Standards of Measure.**

4. **Convert 84 grams to centigrams.**

    A.  0.84 centigrams        B.  8.4 centigrams

    C.  840 centigrams          D.  8,400 centigrams

    The correct answer is **D.** The correct solution is 8,400 centigrams. $84 \text{ g} \times \frac{100 \text{ cg}}{1 \text{ g}} = 8,400$ cg.

    **See Lesson: Standards of Measure.**

# Conversions between Standard and Metric Systems

The table shows the common conversions of length, volume, and weight between the standard and metric systems.

| Measurement | Conversion |
|---|---|
| Centimeters (cm) and inches (in.) | 2.54 centimeters equals 1 inch |
| Meters (m) and feet (ft.) | 1 meter equals 3.28 feet |
| Kilometers (km) and miles (mi.) | 1.61 kilometers equals 1 mile |
| Quarts (qt.) and liters (L) | 1.06 quarts equals 1 liter |
| Liters (L) and gallons (gal.) | 3.79 liters equals 1 gallon |
| Grams (g) and ounces (oz.) | 28.3 grams equals 1 ounce |
| Kilograms (kg) and pounds (lb.) | 2.2 kilograms equals 1 pound |

There are many additional conversion factors, but this lesson uses only the common ones. Most factors have been rounded to the nearest hundredth for accuracy.

**STEP BY STEP**

**Step 1.** Choose the appropriate conversion factor within each system, if necessary.

**Step 2.** Choose the appropriate conversion factor from the standard and metric conversion.

**Step 3.** Multiply and simplify to the nearest hundredth.

## Examples

1. **Convert 12 inches to centimeters.**

   A.  4.72 centimeters

   B.  14.54 centimeters

   C.  28.36 centimeters

   D.  30.48 centimeters

   The correct answer is **D.** The correct solution is 30.48 centimeters. $12 \text{ in} \times \frac{2.54 \text{ cm}}{1 \text{ in}} = 30.48$ cm.
   **See Lesson: Standards of Measure.**

2. **Convert 8 kilometers to feet.**

   A.  13,118.01 feet

   B.  26,236.02 feet

   C.  34,003.20 feet

   D.  68,006.40 feet

   The correct answer is **B.** The correct solution is 26,236.02 feet. $8 \text{ km} \times \frac{1 \text{ mi}}{1.61 \text{ km}} \times \frac{5,280 \text{ ft}}{1 \text{ mi}} = \frac{42,240}{1.61} = 26,236.02$ ft.
   **See Lesson: Standards of Measure.**

3. **Convert 2 gallons to milliliters.**

   A.  527 milliliters

   B.  758 milliliters

   C.  5,270 milliliters

   D.  7,580 milliliters

   The correct answer is **D.** The correct solution is 7,580 milliliters. $2 \text{ gal} \times \frac{3.79 \text{ L}}{1 \text{ gal}} \times \frac{1,000 \text{ ml}}{1 \text{ L}} = 7,580$ mL.
   **See Lesson: Standards of Measure.**

4. **Convert 16 kilograms to pounds.**

    A. 7.27 pounds

    C. 19.27 pounds

    B. 18.2 pounds

    D. 35.2 pounds

The correct answer is **D.** The correct solution is 35.2 pounds. $16 \text{ kg} \times \frac{2.2 \text{ lb}}{1 \text{ kg}} = 35.2 \text{ lb}$.

**See Lesson: Standards of Measure.**

# Time Conversions

Two ways to keep time are 12-hour clock time using a.m. and p.m. and military time based on a 24-hour clock. Keep these three key points in mind:

**KEEP IN MIND**

Midnight (12:00 a.m.) is 2400 or 0000 in military time.

- The hours from 1:00 a.m. to 12:59 p.m. are the same in both methods. For example, 9:15 a.m. in 12-hour clock time is 0915 in military time.

- From 1:00 p.m. to 11:59 p.m., add 12 hours to obtain military time. For example, 4:07 p.m. in 12-hour clock time is 1607 in military time.

- From 12:01 a.m. to 12:59 a.m. in 12-hour clock time, military time is from 0001 to 0059.

## Example

**Identify 9:27 p.m. in military time.**

    A. 0927        B. 1927        C. 2127        D. 2427

The correct answer is **C.** The correct solution is 2127. Add 1200 to the time, $1200 + 927 = 2127$.

**See Lesson: Standards of Measure.**

## Let's Review!

- To convert from one unit to another, choose the appropriate conversion factors.

- In many cases, it is necessary to use multiple conversion factors.

# Chapter 1 Numbers, Basic Operations, and Measurement Practice Quiz

1. **What is 604 – 561?**

   A. 34

   B. 43

   C. 53

   D. 143

2. **What is 45 + 782 + 3?**

   A. 785

   B. 827

   C. 830

   D. 1,000

3. **Evaluate the expression (–224) ÷ 14.**

   A. –210

   B. –16

   C. 16

   D. 210

4. **Which statement about multiplication is true?**

   A. The order of two factors in multiplication has no effect on the product.

   B. The signs of the two factors in multiplication have no effect on the product.

   C. Memorizing a multiplication table is sufficient by itself to determine any product.

   D. None of the above.

5. **Which decimal is the least?**

   A. 5.2304

   B. 5.3204

   C. 5.2403

   D. 5.3024

6. **Change $\frac{5}{11}$ to a decimal. Simplify completely.**

   A. $0.\overline{4}$

   B. $0.\overline{45}$

   C. $0.\overline{5}$

   D. $0.\overline{54}$

# CHAPTER 1 NUMBERS, BASIC OPERATIONS, AND MEASUREMENT PRACTICE QUIZ – ANSWER KEY

**1. B.** The correct solution is 43. Use the subtraction algorithm, which will require borrowing once. **See Lesson: Basic Addition and Subtraction.**

**2. C.** The correct solution is 830. Use the addition algorithm. Add the first two numbers to get 827, then add 3 to get 830. **See Lesson: Basic Addition and Subtraction.**

**3. B.** When dividing signed numbers, remember that if the dividend and divisor have different signs, the quotient is negative. Other than the sign, the process is the same as dividing whole numbers. Use the division algorithm to divide 224 by 14. **See Lesson: Basic Multiplication and Division.**

**4. A.** Regardless of the order of the factors, the product is the same. For instance, 12 × 13 = 13 × 12 = 156. **See Lesson: Basic Multiplication and Division.**

**5. A.** The correct solution is 5.2304 because 5.2304 contains the smallest values in the tenths and the hundredths places. **See Lesson: Decimals and Fractions.**

**6. B.** The correct answer is $0.\overline{45}$ because $\frac{5}{11} = 5.00 \div 11 = 0.\overline{45}$. **See Lesson: Decimals and Fractions.**

# CHAPTER 2 ALGEBRA

## EQUATIONS WITH ONE VARIABLE

This lesson introduces how to solve linear equations and linear inequalities.

## One-Step Linear Equations

A **linear equation** is an equation where two expressions are set equal to each other. The equation is in the form $ax + b = c$, where $a$ is a non-zero constant and $b$ and $c$ are constants. The exponent on a linear equation is always 1, and there is no more than one solution to a linear equation.

There are four properties to help solve a linear equation.

| Property | Definition | Example with Numbers | Example with Variables |
|---|---|---|---|
| Addition Property of Equality | Add the same number to both sides of the equation. | $x - 3 = 9$ <br> $x - 3 + 3 = 9 + 3$ <br> $x = 12$ | $x - a = b$ <br> $x - a + a = b + a$ <br> $x = a + b$ |
| Subtraction Property of Equality | Subtract the same number from both sides of the equation. | $x + 3 = 9$ <br> $x + 3 - 3 = 9 - 3$ <br> $x = 6$ | $x + a = b$ <br> $x + a - a = b - a$ <br> $x = b - a$ |
| Multiplication Property of Equality | Multiply both sides of the equation by the same number. | $\frac{x}{3} = 9$ <br> $\frac{x}{3} \times 3 = 9 \times 3$ <br> $x = 27$ | $\frac{x}{a} = b$ <br> $\frac{x}{a} \times a = b \times a$ <br> $x = ab$ |
| Division Property of Equality | Divide both sides of the equation by the same number. | $3x = 9$ <br> $\frac{3x}{3} = \frac{9}{3}$ <br> $x = 3$ | $ax = b$ <br> $\frac{ax}{a} = \frac{b}{a}$ <br> $x = \frac{b}{a}$ |

## Example

**Solve the equation for the unknown, $\frac{w}{2} = -6$.**

A.  −12

B.  −8

C.  −4

D.  −3

The correct answer is **A.** The correct solution is −12 because both sides of the equation are multiplied by 2. **See Lesson: Equations with One Variable.**

# Two-Step Linear Equations

A two-step linear equation is in the form $ax + b = c$, where $a$ is a non-zero constant and $b$ and $c$ are constants. There are two basic steps in solving this equation.

| STEP BY STEP | |
| --- | --- |
| Step 1. | Use addition and subtraction properties of an equation to move the variable to one side of the equation and all number terms to the other side of the equation. |
| Step 2. | Use multiplication and division properties of an equation to remove the value in front of the variable. |

## Examples

1. **Solve the equation for the unknown, $\frac{x}{-2} - 3 = 5$.**

   A. −16       B. −8       C. 8       D. 16

   The correct answer is **A.** The correct solution is −16.

   $\frac{x}{-2} = 8$       Add 3 to both sides of the equation.

   $x = -16$       Multiply both sides of the equation by −2.

   **See Lesson: Equations with One Variable.**

2. **Solve the equation for the unknown, $4x + 3 = 8$.**

   A. −2       B. $-\frac{5}{4}$       C. $\frac{5}{4}$       D. 2

   The correct answer is **C.** The correct solution is $\frac{5}{4}$.

   $4x = 5$       Subtract 3 from both sides of the equation.

   $x = \frac{5}{4}$       Divide both sides of the equation by 4.

   **See Lesson: Equations with One Variable.**

3. **Solve the equation for the unknown w, $P = 2l + 2w$.**

   A. $2P - 2l = w$       B. $\frac{P-2l}{2} = w$       C. $2P + 2l = w$       D. $\frac{P+2l}{2} = w$

   The correct answer is **B.** The correct solution is $\frac{P-2l}{2} = w$.

   $P - 2l = 2w$       Subtract 2l from both sides of the equation.

   $\frac{P-2l}{2} = w$       Divide both sides of the equation by 2.

   **See Lesson: Equations with One Variable.**

# Multi-Step Linear Equations

In these basic examples of linear equations, the solution may be evident, but these properties demonstrate how to use an opposite operation to solve for a variable. Using these properties, there are three steps in solving a complex linear equation.

> **STEP BY STEP**
>
> **Step 1.** Simplify each side of the equation. This includes removing parentheses, removing fractions, and adding like terms.
>
> **Step 2.** Use addition and subtraction properties of an equation to move the variable to one side of the equation and all number terms to the other side of the equation.
>
> **Step 3.** Use multiplication and division properties of an equation to remove the value in front of the variable.

In Step 2, all of the variables may be placed on the left side or the right side of the equation. The examples in this lesson will place all of the variables on the left side of the equation.

When solving for a variable, apply the same steps as above. In this case, the equation is not being solved for a value, but for a specific variable.

## Examples

1. **Solve the equation for the unknown, $2(4x + 1) - 5 = 3 - (4x - 3)$.**

   A. $\frac{1}{4}$  B. $\frac{3}{4}$  C. $\frac{4}{3}$  D. 4

   The correct answer is **B.** The correct solution is $\frac{3}{4}$.

   | | |
   |---|---|
   | $8x + 2 - 5 = 3 - 4x + 3$ | Apply the distributive property. |
   | $8x - 3 = -4x + 6$ | Combine like terms on both sides of the equation. |
   | $12x - 3 = 6$ | Add 4x to both sides of the equation. |
   | $12x = 9$ | Add 3 to both sides of the equation. |
   | $x = \frac{3}{4}$ | Divide both sides of the equation by 12. |

   **See Lesson: Equations with One Variable.**

2. **Solve the equation for the unknown, $\frac{2}{3}x + 2 = -\frac{1}{2}x + 2(x + 1)$.**

   A. 0  B. 1  C. 2  D. 3

   The correct answer is **A.** The correct solution is 0.

   | | |
   |---|---|
   | $\frac{2}{3}x + 2 = -\frac{1}{2}x + 2x + 2$ | Apply the distributive property. |
   | $4x + 12 = -3x + 12x + 12$ | Multiply all terms by the least common denominator of 6 to eliminate the fractions. |
   | $4x + 12 = 9x + 12$ | Combine like terms on the right side of the equation. |
   | $-5x = 12$ | Subtract 9x from both sides of the equation. |
   | $-5x = 0$ | Subtract 12 from both sides of the equation. |
   | $x = 0$ | Divide both sides of the equation by $-5$. |

   **See Lesson: Equations with One Variable.**

3. **Solve the equation for the unknown for x, $y - y_1 = m(x - x_1)$.**

   A.   $y - y_1 + mx_1$             B.   $my - my_1 + mx_1$          C.   $\frac{y - y_1 + x_1}{m}$           D.   $\frac{y - y_1 + mx_1}{m}$

The correct answer is **D**. The correct solution is $\frac{y - y_1 + mx_1}{m}$.

| | |
|---|---|
| $y - y_1 = mx - mx_1$ | Apply the distributive property. |
| $y - y_1 + mx_1 = mx$ | Add $mx_1$ to both sides of the equation. |
| $\frac{y - y_1 + mx_1}{m} = x$ | Divide both sides of the equation by m. |

**See Lesson: Equations with One Variable.**

# Solving Linear Inequalities

A **linear inequality** is similar to a linear equation, but it contains an inequality sign ($<, >, \leq, \geq$). Many of the steps for solving linear inequalities are the same as for solving linear equations. The major difference is that the solution is an infinite number of values. There are four properties to help solve a linear inequality.

| Property | Definition | Example |
|---|---|---|
| Addition Property of Inequality | Add the same number to both sides of the inequality. | $x - 3 < 9$ <br> $x - 3 + 3 < 9 + 3$ <br> $x < 12$ |
| Subtraction Property of Inequality | Subtract the same number from both sides of the inequality. | $x + 3 > 9$ <br> $x + 3 - 3 > 9 - 3$ <br> $x > 6$ |
| Multiplication Property of Inequality (when multiplying by a positive number) | Multiply both sides of the inequality by the same number. | $\frac{x}{3} \geq 9$ <br> $\frac{x}{3} \times 3 \geq 9 \times 3$ <br> $x \geq 27$ |
| Division Property of Inequality (when multiplying by a positive number) | Divide both sides of the inequality by the same number. | $3x \leq 9$ <br> $\frac{3x}{3} \leq \frac{9}{3}$ <br> $x \leq 3$ |
| Multiplication Property of Inequality (when multiplying by a negative number) | Multiply both sides of the inequality by the same number. | $\frac{x}{-3} \geq 9$ <br> $\frac{x}{-3} \times -3 \geq 9 \times -3$ <br> $x \leq -27$ |
| Division Property of Inequality (when multiplying by a negative number) | Divide both sides of the inequality by the same number. | $-3x \leq 9$ <br> $\frac{-3x}{-3} \leq \frac{9}{-3}$ <br> $x \geq -3$ |

Multiplying or dividing both sides of the inequality by a negative number reverses the sign of the inequality.

In these basic examples, the solution may be evident, but these properties demonstrate how to use an opposite operation to solve for a variable. Using these properties, there are three steps in solving a complex linear inequality.

> **STEP BY STEP**
>
> **Step 1.** Simplify each side of the inequality. This includes removing parentheses, removing fractions, and adding like terms.
>
> **Step 2.** Use addition and subtraction properties of an inequality to move the variable to one side of the equation and all number terms to the other side of the equation.
>
> **Step 3.** Use multiplication and division properties of an inequality to remove the value in front of the variable. Reverse the inequality sign if multiplying or dividing by a negative number.

In Step 2, all of the variables may be placed on the left side or the right side of the inequality. The examples in this lesson will place all of the variables on the left side of the inequality.

## Examples

1. **Solve the inequality for the unknown, $3(2 + x) < 2(3x - 1)$.**

   A. $x < -\frac{8}{3}$       B. $x > -\frac{8}{3}$       C. $x < \frac{8}{3}$       D. $x > \frac{8}{3}$

   The correct answer is **D.** The correct solution is $x > \frac{8}{3}$.

   | | |
   |---|---|
   | $6 + 3x < 6x - 2$ | Apply the distributive property. |
   | $6 - 3x < -2$ | Subtract 6x from both sides of the inequality. |
   | $-3x < -8$ | Subtract 6 to both sides of the inequality. |
   | $x > \frac{8}{3}$ | Divide both sides of the inequality by 3. |

   **See Lesson: Equations with One Variable.**

2. **Solve the inequality for the unknown, $\frac{1}{2}(2x - 3) \geq \frac{1}{4}(2x + 1) - 2$**

   A. $x > -7$       B. $x > -3$       C. $x \geq -\frac{3}{2}$       D. $x \geq -\frac{1}{2}$

   The correct answer is **D.** The correct solution is $x \geq -\frac{1}{2}$.

   | | |
   |---|---|
   | $2(2x - 3) \geq 2x + 1 - 8$ | Multiply all terms by the least common denominator of 4 to eliminate the fractions. |
   | $4x - 6 \geq 2x + 1 - 8$ | Apply the distributive property. |
   | $4x - 6 \geq 2x - 7$ | Combine like terms on the right side of the inequality. |
   | $2x - 6 \geq -7$ | Subtract 2x from both sides of the inequality. |
   | $2x \geq -1$ | Add 6 to both sides of the inequality. |
   | $x \geq -\frac{1}{2}$ | Divide both sides of the inequality by 2. |

   **See Lesson: Equations with One Variable.**

## Let's Review!

- A linear equation is an equation with one solution. Using opposite operations solves a linear equation.
- The process to solve a linear equation or inequality is to eliminate fractions and parentheses and combine like terms on the same side of the sign. Then, solve the equation or inequality by using inverse operations.

# EQUATIONS WITH TWO VARIABLES

This lesson discusses solving a system of linear equations by substitution, elimination, and graphing, as well as solving a simple system of a linear and a quadratic equation.

## Solving a System of Equations by Substitution

A **system of linear equations** is a set of two or more linear equations in the same variables. A solution to the system is an ordered pair that is a solution in all the equations in the system. The ordered pair (1, -2) is a solution for the system of equations $\begin{matrix} 2x + y = 0 \\ -x + 2y = -5 \end{matrix}$ because $\begin{matrix} 2(1) + (-2) = 0 \\ -1 + 2(-2) = -5 \end{matrix}$ makes both equations true.

One way to solve a system of linear equations is by substitution.

> **STEP BY STEP**
>
> **Step 1.** Solve one equation for one of the variables.
>
> **Step 2.** Substitute the expression from Step 1 into the other equation and solve for the other variable.
>
> **Step 3.** Substitute the value from Step 2 into one of the original equations and solve.

All systems of equations can be solved by substitution for any one of the four variables in the problem. The most efficient way of solving is locating the $1x$ or $1y$ in the equations because this eliminates the possibility of having fractions in the equations.

## Examples

1. **Solve the system of equations,** $\begin{matrix} x = y + 6 \\ 4x + 5y = 60 \end{matrix}$.

    A.   (10, 12)          B.   (6, 12)          C.   (6, 4)          D.   (10, 4)

    The correct answer is **D.** The correct solution is (10, 4).
    The first equation is already solved for $x$.

    | | |
    |---|---|
    | $4(y + 6) + 5y = 60$ | Substitute $y + 6$ in for $x$ in the first equation. |
    | $4y + 24 + 5y = 60$ | Apply the distributive property. |
    | $9y + 24 = 60$ | Combine like terms on the left side of the equation. |
    | $9y = 36$ | Subtract 24 from both sides of the equation. |
    | $y = 4$ | Divide both sides of the equation by 9. |
    | $x = 4 + 6$ | Substitute 4 in the first equation for $y$. |
    | $x = 10$ | Simplify using order of operations |

    **See Lesson: Equations with Two Variables.**

2. **Solve the system of equations,** $\begin{array}{l} 3x + 2y = 41 \\ -4x + y = -18 \end{array}$.

A. (5, 13)  B. (6, 6)  C. (7, 10)  D. (10, 7)

The correct answer is **C**. The correct solution is (7, 10).

| | |
|---|---|
| $y = 4x - 18$ | Solve the second equation for $y$ by adding $4x$ to both sides of the equation. |
| $3x + 2(4x - 18) = 41$ | Substitute $4x - 18$ in for $y$ in the first equation. |
| $3x + 8x - 36 = 41$ | Apply the distributive property. |
| $11x - 36 = 41$ | Combine like terms on the left side of the equation. |
| $11x = 77$ | Add 36 to both sides of the equation. |
| $x = 7$ | Divide both sides of the equation by 11. |
| $-4(7) + y = -18$ | Substitute 7 in the second equation for $x$. |
| $-28 + y = -18$ | Simplify using order of operations. |
| $y = 10$ | Add 28 to both sides of the equation. |

**See Lesson: Equations with Two Variables.**

# Solving a System of Equations by Elimination

Another way to solve a system of linear equations is by elimination.

> **STEP BY STEP**
>
> **Step 1.** Multiply, if necessary, one or both equations by a constant so at least one pair of like terms has opposite coefficients.
>
> **Step 2.** Add the equations to eliminate one of the variables.
>
> **Step 3.** Solve the resulting equation.
>
> **Step 4.** Substitute the value from Step 3 into one of the original equations and solve for the other variable.

All system of equations can be solved by the elimination method for any one of the four variables in the problem. One way of solving is locating the variables with opposite coefficients and adding the equations. Another approach is multiplying one equation to obtain opposite coefficients for the variables.

# Examples

1. **Solve the system of equations,** $\begin{aligned} 3x + 5y &= 28 \\ -4x - 5y &= -34 \end{aligned}$.

   A. $(12, 6)$      B. $(6, 12)$      C. $(6, 2)$      D. $(2, 6)$

   The correct answer is **C**. The correct solution is $(6, 2)$.

   | | |
   |---|---|
   | $-x = -6$ | Add the equations. |
   | $x = 6$ | Divide both sides of the equation by -1. |
   | $3(6) + 5y = 28$ | Substitute 6 in the first equation for $x$. |
   | $18 + 5y = 28$ | Simplify using order of operations. |
   | $5y = 10$ | Subtract 18 from both sides of the equation. |
   | $y = 2$ | Divide both sides of the equation by 5. |

   **See Lesson: Equations with Two Variables.**

2. **Solve the system of equations,** $\begin{aligned} -5x + 5y &= 0 \\ 2x - 3y &= -3 \end{aligned}$.

   A. $(2, 2)$      B. $(3, 3)$      C. $(6, 6)$      D. $(9, 9)$

   The correct answer is **B**. The correct solution is $(3, 3)$.

   | | |
   |---|---|
   | $-10x + 10y = 0$ | Multiply all terms in the first equation by 2. |
   | $10x - 15y = -15$ | Multiply all terms in the second equation by 5. |
   | $-5y = -15$ | Add the equations. |
   | $y = 3$ | Divide both sides of the equation by -5. |
   | $2x - 3(3) = -3$ | Substitute 3 in the second equation for $y$. |
   | $2x - 9 = -3$ | Simplify using order of operations. |
   | $2x = 6$ | Add 9 to both sides of the equation. |
   | $x = 3$ | Divide both sides of the equation by 2. |

   **See Lesson: Equations with Two Variables.**

# Solving a System of Equations by Graphing

Graphing is a third method of a solving system of equations. The point of intersection is the solution for the graph. This method is a great way to visualize each graph on a coordinate plane.

| **STEP BY STEP** | |
|---|---|
| **Step 1.** | Graph each equation in the coordinate plane. |
| **Step 2.** | Estimate the point of intersection. |
| **Step 3.** | Check the point by substituting for $x$ and $y$ in each equation of the original system. |

The best approach to graphing is to obtain each line in slope-intercept form. Then, graph the $y$-intercept and use the slope to find additional points on the line.

Example

**Solve the system of equations by graphing,** $\begin{array}{l} y = 3x - 2 \\ y = x - 4 \end{array}$ .

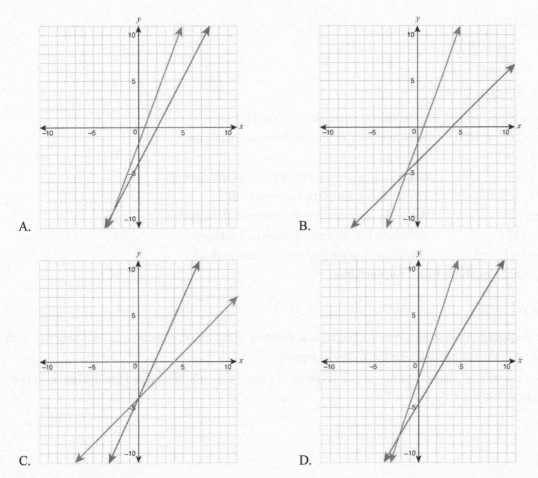

A.          B.

C.          D.

The correct answer is **B.** The correct graph has the two lines intersect at (-1, -5). **See Lesson: Equations with Two Variables.**

# Solving a System of a Linear Equation and an Equation of a Circle

There are many other types of systems of equations. One example is the equation of a line $y = mx$ and the equation of a circle $x^2 + y^2 = r^2$ where $r$ is the radius. With this system of equations, there can be two ordered pairs that intersect between the line and the circle. If there is one ordered pair, the line is tangent to the circle.

**KEEP IN MIND**

There will be two solutions in many cases with the system of a linear equation and an equation of a circle

This system of equations is solved by substituting the expression $mx$ in for $y$ in the equation of a circle. Then, solve the equation for $x$. The values for $x$ are substituted into the linear equation to find the value for $y$.

# Example

**Solve the system of equations,** $\begin{array}{l} y = -3x \\ x^2 + y^2 = 10 \end{array}$.

A.  (1, 3) and (-1, -3)

B.  (1, -3) and (-1, 3)

C.  (-3, 10) and (3, -10)

D.  (3, 10) and (-3, -10)

The correct answer is **B.** The correct solutions are (1, -3) and (-1, 3).

| | |
|---|---|
| $x^2 + (-3x)^2 = 10$ | Substitute $-3x$ in for $y$ in the second equation. |
| $x^2 + 9x^2 = 10$ | Apply the exponent. |
| $10x^2 = 10$ | Combine like terms on the left side of the equation. |
| $x^2 = 1$ | Divide both sides of the equation by 10. |
| $x = \pm 1$ | Apply the square root to both sides of the equation. |
| $y = -3(1) = -3$ | Substitute 1 in the first equation and multiply. |
| $y = -3(-1) = 3$ | Substitute -1 in the first equation and multiply. |

**See Lesson: Equations with Two Variables.**

# Let's Review!

- There are three ways to solve a system of equations: graphing, substitution, and elimination. Using any method will result in the same solution for the system of equations.

- Solving a system of a linear equation and an equation of a circle uses substitution and usually results in two solutions.

# SOLVING REAL WORLD MATHEMATICAL PROBLEMS

This lesson introduces solving real-world mathematical problems by using estimation and mental computation. This lesson also includes real-world applications involving integers, fractions, and decimals.

## Estimating

**Estimations** are rough calculations of a solution to a problem. The most common use for estimation is completing calculations without a calculator or other tool. There are many estimation techniques, but this lesson focuses on integers, decimals, and fractions.

To round a whole number, round the value to the nearest ten or hundred. The number 142 rounds to 140 for the nearest ten and to 100 for the nearest hundred. The context of the problem determines the place value to which to round.

> **KEEP IN MIND**
> An estimation is an educated guess at the solution to a problem.

In most problems with fractions and decimals, the context of the problem requires rounding to the nearest whole number. Rounding these values makes calculation easier and provides an accurate estimation to the solution of the problem.

Other estimation strategies include the following:

- Using friendly or compatible numbers
- Using numbers that are easy to compute
- Adjusting numbers after rounding

## Example

**There are 168 hours in a week. Carson does the following:**

- **Sleeps 7.5 hours each day of the week**
- **Goes to school 6.75 hours five days a week**
- **Practices martial arts and basketball 1.5 hours each three times a week**
- **Reads and studies 1.75 hours every day**
- **Eats 1.5 hours every day**

**Estimate the remaining number of hours.**

A. 30          B. 35          C. 40          D. 45

The correct answer is **C**. The correct solution is 40. He sleeps about 56 hours, goes to school for 35 hours, practices for 9 hours, read and studies for about 14 hours, and eats about 14 hours. This is 128 hours. Therefore, Carson has about 40 hours remaining. **See Lesson: Solving Real World Mathematical Problems.**

# Real World Integer Problems

The following five steps can make solving word problems easier:

1. Read the problem for understanding.

2. Visualize the problem by drawing a picture or diagram.

3. Make a plan by writing an expression to represent the problem.

4. Solve the problem by applying mathematical techniques.

5. Check the answer to make sure it answers the question asked.

> **BE CAREFUL!**
> Make sure that you read the problem fully before visualizing and making a plan.

In basic problems, the solution may be evident, but make sure to demonstrate knowledge of writing the expression. In multi-step problems, first make a plan with the correct expression. Then, apply the correct calculation.

## Examples

1. **The temperature on Monday was −9°F, and on Tuesday it was 8°F. What is the difference in temperature, in °F?**

   A.  −17°        B.  −1°        C.  1°        D.  17°

   The correct answer is **D**. The correct solution is 17° because $8 - (-9) = 17°F$. **See Lesson: Solving Real World Mathematical Problems.**

2. **A golfer's last 12 rounds were −2, +4, −3, −1, +5, +3, −4, −5, −2, −6, −1, and 0. What is the average of these rounds?**

   A.  −12        B.  −1        C.  1        D.  12

   The correct answer is **B**. The correct solution is −1. The total of the scores is −12. The average is −12 divided by 12, which is −1. **See Lesson: Solving Real World Mathematical Problems.**

# Real World Fraction and Decimal Problems

The five steps in the previous section are applicable to solving real-world fraction and decimal problems. The expressions with one step require only one calculation: addition, subtraction, multiplication, or division. The problems with multiple steps require writing out the expressions and performing the correct calculations.

> **KEEP IN MIND**
> Estimating the solution first can help determine if a calculation is completed correctly.

## Examples

1. **The length of a room is $7\frac{2}{3}$ feet. When the length of the room is doubled, what is the new length in feet?**

   A. $14\frac{2}{3}$ B. $15\frac{1}{3}$ C. $15\frac{2}{3}$ D. $16\frac{1}{3}$

   The correct answer is **B**. The correct solution is $15\frac{1}{3}$. The length is multiplied by 2, $7\frac{2}{3} \times 2 = \frac{23}{3} \times \frac{2}{1} = \frac{46}{3} = 15\frac{1}{3}$ feet. **See Lesson: Solving Real World Mathematical Problems.**

2. **A fruit salad is a mixture of $1\frac{3}{4}$ pounds of apples, $2\frac{1}{4}$ pounds of grapes, and $1\frac{1}{4}$ pounds of bananas. After the fruit is mixed, $1\frac{1}{2}$ pounds are set aside, and the rest is divided into three containers. What is the weight in pounds of one container?**

   A. $1\frac{1}{5}$ B. $1\frac{1}{4}$ C. $1\frac{1}{3}$ D. $1\frac{1}{2}$

   The correct answer is **B**. The correct solution is $1\frac{1}{4}$. The amount available for the containers is $1\frac{3}{4} + 2\frac{1}{4} + 1\frac{1}{4} - 1\frac{1}{2} = 5\frac{1}{4} - 1\frac{1}{2} = 5\frac{1}{4} - 1\frac{2}{4} = 4\frac{5}{4} - 1\frac{2}{4} = 3\frac{3}{4}$. This amount is divided into three containers, $3\frac{3}{4} \div 3 = \frac{15}{4} \times \frac{15}{12} = 1\frac{3}{12} = 1\frac{1}{4}$ pounds. **See Lesson: Solving Real World Mathematical Problems.**

3. **In 2016, a town had 17.4 inches of snowfall. In 2017, it had 45.2 inches of snowfall. What is the difference in inches?**

   A. 27.2 B. 27.8 C. 28.2 D. 28.8

   The correct answer is **B**. The correct solution is 27.8 because $45.2 - 17.4 = 27.8$ inches. **See Lesson: Solving Real World Mathematical Problems.**

4. **Mike bought items that cost \$4.78, \$3.49, \$6.79, \$9.78, and \$14.05. He had a coupon worth \$5.00. If he paid with a \$50.00 bill, then how much change does he receive?**

   A. \$16.11 B. \$18.11 C. \$21.11 D. \$23.11

   The correct answer is **A**. The correct solution is \$16.11. The total bill is \$38.89, less the coupon is \$33.89. The amount of change is \$50.00 - \$33.89 = \$16.11. **See Lesson: Solving Real World Mathematical Problems.**

## Let's Review!

- Using estimation is beneficial to determine an approximate solution to the problem when the numbers are complex.
- When solving a word problem with integers, fractions, or decimals, first read and visualize the problem. Then, make a plan, solve, and check the answer.'

# ALGEBRA: POWERS, EXPONENTS, ROOTS, AND RADICALS

This lesson introduces how to apply the properties of exponents and examines square roots and cube roots. It also discusses how to estimate quantities using integer powers of 10.

## Properties of Exponents

An expression that is a repeated multiplication of the same factor is a **power**. The **exponent** is the number of times the **base** is multiplied. For example, $6^2$ is the same as 6 times 6, or 36. There are many rules associated with exponents.

| Property | Definition | Examples |
|---|---|---|
| Product Rule (Same Base) | $a^m \times a^n = a^{m+n}$ | $4^1 \times 4^4 = 4^{1+4} = 4^5 = 1024$<br>$x^1 \times x^4 = x^{1+4} = x^5$ |
| Product Rule (Different Base) | $a^m \times b^m = (a \times b)^m$ | $2^2 \times 3^2 = (2 \times 3)^2 = 6^2 = 36$<br>$3^3 \times x^3 = (3 \times x)^3 = (3x)^3 = 27x^3$ |
| Quotient Rule (Same Base) | $\dfrac{a^m}{a^n} = a^{m-n}$ | $\dfrac{4^4}{4^2} = 4^{4-2} = 4^2 = 16$<br>$\dfrac{x^6}{x^3} = x^{6-3} = x^3$ |
| Quotient Rule (Different Base) | $\dfrac{a^m}{b^m} = \left(\dfrac{a}{b}\right)^m$ | $\dfrac{4^4}{3^4} = \left(\dfrac{4}{3}\right)^4$<br>$\dfrac{x^6}{y^6} = \left(\dfrac{x}{y}\right)^6$ |
| Power of a Power Rule | $(a^m)^n = a^{mn}$ | $(2^2)^3 = 2^{2\times3} = 2^6 = 64$<br>$(x^5)^8 = x^{5\times8} = x^{40}$ |
| Zero Exponent Rule | $a^0 = 1$ | $64^0 = 1$<br>$y^0 = 1$ |
| Negative Exponent Rule | $a^{-m} = \dfrac{1}{a^m}$ | $3^{-3} = \dfrac{1}{3^3} = \dfrac{1}{27}$<br>$\dfrac{1}{x^{-3}} = x^3$ |

For many exponent expressions, it is necessary to use multiplication rules to simplify the expression completely.

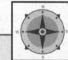

**KEEP IN MIND**

The expressions $(-2)^2 = (-2) \times (-2) = 4$ and $-2^2 = -(2 \times 2) = -4$ have different results because of the location of the negative signs and parentheses. For each problem, focus on each detail to simplify completely and correctly.

## Examples

1. **Simplify** $(3^2)^3$.

   A. 18        B. 216        C. 243        D. 729

   The correct answer is **D**. The correct solution is 729 because $(3^2)^3 = 3^{2 \times 3} = 3^6 = 729$. **See Lesson: Powers, Exponents, Roots, and Radicals.**

2. **Simplify** $(2x^2)^4$.

   A. $2x^8$        B. $4x^4$        C. $8x^6$        D. $16x^8$

   The correct answer is **D**. The correct solution is $16x^8$ because $(2x^2)^4 = 2^4(x^2)^4 = 2^4 x^{2 \times 4} = 16x^8$.
   **See Lesson: Powers, Exponents, Roots, and Radicals.**

3. **Simplify** $\left(\frac{x^{-2}}{y^2}\right)^3$.

   A. $\frac{1}{x^6 y^6}$        B. $\frac{x^6}{y^6}$        C. $\frac{y^6}{x^6}$        D. $x^6 y^6$

   The correct answer is **A**. The correct solution is $\frac{1}{x^6 y^6}$ because $\left(\frac{x^{-2}}{y^2}\right)^3 = \left(\frac{1}{x^2 y^2}\right)^3 = \frac{1}{x^{2 \times 3} y^{2 \times 3}} = \frac{1}{x^6 y^6}$.
   **See Lesson: Powers, Exponents, Roots, and Radicals.**

# Square Root and Cube Roots

The **square** of a number is the number raised to the power of 2. The **square root** of a number, when the number is squared, gives that number. $10^2 = 100$, so the square of 100 is 10, or $\sqrt{100} = 10$. **Perfect squares** are numbers with whole number square roots, such as 1, 4, 9, 16, and 25.

Squaring a number and taking a square root are opposite operations, meaning that the operations undo each other. This means that $\sqrt{x^2} = x$ and $(\sqrt{x})^2 = x$. When solving the equation $x^2 = p$, the solutions are $x = \pm\sqrt{p}$ because a negative value squared is a positive solution.

**KEEP IN MIND**

Most square roots and cube roots are not perfect roots.

The **cube** of a number is the number raised to the power of 3. The **cube root** of a number, when the number is cubed, gives that number. $10^3 = 1000$, so the cube of 1,000 is 100, or $\sqrt[3]{1000} = 10$. **Perfect cubes** are numbers with whole number cube roots, such as 1, 8, 27, 64, and 125.

Cubing a number and taking a cube root are opposite operations, meaning that the operations undo each other. This means that $\sqrt[3]{x^3} = x$ and $(\sqrt[3]{x})^3 = x$. When solving the equation $x^3 = p$, the solution is $x = \sqrt[3]{p}$.

If a number is not a perfect square root or cube root, the solution is an approximation. When this occurs, the solution is an irrational number. For example, $\sqrt{2}$ is the irrational solution to $x^2 = 2$.

## Examples

1. **Solve $x^2 = 121$.**

   A. $-10, 10$       B. $-11, 11$       C. $-12, 12$       D. $-13, 13$

   The correct answer is **B.** The correct solution is $-11, 11$ because the square root of 121 is 11. The values of $-11$ and 11 make the equation true. **See Lesson: Powers, Exponents, Roots, and Radicals.**

2. **Solve $x^3 = 125$.**

   A. 1       B. 5       C. 10       D. 25

   The correct answer is **B.** The correct solution is 5 because the cube root of 125 is 5. **See Lesson: Powers, Exponents, Roots, and Radicals.**

# Express Large or Small Quantities as Multiples of 10

**Scientific notation** is a large or small number written in two parts. The first part is a number between 1 and 10. In these problems, the first digit will be a single digit. The number is followed by a multiple to a power of 10. A positive integer exponent means the number is greater than 1, while a negative integer exponent means the number is smaller than 1.

The number $3 \times 10^4$ is the same as $3 \times 10,000 = 30,000$.

The number $3 \times 10^{-4}$ is the same as $3 \times 0.0001 = 0.0003$.

For example, the population of the United States is about $3 \times 10^8$, and the population of the world is about $7 \times 10^9$. The population of the United States is 300,000,000, and the population of the world is 7,000,000,000. The world population is about 20 times larger than the population of the United States.

## Examples

1. **The population of China is about $1 \times 10^9$, and the population of the United States is about $3 \times 10^8$. How many times larger is the population of China than the population of the United States?**

   A. 2       B. 3       C. 4       D. 5

   The correct answer is **B.** The correct solution is 3 because the population of China is about 1,000,000,000 and the population of the United States is about 300,000,000. So the population is about 3 times larger. **See Lesson: Powers, Exponents, Roots, and Radicals.**

2. **A red blood cell has a length of $8 \times 10^{-6}$ meter, and a skin cell has a length of $3 \times 10^{-5}$ meter. How many times larger is the skin cell?**

   A. 1       B. 2       C. 3       D. 4

   The correct answer is **D.** The correct solution is 4 because $3 \times 10^{-5}$ is 0.00003 and $8 \times 10^{-6}$ is 0.000008. So, the skin cell is about 4 times larger. **See Lesson: Powers, Exponents, Roots, and Radicals.**

## Let's Review!

- The properties and rules of exponents are applicable to generate equivalent expressions.
- Only a few whole numbers out of the set of whole numbers are perfect squares. Perfect cubes can be positive or negative.
- Numbers expressed in scientific notation are useful to compare large or small numbers.

# POLYNOMIALS

This lesson introduces adding, subtracting, and multiplying polynomials. It also explains polynomial identities that describe numerical expressions.

## Adding and Subtracting Polynomials

A **polynomial** is an expression that contains exponents, variables, constants, and operations. The exponents of the variables are only whole numbers, and there is no division by a variable. The operations are addition, subtraction, multiplication, and division. Constants are terms without a variable. A polynomial of one term is a **monomial**; a polynomial of two terms is a **binomial**; and a polynomial of three terms is a **trinomial.**

To add polynomials, combine like terms and write the solution from the term with the highest exponent to the term with the lowest exponent. To simplify, first rearrange and group like terms. Next, combine like terms.

> **KEEP IN MIND**
>
> The solution is an expression, and a value is not calculated for the variable.

$$(3x^2 + 5x - 6) + (4x^3 - 3x + 4)$$
$$= 4x^3 + 3x^2 + (5x - 3x) + (-6 + 4)$$
$$= 4x^3 + 3x^2 + 2x - 2$$

To subtract polynomials, rewrite the second polynomial using an additive inverse. Change the minus sign to a plus sign, and change the sign of every term inside the parentheses. Then, add the polynomials.

$$(3x^2 + 5x - 6) - (4x^3 - 3x + 4) = (3x^2 + 5x - 6) + (-4x^3 + 3x - 4) = -4x^3 + 3x^2 + (5x + 3x) + (-6 - 4)$$
$$= -4x^3 + 3x^2 + 8x - 10$$

## Examples

1. **Perform the operation, $(2y^2 - 5y + 1) + (-3y^2 + 6y + 2)$.**

   A. $y^2 + y + 3$

   B. $-y^2 - y + 3$

   C. $y^2 - y + 3$

   D. $-y^2 + y + 3$

   The correct answer is **D**. The correct solution is $-y^2 + y + 3$.
   $(2y^2 - 5y + 1) + (-3y^2 + 6y + 2) = (2y^2 - 3y^2) + (-5y + 6y) + (1 + 2) = -y^2 + y + 3$
   **See Lesson: Polynomials.**

2. **Perform the operation, $(3x^2y + 4xy - 5xy^2) - (x^2y - 3xy - 2xy^2)$.**

   A. $2x^2y - 7xy + 3xy^2$

   B. $2x^2y + 7xy + 3xy^2$

   C. $2x^2y + 7xy - 3xy^2$

   D. $2x^2y - 7xy - 3xy^2$

   The correct answer is **C**. The correct solution is $2x^2y + 7xy - 3xy^2$.
   $(3x^2y + 4xy - 5xy^2) - (x^2y - 3xy - 2xy^2) = (3x^2y + 4xy - 5xy^2) + (-x^2y + 3xy + 2xy^2) =$
   $(3x^2y - x^2y) + (4xy + 3xy) + (-5xy^2 + 2xy^2) = 2x^2y + 7xy - 3xy^2$
   **See Lesson: Polynomials.**

# Multiplying Polynomials

Multiplying polynomials comes in many forms. When multiplying a monomial by a monomial, multiply the coefficients and apply the multiplication rule for the power of an exponent.

$$4xy(3x^2y) = 12x^3y^2.$$

When multiplying a monomial by a polynomial, multiply each term of the polynomial by the monomial.

> **BE CAREFUL!**
>
> Make sure that you apply the distributive property to all terms in the polynomials.

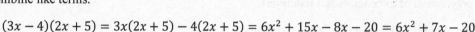

$$4xy(3x^2y - 2xy^2) = 4xy(3x^2y) + 4xy(-2xy^2) = 12x^3y^2 - 8x^2y^3.$$

When multiplying a binomial by a binomial, apply the distributive property and combine like terms.

$$(3x - 4)(2x + 5) = 3x(2x + 5) - 4(2x + 5) = 6x^2 + 15x - 8x - 20 = 6x^2 + 7x - 20$$

When multiplying a binomial by a trinomial, apply the distributive property and combine like terms.

$$(x + 2)(3x^2 - 2x + 3) = (x + 2)(3x^2) + (x + 2)(-2x) + (x + 2)(3) = 3x^3 + 6x^2 - 2x^2 - 4x + 3x + 6$$
$$= 3x^3 + 4x^2 - x + 6$$

## Examples

1. **Multiply, $3xy^2(2x^2y)$.**

   A. $6x^2y^2$ 　　　 B. $6x^3y^2$ 　　　 C. $6x^3y^3$ 　　　 D. $6x^2y^3$

   The correct answer is **C**. The correct solution is $6x^3y^3$. $3xy^2(2x^2y) = 6x^3y^3$. **See Lesson: Polynomials.**

2. **Multiply, $-2xy(3xy - 4x^2y^2)$.**

   A. $-6x^2y^2 + 8x^3y^3$ 　　　　　　 B. $-6x^2y^2 - 8x^3y^3$

   C. $-6xy + 8x^3y^3$ 　　　　　　　 D. $-6xy - 8x^3y^3$

   The correct answer is **A**. The correct solution is $-6x^2y^2 + 8x^3y^3$.

   $$-2xy(3xy - 4x^2y^2) = -2xy(3xy) - 2xy(-4x^2y^2) = -6x^2y^2 + 8x^3y^3$$

   **See Lesson: Polynomials.**

# Polynomial Identities

There are many polynomial identities that show relationships between expressions.

- Difference of two squares: 　　$a^2 - b^2 = (a - b)(a + b)$
- Square of a binomial: 　　　　$(a + b)^2 = a^2 + ab + b^2$
- Square of a binomial: 　　　　$(a - b)^2 = a^2 - ab + b^2$
- Sum of cubes: 　　　　　　　$a^3 + b^3 = (a + b)(a^2 - ab + b^2)$
- Difference of two cubes: 　　　$a^3 - b^3 = (a - b)(a^2 + ab + b^2)$

## Examples

1. **Apply the polynomial identity to rewrite** $x^2 + 6x + 9$.

   A. $x^2 + 9$

   B. $(x^2 + 3)^2$

   C. $(x + 3)^2$

   D. $(3x)^2$

The correct answer is **C.** The correct solution is $(x + 3)^2$. The expression $x^2 + 6x + 9$ is rewritten as $(x + 3)^2$ because the value of $a$ is x and the value of $b$ is 3. **See Lesson: Polynomials.**

2. **Apply the polynomial identity to rewrite** $8x^3 - 1$.

   A. $(2x + 1)(4x^2 + 2x - 1)$

   B. $(2x - 1)(4x^2 - 2x - 1)$

   C. $(2x + 1)(4x^2 - 2x + 1)$

   D. $(2x - 1)(4x^2 + 2x + 1)$

The correct answer is **D.** The correct solution is $(2x - 1)(4x^2 + 2x + 1)$. The expression $8x^3 - 1$ is rewritten as $(2x - 1)(4x^2 + 2x + 1)$ because the value of $a$ is $2x$ and the value of $b$ is 1. **See Lesson: Polynomials.**

## Let's Review!

- Adding, subtracting, and multiplying are commonly applied to polynomials. The key step in applying these operations is combining like terms.
- Polynomial identities require rewriting polynomials into different forms.

# CHAPTER 2 ALGEBRA PRACTICE QUIZ

1. Siobhan walks 1.45 miles to school and then back home each day Monday through Friday. How many miles does she walk each week?

   A. 7.25

   B. 10.15

   C. 14.5

   D. 20.3

2. A store has 75 pounds of bananas. Eight customers buy 3.3 pounds, five customers buy 4.25 pounds, and one customer buys 6.8 pounds. How many pounds are left in stock?

   A. 19.45

   B. 19.55

   C. 20.45

   D. 20.55

3. Solve the equation for the unknown, $3(x + 4) - 1 = 2(x + 3) - 2.$

   A. –7

   B. –2

   C. 2

   D. 7

4. Solve the inequality for the unknown, $2(3x - 1) + 5 \geq 3x - 4 - 4x.$

   A. $x \geq -7$

   B. $x \geq -4$

   C. $x \geq -1$

   D. $x \geq 0$

5. Solve the system of equations, $2x - 3y = -1$ $x + 2y = 24$.

   A. $(7, 10)$

   B. $(10, 7)$

   C. $(6, 8)$

   D. $(8, 6)$

6. Solve the system of equations, $-2x + 2y = 28$ $3x + y = -22$.

   A. $(9, 5)$

   B. $(-9, -5)$

   C. $(9, -5)$

   D. $(-9, 5)$

7. Multiply, $(x - 1)(x^2 + 2x + 3).$

   A. $x^3 + x^2 + x - 3$

   B. $x^3 - x^2 - x - 3$

   C. $x^3 + x^2 - x - 3$

   D. $x^3 - x^2 + x - 3$

8. Perform the operation, $(-3x + 5xy - 6y) - (4x + 2xy - 5y).$

   A. $-7x + 7xy - y$

   B. $-7x + 7xy - 11y$

   C. $-7x + 3xy - y$

   D. $-7x + 3xy - 11y$

9. Solve $x^3 = 64$.

   A. 2

   B. 3

   C. 4

   D. 5

10. Simplify $\frac{x^2 y^{-2}}{x^{-3} y^3}$.

   A. $\frac{x^5}{y^5}$

   B. $\frac{y^5}{x^5}$

   C. $\frac{1}{x^5 y^5}$

   D. $x^5 y^5$

# Chapter 2 Algebra
# Practice Quiz – Answer Key

**1. C.** The correct solution is 14.5 because $1.45(10) = 14.5$ miles. See **Lesson: Solving Real World Mathematical Problems.**

**2. D.** The correct solution is 20.55 because the number of pounds purchased is $8(3.3) + 5(4.25) + 6.8 = 26.4 + 21.25 + 6.8 = 54.45$ pounds. The number of pounds remaining is $75 - 54.45 = 20.55$ pounds. See **Lesson: Solving Real World Mathematical Problems.**

**3. A.** The correct solution is $-7$.

| | |
|---|---|
| $3x + 12 - 1 = 2x + 6 - 2$ | Apply the distributive property. |
| $3x + 11 = 2x + 4$ | Combine like terms on both sides of the equation. |
| $x + 11 = 4$ | Subtract 2x from both sides of the equation. |
| $x = -7$ | Subtract 11 from both sides of the equation. |

See **Lesson: Equations with One Variable.**

**4. C.** The correct solution is $x > -1$.

| | |
|---|---|
| $6x - 2 + 5 \geq 3x - 4 - 4x$ | Apply the distributive property. |
| $6x + 3 \geq -x - 4$ | Combine like terms on both sides of the inequality. |
| $7x + 3 \geq -4$ | Add x to both sides of the inequality. |
| $7x \geq -7$ | Subtract 3 from both sides of the inequality. |
| $x \geq -1$ | Divide both sides of the inequality by 7. |

See **Lesson: Equations with One Variable.**

**5. B.** The correct solution is (10, 7).

| | |
|---|---|
| $-2x - 4y = -48$ | Multiply all terms in the second equation by -2. |
| $-7y = -49$ | Add the equations. |
| $y = 7$ | Divide both sides of the equation by -7. |
| $x + 2(7) = 24$ | Substitute 7 in the second equation for $y$. |
| $x + 14 = 24$ | Simplify using order of operations. |
| $x = 10$ | Subtract 14 from both sides of the equation. |

See **Lesson: Equations with Two Variables.**

**6. D.** The correct solution is (-9, 5).

| | |
|---|---|
| $-6x - 2y = 44$ | Multiply all terms in the second equation by -2. |
| $-8x = 72$ | Add the equations. |
| $x = -9$ | Divide both sides of the equation by -8. |
| $3(-9) + y = -22$ | Substitute -9 in the second equation for $x$. |
| $-27 + y = -22$ | Simplify using order of operations. |
| $y = 5$ | Add 27 to both sides of the equation. |

See **Lesson: Equations with Two Variables.**

**7. A.** The correct solution is $x^3 + x^2 + x - 3$.

$$(x - 1)(x^2 + 2x + 3) = (x - 1)(x^2) + (x - 1)(2x) + (x - 1)(3) = x^3 - x^2 + 2x^2 - 2x + 3x - 3 = x^3 + x^2 + x - 3$$

See **Lesson: Polynomials.**

**8. C.** The correct solution is $-7x + 3xy - y$.

$$(-3x + 5xy - 6y) - (4x + 2xy - 5y) = (-3x + 5xy - 6y) + (-4x - 2xy + 5y)$$
$$= (-3x - 4x) + (5xy - 2xy) + (-6y + 5y) = -7x + 3xy - y$$

See **Lesson: Polynomials.**

**9. C.** The correct solution is 4 because the cube root of 64 is 4. See **Lesson: Powers, Exponents, Roots, and Radicals.**

**10. A.** The correct solution is $\frac{x^5}{y^5}$ because $\frac{x^2 y^{-2}}{x^{-3} y^3} = x^{2-(-3)} y^{-2-3} = x^5 y^{-5} = \frac{x^5}{y^5}$. See **Lesson: Powers, Exponents, Roots, and Radicals.**

# SECTION II
# READING COMPREHENSION

# Reading: 47 questions, 50 minutes

**Areas assessed:** Key Ideas and Details, Craft and Structure, Integration of Knowledge and Ideas

## *READING TIPS*

- If the question doesn't reference something in one of the answers, that answer is probably incorrect. Check to see what is/isn't referenced and choose the best answer from there.

- Do not assume facts about questions. Often, if information is not provided in the question, it will not be relevant. Stick to the facts that are provided.

- Some questions will focus on your ability to determine the difference between opinion and fact. Practice recognizing the difference between fact (the grass is green) and opinion (the grass smells nice).

- Read carefully and slowly. Questions may be confusing if you read too quickly.

- If you think that 2 answers could be correct, ask yourself, "What is it REALLY asking?"

- Study and know different types of writing styles. You may be asked to identify. i.e. narrative, expository, entertaining, analytical, or persuasive writing.

- Know how to identify first person (I), second person (You), third person (Narration).

- Use only the information you are given, if it is not stated in the text then don't assume it to be relevant.

- Use Process of Elimination. Eliminate answers you know are wrong and work your way to one, final answer.

- Know how to use an index, dictionary, almanac, encyclopedia, and glossary.

- Try to improve your reading speed and comprehension in advance. You want to ensure that you can finish the section before the time is up.

- Pay attention to the wording in questions. The wording in the question itself will usually provide helpful hints that can lead you toward the correct answer.

# CHAPTER 3 READING COMPREHENSION

# MAIN IDEAS, TOPIC SENTENCES, AND SUPPORTING DETAILS

To read effectively, you need to know how to identify the most important information in a text. You must also understand how ideas within a text relate to one other.

## Main Ideas

The central or most important idea in a text is the **main idea**. As a reader, you need to avoid confusing the main idea with less important details that may be interesting but not central to the author's point.

The **topic** of a text is slightly different than the main idea. The topic is a word or phrase that describes roughly what a text is about. A main idea, in contrast, is a complete sentence that states the topic and explains what an author wants to say about it.

All types of texts can contain main ideas. Read the following informational paragraph and try to identify the main idea:

> The immune system is the body's defense mechanism. It fights off harmful bacteria, viruses, and substances that attack the body. To do this, it uses cells, tissues, and organs that work together to resist invasion.

The topic of this paragraph is the immune system. The main idea can be expressed in a sentence like this: "This paragraph defines and describes the immune system." Ideas about organisms and substances that invade the body are not the central focus. The topic and main idea must always be directly related to every sentence in the text, as the immune system is here.

Read the persuasive paragraph below and consider the topic and main idea:

> Football is not a healthy activity for kids. It causes head injuries that harm the ability to learn and achieve. It causes painful bodily injuries that can linger into adulthood. It teaches aggressive behavioral habits that make life harder for players after they have left the field.

The topic of this paragraph is youth football, and the main idea is that kids should not play the game. Note that if you are asked to state the main idea of a persuasive text, it is your job to be objective. This means you should describe the author's opinion, not make an argument of your own in response.

Both of the example paragraphs above state their main idea explicitly. Some texts have an implicit, or suggested, main idea. In this case, you need to figure out the main idea using the details as clues.

**FOR EXAMPLE**

The following fictional paragraph has an implicit main idea:

Daisy parked her car and sat gripping the wheel, not getting out. A few steps to the door. A couple of knocks. She could give him the news in two words. She'd already decided what she was going to do, so it didn't matter what he said, not really. Still, she couldn't make her feet carry her to the door.

The main idea here is that Daisy feels reluctant to speak to someone. This point is not stated outright, but it is clear from the details of Daisy's thoughts and actions.

# Topic Sentences

Many paragraphs identify the topic and main idea in a single sentence. This is called a **topic sentence,** and it often appears at the beginning of a paragraph. However, a writer may choose to place a topic sentence anywhere in the text.

Some paragraphs contain an introductory sentence to grab the reader's attention before clearly stating the topic. A paragraph may begin by asking a rhetorical question, presenting a striking idea, or showing why the topic is important. When authors use this strategy, the topic sentence usually comes second:

Have you ever wondered how your body fights off a nasty cold? **It uses a complex defense mechanism called the immune system.** The immune system fights off harmful bacteria, viruses, and substances that attack the body. To do this, it uses cells, tissues, and organs that work together to resist invasion.

Here, the first sentence grabs the attention, and the second, **boldfaced** topic sentence states the main idea. The remaining sentences provide further information, explaining what the immune system does and identifying its basic components.

**COMPARE!**

The informational paragraph above contains a question that grabs the attention at the beginning. The writer could convey the same information with a little less flair by omitting this device. The version you read in Section 1 does exactly this. (The topic sentence below is **boldfaced.**)

**The immune system is the body's defense mechanism.** It fights off harmful bacteria, viruses, and substances that attack the body. To do this, it uses cells, tissues, and organs that work together to resist invasion.

Look back at the football paragraph from Section 1. Which sentence is the topic sentence?

Sometimes writers wait until the end of a paragraph to reveal the main idea in a topic sentence. When you're reading a paragraph that is organized this way, you may feel like you're reading a bit of a puzzle. It's not fully clear what the piece is about until you get to the end:

It causes head injuries that harm the ability to learn and achieve. It causes painful bodily injuries that can linger through the passage of years. It teaches aggressive behavioral habits that make life harder for players after they have left the field. **Football is not a healthy activity for kids.**

Note that the topic—football—is not actually named until the final, **boldfaced** topic sentence. This is a strong hint that this final sentence is the topic sentence. Other paragraphs with this structure may contain several examples or related ideas and then tie them together with a summary statement near the end.

# Supporting Details

The **supporting details** of a text develop the main idea, contribute further information, or provide examples.

All of the supporting details in a text must relate back to the main idea. In a text that sets out to define and describe the immune system, the supporting details could explain how the immune system works, define parts of the immune system, and so on.

> **Main Idea:** The immune system is the body's defense mechanism.
>
> **Supporting Detail:** It fights off harmful bacteria, viruses, and substances that attack the body.
>
> **Supporting Detail:** To do this, it uses cells, tissues, and organs that work together to resist invasion.

The above text could go on to describe white blood cells, which are a vital part of the body's defense system against disease. However, the supporting details in such a text should *not* drift off into descriptions of parts of the body that make no contribution to immune response.

Supporting details may be facts or opinions. A single text can combine both facts and opinions to develop a single main idea.

> **Main Idea:** Football is not a healthy activity for kids.
>
> **Supporting Detail:** It teaches aggressive behavioral habits that make life harder for players after they have left the field.
>
> **Supporting Detail:** In a study of teenage football players by Dr. Sophia Ortega at Harvard University, 28% reported involvement in fights or other violent incidents, compared with 19% of teenage boys who were not involved in sports.

The first supporting detail above states an opinion. The second is still related to the main idea, but it provides factual information to back up the opinion. Further development of this paragraph could contain other types of facts, including information about football injuries and anecdotes about real players who got hurt playing the game.

## Let's Review!

- The main idea is the most important piece of information in a text.
- The main idea is often expressed in a topic sentence.
- Supporting details develop the main idea, contribute further information, or provide examples.

# SUMMARIZING TEXT AND USING TEXT FEATURES

Effective readers need to know how to identify and restate the main idea of a text through summary. They must also follow complex instructions, figure out the sequence of events in a text that is not presented in order, and understand information presented in graphics.

## Summary Basics

A **summary** is a text that restates the ideas from a different text in a new way. Every summary needs to include the main idea of the original. Some summaries may include information about the supporting details as well.

The content and level of detail in a summary vary depending on the purpose. For example, a journalist may summarize a recent scientific study in a newspaper profile of its authors. A graduate student might briefly summarize the same study in a paper questioning its conclusions. The journalist's version would likely use fairly simple language and restate only the main points. The student's version would likely use specialized scientific vocabulary and include certain supporting details, especially the ones most applicable to the argument the student intends to make later.

The language of a summary must be substantially different from the original. It should not retain the structure and word choice of the source text. Rather, it should provide a completely new way of stating the ideas.

Read the passage below and the short summary that follows:

> **Original:** There is no need for government regulations to maintain a minimum wage because free market forces naturally adjust wages on their own. Workers are in short supply in our thriving economy, and businesses must offer fair wages and working conditions to attract labor. Business owners pay employees well because common sense dictates that they cannot succeed any other way.

> **Effective Summary:** The author argues against minimum wage laws. He claims free market forces naturally keep wages high in a healthy economy with a limited labor supply.

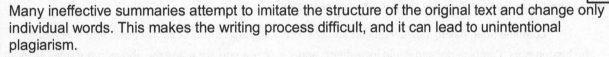

---

**KEY POINT!**

Many ineffective summaries attempt to imitate the structure of the original text and change only individual words. This makes the writing process difficult, and it can lead to unintentional plagiarism.

**Ineffective Summary (Plagiarism):** It is unnecessary for government regulations to create a minimum wage because capitalism adjusts wages without help. Good labor is rare in our excellent economy, and businesses need to offer fair wages and working conditions in order to attract workers.

The above text is an example of structural plagiarism. Summary writing does not just involve rewriting the original words one by one. An effective summary restates the main ideas of the text in a wholly original way.

---

The effective summary above restates the main ideas in a new but objective way. Objectivity is a key quality of an effective summary. A summary does not exaggerate, judge, or distort the author's original ideas.

> **Not a Summary:** The author makes a wild and unsupportable claim that minimum wage laws are unnecessary because market forces keep wages high without government intervention.

Although the above text might be appropriate in persuasive writing, it makes its own claims and judgments rather than simply restating the original author's ideas. It would not be an effective sentence in a summary.

In some cases, particularly dealing with creative works like fiction and poetry, summaries may mention ideas that are clearly implied but not stated outright in the original text. For example, a mobster in a thriller novel might turn to another character and say menacingly, "I wouldn't want anything to happen to your sweet little kids." A summary of this passage could objectively say the mobster had threatened the other character. But everything in the summary needs to be clearly supportable in the text. The summary could not go on to say how the other character feels about the threat unless the author describes it.

# Attending to Sequence and Instructions

Events happen in a sequence. However, many written texts present events out of order to create an effect on the reader. Nonfiction writers such as journalists and history writers may use this strategy to create surprise or bring particular ideas to the forefront. Fiction writers may interrupt the flow of a plot to interweave bits of a character's history or to provide flashes of insight into future events. Readers need to know how to untangle this presentation of events and figure out what actually happened first, second, and third. Consider the following passage:

> The man in dark glasses was looking for something. He checked his pockets. He checked his backpack. He walked back to his car, unlocked the doors, and inspected the area around the seats. Shaking his head, he re-locked the doors and rubbed his forehead in frustration. When his hand bumped his sunglasses, he finally realized where he had put them.

This passage does not mention putting the sunglasses on until the end, but it is clear from context that the man put them on first, before beginning his search. You can keep track of sequence by paying attention to time words like *when* and *before,* noticing grammatical constructions *he had* that indicate when events happened, and making common sense observations like the fact that the man is wearing his dark glasses in the first sentence.

Sequence is also an important aspect of reading technical and functional documents such as recipes and other instructions. If such documents present many steps in a large text block without illustrations or visual breaks, you may need to break them down and categorize them yourself. Always read all the steps first and think about how to follow them before jumping in. To see why, read the pancake recipe below:

> Combine flour, baking powder, sugar, and salt. Break the eggs into a separate bowl. Add milk and oil to the beaten eggs. Combine dry and liquid ingredients and stir. While you are doing the above, put a small amount of oil into a pan and heat it on medium heat. When it is hot, spoon batter onto the pan.

To follow directions like these effectively, a reader must break them down into categories, perhaps even rewriting them in a numbered list and noting when to start steps like heating the pan, which may be worth doing in a different order than it appears above.

# Interpreting Graphics

Information is often presented in pictures, graphs, or diagrams. These **graphic elements** may provide information to back up an argument, illustrate factual information or instructions, or present key facts and statistics.

When you read charts and graphs, it is important to look carefully at all the information presented, including titles and labels, to be sure that you are interpreting the visuals correctly.

## Diagram

A diagram presents a picture with labels that shows the parts of an object or functions of a mechanism. The diagram of a knee joint below shows the parts of the knee. Like many diagrams, it is placed in relation to a larger object—in this case, a leg—to clarify how the labeled parts fit into a larger context.

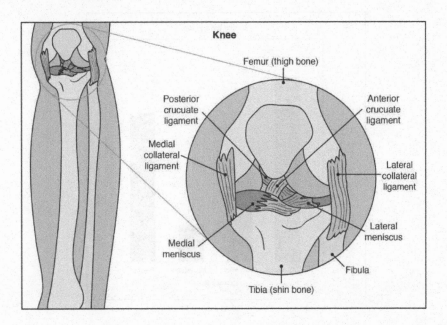

## Flowchart

A flowchart shows a sequence of actions or decisions involved in a complex process. A flowchart usually begins with an oval-shaped box that asks a yes-no question or gives an instruction. Readers follow arrows indicating possible responses. This helps readers figure out how to solve a problem, or it illustrates how a complex system works.

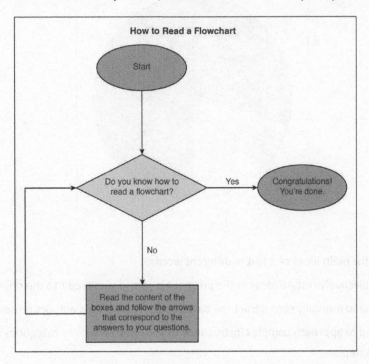

# Bar Graph

A bar graph uses bars of different sizes to represent numbers. Larger bars show larger numbers to convey the magnitude of differences between two numeric values at a glance. In this case, each rectangle shows the number of candy bars of different types that a particular group of people ate.

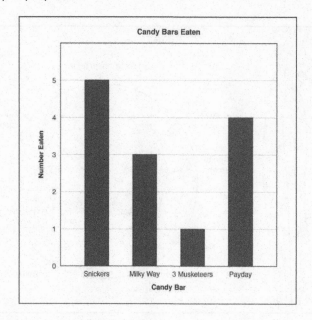

# Pie Chart

A pie chart is useful for representing all of something—in this case, the whole group of people surveyed about their favorite kind of pie. Larger wedges mean larger percentages of people liked a particular kind of pie. Percentage values may be written directly on the chart or in a key to the side.

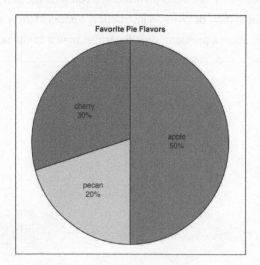

# Let's Review!

- A summary restates the main ideas of a text in different words.
- A summary should objectively restate ideas in the present tense and give credit to the original author.
- Effective readers need to mentally reconstruct the basic sequence of events authors present out of order.
- Effective readers need to approach complex instructions by grouping steps into categories or considering how best to approach the steps.
- Information may be presented graphically in the form of diagrams, flowcharts, graphs, or charts.

# TONE AND MOOD, AND TRANSITION WORDS

Authors use language to show their emotions and to make readers feel something too. They also use transition words to help guide the reader from one idea to the next.

## Tone and Mood

The **tone** of a text is the author's or speaker's attitude toward the subject. The tone may reflect any feeling or attitude a person can express: happiness, excitement, anger, boredom, or arrogance.

Readers can identify tone primarily by analyzing word choice. The reader should be able to point to specific words and details that help to establish the tone.

> **Example:** The train rolled past miles and miles of cornfields. The fields all looked the same. They swayed the same. They produced the same dull nausea in the pit of my stomach. I'd been sent out to see the world, and so I looked, obediently. What I saw was sameness.

Here, the author is expressing boredom and dissatisfaction. This is clear from the repetition of words like "same" and "sameness." There's also a sense of unpleasantness from phrases like "dull nausea" and passivity from words like "obediently."

Sometimes an author uses an ironic tone. Ironic texts often mean the opposite of what they actually say. To identify irony, you need to rely on your prior experience and common sense to help you identify texts with words and ideas that do not quite match.

> **Example:** With that, the senator dismissed the petty little problem of mass shootings and returned to the really important issue: his approval ratings.

Here the author flips around the words most people would usually use to discuss mass murder and popularity. By calling a horrific issue "petty" and a trivial issue "important," the author highlights what she sees as a politician's backwards priorities. Except for the phrase "mass shootings," the words here are light and airy—but the tone is ironic and angry.

A concept related to tone is **mood**, or the feelings an author produces in the reader. To determine the mood of a text, a reader can consider setting and theme as well as word choice and tone. For example, a story set in a haunted house may produce an unsettled or frightened feeling in a reader.

Tone and mood are often confused. This is because they are sometimes the same. For instance, in an op-ed article that describes children starving while food aid lies rotting, the author may use an outraged tone and simultaneously arouse an outraged mood in the reader.

However, tone and mood can be different. When they are, it's useful to have different words to distinguish between the author's attitude and the reader's emotional reaction.

> **Example:** I had to fly out of town at 4 a.m. for my trip to the Bahamas, and my wife didn't even get out of bed to make me a cup of coffee. I told her to, but she refused just because she'd been up five times with our newborn. I'm only going on vacation for one week, and she's been off work for a month! She should show me a little consideration.

Here, the tone is indignant. The mood will vary depending on the reader, but it is likely to be unsympathetic.

# Transitions

Authors use connecting words and phrases, or **transitions**, to link ideas and help readers follow the flow of their thoughts. The number of possible ways to transition between ideas is almost limitless.

Below are a few common transition words, categorized by the way they link ideas.

| Transitions | Examples |
|---|---|
| **Time and sequence** transitions orient the reader within a text. They can also help show when events happened in time. | *First, second, next, now, then, at this point, after, afterward, before this, previously, formerly, thereafter, finally, in conclusion* |
| **Addition or emphasis** transitions let readers know the author is building on an established line of thought. Many place extra stress on an important idea. | *Moreover, also, likewise, furthermore, above all, indeed, in fact* |
| **Example** transitions introduce ideas that illustrate a point. | *For example, for instance, to illustrate, to demonstrate* |
| **Causation** transitions indicate a cause-and-effect relationship. | *As a result, consequently, thus* |
| **Contrast** transitions indicate a difference between ideas. | *Nevertheless, despite, in contrast, however* |

Transitions may look different depending on their function within the text. Within a paragraph, writers often choose short words or expressions to provide transitions and smooth the flow. Between paragraphs or larger sections of text, transitions are usually longer. They may use some of the key words or ideas above, but the author often goes into detail restating larger concepts and explaining their relationships more thoroughly.

> **Between Sentences:** Students who cheat do not learn what they need to know. *As a result,* they get farther behind and face greater temptation to cheat in the future.

> **Between Paragraphs:** *As a result of the cheating behaviors described above,* students find themselves in a vicious cycle.

Longer transitions like the latter example may be useful for keeping the reader clued in to the author's focus in an extended text. But long transitions should have clear content and function. Some long transitions, such as the very wordy "due to the fact that" take up space without adding more meaning and are considered poor style.

## Let's Review!

- Tone is the author's or speaker's attitude toward the subject.
- Mood is the feeling a text creates in the reader.
- Transitions are connecting words and phrases that help readers follow the flow of a writer's thoughts.

# UNDERSTANDING THE AUTHOR'S PURPOSE, POINT OF VIEW, AND RHETORICAL STRATEGIES

In order to understand, analyze, and evaluate a text, readers must know how to identify the author's purpose and point of view. Readers also need to attend to an author's language and rhetorical strategies.

## Author's Purpose

When writers put words on paper, they do it for a reason. This reason is the author's **purpose**. Most writing exists for one of three purposes: to inform, to persuade, or to entertain.

---

**TEST TIP**

You may have learned about a fourth purpose for writing: conveying an emotional experience. Many poems as well as some works of fiction, personal essays, and memoirs are written to give the reader a sense of how an event or moment might feel. This type of text is rarely included on placement tests, and if it is, it tends to be lumped in with literature meant to entertain.

---

If a text is designed to share knowledge, its purpose is to **inform**. Informational texts include technical documents, cookbooks, expository essays, journalistic newspaper articles, and many nonfiction books. Informational texts are based on facts and logic, and they usually attempt an objective tone. The style may otherwise vary; some informational texts are quite dry, whereas others have an engaging style.

If a text argues a point, its purpose is to **persuade**. A persuasive text attempts to convince a reader to believe a certain point of view or take a certain action. Persuasive texts include op-ed newspaper articles, book and movie reviews, project proposals, and argumentative essays. Key signs of persuasive texts include judgments, words like *should,* and other signs that the author is sharing opinions.

If a text is primarily for fun, its purpose is to **entertain**. Entertaining texts usually tell stories or present descriptions. Entertaining texts include novels, short stories, memoirs, and some poems. Virtually all stories are lumped into this category, even if they describe unpleasant experiences.

---

**CONNECTIONS**

You may have read elsewhere that readers can break writing down into the following basic categories. These categories are often linked to the author's purpose.

**Narrative** writing tells a story and is usually meant to entertain.
**Expository** writing explains an idea and is usually meant to inform.
**Technical** writing explains a mechanism or process and is usually meant to inform.
**Persuasive** writing argues a point and, as the label suggests, is meant to persuade.

---

A text can have more than one purpose. For example, many traditional children's stories come with morals or lessons. These are meant both to entertain children and persuade them to behave in ways society considers appropriate. Also, commercial nonfiction texts like popular science books are often written in an engaging or humorous style. The purpose of such a text is to inform while also entertaining the reader.

# Point of View

Every author has a general outlook or set of opinions about the subject. These make up the author's **point of view**.

To determine point of view, a reader must recognize implicit clues in the text and use them to develop educated guesses about the author's worldview. In persuasive texts, the biggest clue is the author's explicit argument. From considering this argument, a reader can usually make some inferences about point of view. For instance, if an author argues that parents should offer kids opportunities to exercise throughout the day, it would be reasonable to infer that the author has an overall interest in children's health, and that he or she is troubled by the idea of kids pursuing sedentary behaviors like TV watching.

It is more challenging to determine point of view in a text meant to inform. Because the writer does not present an explicit argument, readers must examine assumptions and word choice to determine the writer's point of view.

> **Example:** Models suggest that at the current rate of global warming, hurricanes in 2100 will move 9 percent slower and drop 24 percent more rain. Longer storm durations and rainfall rates will likely translate to increased economic damage and human suffering.

It is reasonable to infer that the writer of this passage has a general trust for science and scientists. This writer assumes that global warming is happening, so it is clear he or she is not a global warming denier. Although the writer does not suggest a plan to prevent future storm damage, the emphasis on negative effects and the use of negative words like "damage" and "suffering" suggest that the author is worried about global warming.

Texts meant to entertain also contain clues about the author's point of view. That point of view is usually evident from the themes and deeper meanings. For instance, a memoirist who writes an upbeat story about a troubled but loving family is likely to believe strongly in the power of love. Note, however, that in this type of work, it is not possible to determine point of view merely from one character's words or actions. For instance, if a character says, "Your mother's love doesn't matter much if she can't take care of you," the reader should *not* automatically assume the writer agrees with that statement. Narrative writers often present a wide range of characters with varying outlooks on life. A reader can only determine the author's point of view by considering the work as a whole. The attitudes that are most emphasized and the ones that win out in the end are likely to reflect the author's point of view.

# Rhetorical Strategies

**Rhetorical strategies** are the techniques an author uses to support an argument or develop a main idea. Effective readers need to study the language of a text and determine how the author is supporting his or her points.

One strategy is to appeal to the reader's reason. This is the foundation of effective writing, and it simply means that the writer relies on factual information and the logical conclusions that follow from it. Even persuasive writing uses this strategy by presenting facts and reasons to back up the author's opinions.

> **Ineffective:** Everyone knows *Sandra and the Lumps* is the best band of the new millennium.

> **Effective:** The three most recent albums by *Sandra and the Lumps* are the first, second, and third most popular records released since the turn of the millennium.

Another strategy is to establish trust. A writer can do this by choosing credible sources and by presenting ideas in a clear and professional way. In persuasive writing, writers may show they are trustworthy by openly acknowledging that some people hold contradicting opinions and by responding fairly to those positions. Writers should never attack or misrepresent their opponents' position.

**Ineffective:** People who refuse to recycle are too lazy to protect their children's future.

**Effective:** According to the annual Throw It Out Questionnaire, many people dislike the onerous task of sorting garbage, and some doubt that their effort brings any real gain.

A final strategy is to appeal to the reader's emotions. For instance, a journalist reporting on the opioid epidemic could include a personal story about an addict's attempts to overcome substance abuse. Emotional content can add a human dimension to a story that would be missing if the writer only included statistics and expert opinions. But emotions are easily manipulated, so writers who use this strategy need to be careful. Emotions should never be used to distort the truth or scare readers into agreeing with the writer.

**Ineffective:** If you don't take action on gun control, you're basically killing children.

**Effective:** Julie was puzzling over the Pythagorean Theorem when she heard the first gunshot.

## Let's Review!

- Every text has a purpose.
- Most texts are meant to inform, persuade, or entertain.
- Texts contain clues that imply an author's outlook or set of opinions about the subject.
- Authors use rhetorical strategies to appeal to reason, establish trust, or invoke emotions.

# FACTS, OPINIONS, AND EVALUATING AN ARGUMENT

Nonfiction writing is based on facts and real events, but most nonfiction nevertheless expresses a point of view. Effective readers must evaluate the author's point of view and form their own conclusions about the points in the text.

## Fact and Opinion

Many texts make an **argument.** In this context, the word *argument* has nothing to do with anger or fighting. It simply means the author is trying to convince readers of something.

Arguments are present in a wide variety of texts. Some relate to controversial issues, for instance by advocating support for a political candidate or change in laws. Others may defend a certain interpretation of facts or ideas. For example, a literature paper may argue that an author's story suggests a certain theme, or a science paper may argue for a certain interpretation of data. An argument may also present a plan of action such as a business strategy.

To evaluate an argument, readers must distinguish between **fact** and **opinion**. A fact is verifiably true. An opinion is someone's belief.

> **Fact:** Seattle gets an average of 37 inches of rain per year.

> **Opinion:** The dark, rainy, cloudy weather makes Seattle an unpleasant place to live in winter.

Meteorologists measure rainfall directly, so the above fact is verifiably true. The statement "it is unpleasant" clearly reflects a feeling, so the second sentence is an opinion.

The difference between fact and opinion is not always straightforward. For instance, a text may present a fact that contains an opinion within it:

> **Fact:** Nutritionist Fatima Antar questions the wisdom of extreme carbohydrate avoidance.

Assuming the writer can prove that this sentence genuinely reflects Fatima Antar's beliefs, it is a factual statement of her point of view. The reader may trust that Fatima Antar really holds this opinion, whether or not the reader is convinced by it.

If a text makes a judgment, it is not a fact:

> **Opinion:** The patient's seizure drug regimen caused horrendous side effects.

The above sentence uses language that different people would interpret in different ways. Because people have varying ideas about what they consider "horrendous," this sentence is an opinion as it is written, even though the actual side effects and the patient's opinion of them could both be verified.

**COMPARE!**

Small changes to the statement about seizure drugs could turn it into a factual statement:

**Fact:** The patient's seizure drug regiment caused side effects such as migraines, confusion, and dangerously high blood pressure.

The above statement can be verified because the patient and other witnesses could confirm the exact nature of her symptoms. This makes it a fact.

**Fact:** The patient reported that her seizure drug regimen caused horrendous side effects.

This statement can also be verified because the patient can verify that she considers the side effects horrendous. By framing the statement in this way, the writer leaves nothing up to interpretation and is clearly in the realm of fact.

The majority of all arguments contain both facts and opinions, and strong arguments may contain both fact and opinion elements. It is rare for an argument to be composed entirely of facts, but it can happen if the writer is attempting to convince readers to accept factual information that is little-known or widely questioned. Most arguments present an author's opinion and use facts, reasoning, and expert testimony to convince readers.

## Evaluating an Argument

Effective readers must evaluate an argument and decide whether or not it is valid. To do this, readers must consider every claim the author presents, including both the main argument and any supporting statements. If an argument is based on poor reasoning or insufficient evidence, it is not valid—even if you agree with the main idea.

**KEY POINT!**

Most of us want to agree with arguments that reflect our own beliefs. But it is inadvisable to accept an argument that is not properly rooted in good reasoning. Consider the following statements about global climate change:

**Poor Argument:** It just snowed fifteen inches! How can anyone say the world is getting warmer?
**Poor Argument:** It's seventy degrees in the middle of February! How can anyone deny global warming?

Both of these arguments are based on insufficient evidence. Each relies on *one* weather event in *one* location to support an argument that the entire world's climate is or is not changing. There is not nearly enough information here to support an argument on either side.

Beware of any argument that presents opinion information as fact.

> **False Claim of Fact**: I know vaccines cause autism because my niece began displaying autism symptoms after receiving her measles vaccine.

The statement above states a controversial idea as fact without adequate evidence to back it up. Specifically, it makes a false claim of cause and effect about an incident that has no clear causal relationship.

Any claim that is not supported by sufficient evidence is an example of **faulty reasoning**.

| Type of Faulty Reasoning | Definition | Example | Explanation |
|---|---|---|---|
| Circular Reasoning | Restating the argument in different words instead of providing evidence | Baseball is the best game in the world because it is more fun than any other game. | Here, everything after the word *because* says approximately the same thing as everything before it. It looks like the author is providing a reason, but no evidence has actually been offered. |
| Either/Or Fallacy | Presenting an issue as if it involves only two choices when in fact it is not so simple | Women should focus on motherhood, not careers. | This statement assumes that women cannot do both. It also assumes that no woman needs a career in order to provide for her children. |
| Overgeneralizations | Making a broad claim based on too little evidence | All elderly people have negative stereotypes of teenagers. | This statement lumps a whole category of people into a group and claims the whole group shares the same belief—always an unlikely prospect. |

Most texts about evaluating arguments focus on faulty reasoning and false statements of fact. But arguments that attempt to misrepresent facts as opinions are equally suspicious. A careful reader should be skeptical of any text that denies clear physical evidence or questions the truth of events that have been widely verified.

# Assumptions and Biases

A well-reasoned argument should be supported by facts, logic, and clearly explained opinions. But most arguments are also based on **assumptions,** or unstated and unproven ideas about what is true. Consider the following argument:

> **Argument:** To improve equality of opportunity for all children, schools in underprivileged areas should receive as much taxpayer funding as schools in wealthy districts.

This argument is based on several assumptions. First is the assumption that all children should have equal opportunities. Another is that taxpayer-funded public schools are the best way to provide these opportunities. Whether or not you disagree with either of these points, it is worth noting that the second idea in particular is not the only way to proceed. Readers who examine the assumptions behind an argument can sometimes find points of disagreement even if an author's claims and logic are otherwise sound.

Examining an author's assumptions can also reveal a writer's biases. A **bias** is a preconceived idea that makes a person more likely to show unfair favor for certain thoughts, people, or groups. Because every person has a different experience of the world, every person has a different set of biases. For example, a person who has traveled widely may feel differently about world political events than someone who has always lived in one place.

Virtually all writing is biased to some degree. However, effective writing attempts to avoid bias as much as possible. Writing that is highly biased may be based on poor assumptions that render the entire argument invalid.

Highly biased writing often includes overgeneralizations. Words like *all, always, never,* and so on may indicate that the writer is overstating a point. While these words can exist in true statements, unbiased writing is more likely to qualify ideas using words like *usually, often,* and *rarely.*

Another quality of biased writing is excessively emotional word choice. When writers insult people who disagree with them or engage the emotions in a way that feels manipulative, they are being biased.

**Biased:** Power-hungry politicians don't care that their standardized testing requirements are producing a generation of overanxious, incurious, impractical kids.

**Less biased:** Politicians need to recognize that current standardized testing requirements are causing severe anxiety and other negative effects in children.

Biased writing may also reflect stereotypical thinking. A **stereotype** is a particularly harmful type of bias that applies specifically to groups of people. Stereotypical thinking is behind racism, sexism, homophobia, and so on. Even people who do not consider themselves prejudiced can use language that reflects common stereotypes. For example, the negative use of the word *crazy* reflects a stereotype against people with mental illnesses.

Historically, writers in English have used male nouns and pronouns to indicate all people. Revising such language for more inclusivity is considered more effective in contemporary writing.

**Biased:** The history of the human race proves that man is a violent creature.

**Less biased:** The history of the human race proves that people are violent.

## Let's Review!

- A text meant to convince someone of something is making an argument.
- Arguments may employ both facts and opinions.
- Effective arguments must use valid reasoning.
- Arguments are based on assumptions that may be reasonable or highly biased.
- Almost all writing is biased to some degree, but strong writing makes an effort to eliminate bias.

# UNDERSTANDING PRIMARY SOURCES, MAKING INFERENCES, AND DRAWING CONCLUSIONS

Effective readers must understand the difference between types of sources and choose credible sources of information to support research. Readers must also consider the content of their reading materials and draw their own conclusions.

## Primary Sources

When we read and research information, we must differentiate between different types of sources. Sources are often classified depending on how close they are to the original creation or discovery of the information they present.

**Primary sources** include firsthand witness accounts of events, research described by the people who conducted it, and any other original information. Contemporary researchers can often access mixed media versions of primary sources such as video and audio recordings, photographs of original work, and so on. Note that original content is still considered primary even if it is reproduced online or in a book.

> **Examples:** Diaries, scientific journal articles, witness testimony, academic conference presentations, business memos, speeches, letters, interviews, and original literature and artwork.

**Secondary sources** respond to, analyze, summarize, or comment on primary sources. They add value to a discussion of the topic by giving readers new ways to think about the content. However, they may also introduce errors or layers of bias. Secondary sources may be very good sources of information, but readers must evaluate them carefully.

> **Examples:** Biographies, books and articles that summarize research for wider audiences, analyses of original literature and artwork, histories, political commentary.

**Tertiary sources** compile information in a general, highly summarized, and sometimes simplified way. Their purpose is not to add anything to the information, but rather to present the information in an accessible manner, often for audiences who are only beginning to familiarize themselves with a topic.

> **Examples:** Encyclopedias, guidebooks, literature study guides.

### Source Materials in Action

Primary sources are often considered most trustworthy because they are closest to the original material and least likely to contain errors. However, readers must take a common sense approach to evaluating trustworthiness. For example, a single letter written by one biased witness of a historical event may not provide as much insight into what really happened as a secondary account by a historian who has considered the points of view of a dozen firsthand witnesses.

Tertiary sources are useful for readers attempting to gain a quick overview of understanding about a subject. They are also a good starting point for readers looking for keywords and subtopics to use for further research of a subject. However, they are not sufficiently detailed or credible to support an article, academic paper, or other document intended to add valuable analysis and commentary on a subject.

## Evaluating Credibility

Not everything you read is equally trustworthy. Many sources contain mistakes, faulty reasoning, or deliberate misinformation designed to manipulate you. Effective readers seek out information from **credible**, or trustworthy, sources.

There is no single formula for determining credibility. Readers must make judgment calls based on individual texts and their purpose.

> **FOR EXAMPLE**
>
> Most sources should attempt to be objective. But if you're reading an article that makes an argument, you do not need to demand perfect objectivity from the source. The purpose of a persuasive article is to defend a point of view. As long as the author does this openly and defends the point of view with facts, logic, and other good argumentative techniques, you may trust the source.
>
> Other sources may seem highly objective but not be credible. For example, some scientific studies meet all the criteria for credibility below except the one about trustworthy publishers. If a study is funded or conducted by a company that stands to profit from it, you should treat the results with skepticism no matter how good the information looks otherwise.

## Sources and References

Credible texts are primary sources or secondary sources that refer to other trustworthy sources. If the author consults experts, they should be named, and their credentials should be explained. Authors should not attempt to hide where they got their information. Vague statements like "studies show" are not as trustworthy as statements that identify who completed a study.

## Objectivity

Credible texts usually make an effort to be objective. They use clear, logical reasoning. They back arguments up with facts, expert opinions, or clear explanations. The assumptions behind the arguments do not contain obvious stereotypes.

Emotional arguments are acceptable in some argumentative writing, but they should not be manipulative. For example, photos of starving children may be acceptable for raising awareness of a famine, but they need to be respectful of both the victims and the audience—not just there for shock value.

## Date of Publication

Information changes quickly in some fields, especially the sciences and technology. When researching a fast-changing topic, look for sources published in the last ten years.

## Author Information

If an author and/or a respected organization take public credit for information, it is more likely to be reliable. Information published anonymously on the Internet may be suspicious because nobody is clearly responsible for mistakes. Authors with strong credentials such as university professors in a given field are more trustworthy than authors with no clear resume.

## Publisher Information

Information published by the government, a university, a major national news organization, or another respected organization is often more credible. On the Internet, addresses ending in .edu or .gov may be more trustworthy than .com addresses. Publishers who stand to profit or otherwise benefit from the content of a text are always questionable.

## Professionalism

Credible sources usually look professional and present information free of grammatical errors or major factual errors.

> **BE CAREFUL!**
> Strong credentials only make a source more trustworthy if the credentials are related to the topic. A Columbia University Professor of Archeology is a credible source on ancient history. But if she writes a parenting article, it's not necessarily more credible than a parenting article by someone without a flashy university title.

# Making Inferences and Drawing Conclusions

In reading—and in life—people regularly make educated guesses based on limited information. When we use the information we have to figure out something nobody has told us directly, we are making an **inference**. People make inferences every day.

**Example:** You hear a loud thump. Then a pained voice says, "Honey, can you bring the first aid kit?"

From the information above, it is reasonable to infer that the speaker is hurt. The thumping noise, the pain in the speaker's voice, and the request for a first aid kit all suggest this conclusion.

When you make inferences from reading, you use clues presented in the text to help you draw logical conclusions about what the author means. Before you can make an inference, you must read the text carefully and understand the explicit, or overt, meaning. Next, you must look for clues to any implied, or suggested, meanings behind the text. Finally, consider the clues in light of your prior knowledge and the author's purpose, and draw a conclusion about the meaning.

As soon as Raizel entered the party, someone handed her a plate. She stared down at the hot dog unhappily.

"What?" asked an unfamiliar woman nearby with an edge to her voice. "You don't eat dead animal?"

From the passage above, it would be reasonable to infer that the unfamiliar woman has a poor opinion of vegetarians. Several pieces of information suggest this: her combative tone, the edge in her voice, and the mocking question at the end.

When you draw inferences from a text, make sure your conclusion is truly indicated by the clues provided.

**BE CAREFUL!**

Before you make a conclusion about a text, consider it in light of your prior knowledge and the clues presented. After reading the paragraph above, you might suspect that Raizel is a vegetarian. But the text does not fully support that conclusion. There are many reasons why Raizel might not want to eat a hot dog. Perhaps she is keeping kosher, or she has social anxiety that makes it difficult to eat at parties, or she simply isn't hungry. The above inference about the unfamiliar woman's dislike for vegetarians is strongly supported. But you'd need further evidence before you could safely conclude that Raizel is actually a vegetarian.

Author Glenda Davis had high hopes for her children's book *Basketball Days*. But when the novel was released with a picture of a girl on the cover, boys refused to pick it up. The author reported this to her publisher, and the paperback edition was released with a new cover—this time featuring a dog and a basketball hoop. After that, many boys read the book. And Davis never heard anyone complain that the main character was a girl.

The text above implies that boys are reluctant to read books with a girl on the cover. A hasty reader might stop reading early and conclude that boys are reluctant to read about girls—but this inference is not suggested by the full text.

## Let's Review!

- Effective readers must consider the credibility of their sources
- Primary sources are usually considered the most trustworthy
- Readers must often make inferences about ideas that are implied but not explicitly stated in a text

# CHAPTER 3 READING COMPREHENSION PRACTICE QUIZ

1. **The author's _____ is the reason for writing.**

   A. purpose

   B. rhetoric

   C. main idea

   D. point of view

2. **Readers can determine tone primarily by examining:**

   A. setting.

   B. word choice.

   C. their feelings.

   D. connecting words.

3. **A topic sentence always expresses:**

   A. an opinion.

   B. the main idea.

   C. the conclusion.

   D. supporting details.

4. **What are graphic elements in a text?**

   A. Ideas arranged sequentially

   B. Main ideas restated differently

   C. Information presented visually

   D. White space between paragraphs

5. **Which phrase describes the set of techniques an author uses to support an argument or develop a main idea?**

   A. Points of view

   B. Logical fallacies

   C. Statistical analyses

   D. Rhetorical strategies

6. **A source is not credible if:**

   A. its publisher is government funded.

   B. any of its sources are primary sources.

   C. any of its sources are secondary sources.

   D. its publisher is profiting from the information.

7. **Transitions tend to be longer and more detailed when they occur between:**

   A. Words

   B. Clauses

   C. Sentences

   D. Paragraphs

8. **Which statement is an opinion?**

   A. Freshman Anita Jones states that excessive homework requirements cause her undue stress.

   B. Students reported symptoms such as headaches, anxiety attacks, and difficulty sleeping.

   C. Excessive homework requirements causes students undue stress and harm their quality of life.

   D. Students who do homework more than three hours per day show elevated cortisol levels compared to students who do no homework.

9. **Readers make inferences when they:**

   A. restate the main idea of a text in different words.

   B. differentiate between primary and secondary sources.

   C. determine that a text is not a credible source of information.

   D. use clues in the text to help them deduce implicit information.

10. **A _____ would be most helpful for helping someone figure out what to do when a computer breaks down**

    A. Diagram

    B. Pie chart

    C. Bar graph

    D. Flowchart

11. **A(n) _____ main idea is suggested, not stated outright.**

    A. explicit

    B. implied

    C. persuasive

    D. informational

12. **What is a bias?**

    A. A preconceived and sometimes unfair belief

    B. A person or group that often faces prejudice

    C. An unstated idea that underlies an argument

    D. A sweeping statement that may not always be true

# CHAPTER 3 READING COMPREHENSION
# PRACTICE QUIZ – ANSWER KEY

**1. A.** The main idea of a text is its key point, and the point of view is the author's outlook on the subject. The purpose is the reason for writing. **See Lesson: Understanding the Author's Purpose, Point of View, and Rhetorical Strategies.**

**2. B.** Word choice, or diction, is the reader's most important tool in determining tone. **See Lesson: Tone and Mood, Transition Words.**

**3. B:** A topic sentence expresses the main idea of the text. **See Lesson: Main Ideas, Topic Sentences, and Supporting Details.**

**4. C.** Graphic elements in a text present information visually in order to back up an argument, illustrate factual information or instructions, or present key facts and statistics. **See Lesson: Summarizing Text and Using Text Features.**

**5. D.** The techniques an author uses to support an argument or develop a main idea are called rhetorical strategies. **See Lesson: Understanding the Author's Purpose, Point of View, and Rhetorical Strategies.**

**6. D.** A text is highly unlikely to be credible if its publisher is an organization that stands to benefit if people believe the information it contains. **See Lesson: Understanding Primary Sources, Making Inferences and Drawing Conclusions.**

**7. D.** Transitions between paragraphs or longer sections of text tend to be detailed and may include a short recap of related ideas from earlier parts of the text. **See Lesson: Tone and Mood, Transition Words.**

**8. C.** Words like "excessive" and "undue" are subject to interpretation and reflect beliefs rather than verifiable facts. However, words like these may appear in factual statements about what people said they felt or believed. **See Lesson: Facts Opinions and Evaluating an Argument**

**9. D.** Readers make inferences when they deduce implicit information in a text. **See Lesson: Understanding Primary Sources Making Inferences and Drawing Conclusions.**

**10. D.** A flowchart could list questions to ask and simple problems to check for when a computer breaks down, helping consumers figure out when they can fix a problem themselves and when they need to visit a repair shop. **See Lesson: Summarizing Text and Using Text Features.**

**11. B.** To imply something is to suggest it rather than stating it explicitly. **See Lesson: Main Ideas, Topic Sentences, and Supporting Details.**

**12. A.** Biases may be stated or unstated, and they are not necessarily sweeping. They are preconceived and sometimes unfair ideas about the world. **See Lesson: Facts Opinions and Evaluating an Argument**

# SECTION III
# VOCABULARY AND
# GENERAL KNOWLEDGE

# Vocabulary and General Knowledge:
## 50 questions, 50 minutes

**Areas assessed:** Vocabulary Acquisition, Roots, Prefixes, Suffixes, and Medical Terminology

### *VOCABULARY AND GENERAL KNOWLEDGE TIPS*

- Even if English is your first language, do not be overly confident.

- Spelling: Important to remember how many repeated letters are in a word. For example, accommodate, foreign, appointments, necessary.

- Learn the meaning of common prefixes and suffixes.

- Study medical terms and formal terms.

- If you are not sure about the meaning of the word, use context clues and process of elimination to come to a final answer.

# CHAPTER 4 VOCABULARY ACQUISITION

## ROOT WORDS, PREFIXES, AND SUFFIXES

A root word is the most basic part of a word. You can create new words by: adding a prefix, a group of letters placed before the root word; or a suffix, a group of letters placed at the end of a root word. In this lesson you will learn about root words, prefixes, suffixes, and how to determine the meaning of a word by analyzing these word parts.

### Root Words

**Root words** are found in everyday language. They are the most basic parts of words. Root words in the English language are mostly derived from Latin or Greek. You can add beginnings (prefixes) and endings (suffixes) to root words to change their meanings. To discover what a root word is, simply remove its prefix and/or suffix. What you are left with is the root word, or the core or basis of the word.

At times, root words can be stand-alone words.

Here are some examples of stand-alone root words:

| STAND-ALONE ROOT WORDS | MEANINGS |
|---|---|
| *dress* | *clothing* |
| *form* | *shape* |
| *normal* | *typical* |
| *phobia* | *fear of* |
| *port* | *carry* |

Most root words, however, are **not** stand-alone words. They are not full words on their own, but they still form the basis of other words when you remove their prefixes and suffixes.

Here are some common root words in the English language:

| ROOT WORDS | MEANINGS | EXAMPLES |
| --- | --- | --- |
| ami, amic | love | amicable |
| anni | year | anniversary |
| aud | to hear | auditory |
| bene | good | beneficial |
| biblio | book | bibliography |
| cap | take, seize | capture |
| cent | one hundred | century |
| chrom | color | chromatic |
| chron | time | chronological |
| circum | around | circumvent |
| cred | believe | credible |
| corp | body | corpse |
| dict | to say | dictate |
| equi | equal | equality |
| fract; rupt | to break | fracture |
| ject | throw | eject |
| mal | bad | malignant |
| min | small | miniature |
| mort | death | mortal |
| multi | many | multiply |
| ped | foot | pedestrian |
| rupt | break | rupture |
| sect | cut | dissect |
| script | write | manuscript |
| sol | sun | solar |
| struct | build | construct |
| terr | earth | terrain |
| therm | heat | thermometer |
| vid, vis | to see | visual |
| voc | voice; to call | vocal |

# Prefixes

**Prefixes** are the letters added to the **beginning** of a root word to make a new word with a different meaning.

Prefixes on their own have meanings, too. If you add a prefix to a root word, it can change its meaning entirely.

Here are some of the most common prefixes, their meanings, and some examples:

| PREFIX | MEANING | EXAMPLE |
|---|---|---|
| auto | *self* | autograph |
| con | *with* | conclude |
| hydro- | *water* | hydrate |
| im-, in-, non-, un- | *not* | unimportant |
| inter- | *between* | international |
| mis- | *incorrect, badly* | mislead |
| over- | *too much* | over-stimulate |
| post- | *after* | postpone |
| pre- | *before* | preview |
| re- | *again* | rewrite |
| sub- | *under, below* | submarine |
| trans- | *across* | transcribe |

Let's look back at some of the root words from Section 1. By adding prefixes to these root words, you can create a completely new word with a new meaning:

| ROOT WORD | PREFIX | NEW WORD | MEANING |
|---|---|---|---|
| dress (*clothing*) | un- (*remove*) | **un**dress | *remove clothing* |
| sect (*cut*) | inter- (*between*) | **inter**sect | *cut across or through* |
| phobia (*fear*) | hydro- (*water*) | **hydro**phobia | *fear of water* |
| script (*write*) | post- (*after*) | **post**script | *additional remark at the end of a letter* |

# Suffixes

**Suffixes** are the letters added to the **end** of a root word to make a new word with a different meaning.

Suffixes on their own have meanings, too. If you add a suffix to a root word, it can change its meaning entirely.

Here are some of the most common suffixes, their meanings, and some examples:

| SUFFIX | MEANING | EXAMPLE |
|---|---|---|
| -able, -ible | *can be done* | agreeable |
| -an, -ean, -ian | *belonging or relating to* | European |
| -ed | *happened in the past* | jogged |
| -en | *made of* | wooden |
| -er | *comparative (more than)* | stricter |
| -est | *comparative (most)* | largest |
| -ful | *full of* | meaningful |
| -ic | *having characteristics of* | psychotic |
| -ion, -tion, -ation, -ition | *act, process* | hospitalization |
| -ist | *person who practices* | linguist |
| -less | *without* | artless |
| -logy | *study of* | biology |

Let's look back at some of the root words from Section 1. By adding suffixes to these root words, you can create a completely new word with a new meaning:

| ROOT WORD | SUFFIX | NEW WORD | MEANING |
|---|---|---|---|
| aud (*to hear*) | -logy (*study of*) | audio**logy** | *the study of hearing* |
| form (*shape*) | -less (*without*) | form**less** | *without a clear shape* |
| port (*carry*) | -able (*can be done*) | port**able** | *able to be carried* |
| normal (*typical*) | -ity (*state of*) | normal**ity** | *condition of being normal* |

# Determining Meaning

Knowing the meanings of common root words, prefixes, and suffixes can help you determine the meaning of unknown words. By looking at a word's individual parts, you can get a good sense of its definition.

If you look at the word *transportation*, you can study the different parts of the word to figure out what it means.

If you were to break up the word you would see the following:

| PREFIX: *trans = across* | ROOT: *port = carry* | SUFFIX: *tion = act or process* |
|---|---|---|

If you put all these word parts together, you can define transportation as: *the act or process of carrying something across*.

Let's define some other words by looking at their roots, prefixes and suffixes:

| WORD | PREFIX | ROOT | SUFFIX | WORKING DEFINITION |
|---|---|---|---|---|
| indestructible | in- (*not*) | struct (*build*) | -able (*can be done*) | Not able to be "un" built (torn down) |
| nonconformist | non- (*not*) con- (*with*) | form (*shape*) | -ist (*person who practices*) | A person who can not be shaped (someone who doesn't go along with the norm) |
| subterranean | sub- (*under, below*) | terr (*earth*) | -ean (*belonging or relating to*) | Relating or belonging to something under the earth |

## Let's Review!

- A root word is the most basic part of a word.
- A prefix is the letters added to beginning of a root word to change the word and its meaning.
- A suffix is the letters added to the end of a root word to change the word and its meaning.
- You can figure out a word's meaning by looking closely at its different word parts (root, prefixes, and suffixes).

# CONTEXT CLUES AND MULTIPLE MEANING WORDS

Sometimes when you read a text, you come across an unfamiliar word. Instead of skipping the word and reading on, it is important to figure out what that word means so you can better understand the text. There are different strategies you can use to determine the meaning of unfamiliar words. This lesson will cover (1) how to determine unfamiliar words by reading context clues, (2) multiple meaning words, and (3) using multiple meaning words properly in context.

## Using Context Clues to Determine Meaning

When reading a text, it is common to come across unfamiliar words. One way to determine the meaning of unfamiliar words is by studying other context clues to help you better understand what the word means.

**Context** means the other words in the sentences around the unfamiliar word.

You can look at these other words to find **clues** or **hints** to help you figure out what the word means.

---

**FOR EXAMPLE**

Look at the following sentence:

Some of the kids in the cafeteria _ostracized_ Janice because she dressed differently; they never allowed her to sit at their lunch table, and they whispered behind her back.

If you did not know what the word _ostracized_ meant, you could look at the **other words** for **clues** to help you.

Here is what we know based on the clues in the sentence:

- Janice dressed differently
- Some kids did not allow her to sit at their table
- They whispered behind her back

We know that the kids **never allowed her to sit at their lunch** table and that they **whispered behind her back**. If you put all these clues together, you can conclude that the other students were **mistreating** Janice by **excluding** her.

Therefore, based on these context clues, _ostracized_ means "excluded from the group."

---

Here's another example:

**EXAMPLE 2**

Look at this next sentence:

Louis's teacher was offended because after she called on him he gave a _flippant_ response instead of a serious answer.

If you did not know what the word _flippant_ meant, you could look at the **other words** for **clues** to help you.

Here is what we know based on the clues in the sentence:

- Louis's teacher was offended
- He gave a flippant response instead of a serious answer

We know that Louis said something that **offended** his teacher. Another keyword in this sentence is the word **instead**. This means that **instead of a serious answer** Louis gave the **opposite** of a serious answer.

Therefore, based on these context clues, _flippant_ means "lacking respect or seriousness."

# Multiple Meaning Words

Sometimes when we read words in a text, we encounter words that have **multiple meanings**.

**Multiple meaning words** are words that have **more than one definition** or meaning.

**FOR EXAMPLE**

The word **current** is a multiple meaning word. Here are the different definitions of _current:_

CURRENT:

1.  adj: happening or existing in the present time

    Example: _It is important to keep up with_ _current_ _events so you know what's happening in the world._

2.  noun: the continuous movement of a body of water or air in a certain direction

    Example: _The river's_ _current_ _was strong as we paddled down the rapids._

3.  noun: a flow of electricity

    Example: _The electrical_ _current_ _was very weak in the house._

Here are some other examples of words with multiple meanings:

| Multiple Meaning Word | Definition #1 | Definition #2 | Definition #3 |
|---|---|---|---|
| Buckle | noun: a metal or plastic device that connects one end of a belt to another | verb: to fasten or attach | verb: to bend or collapse from pressure or heat |
| Cabinet | noun: a piece of furniture used for storing things | noun: a group of people who give advice to a government leader | - |
| Channel | noun: a radio or television station | noun: a system used for sending something | noun: a long, narrow place where water flows |
| Doctor | noun: a person skilled in the science of medicine, dentistry, or one holding a PhD | verb: to change something in a way to trick or deceive | verb: to give medical treatment |
| Grave | noun: a hole in the ground for burying a dead body | adj: very serious | - |
| Hamper | noun: a large basket used for holding dirty clothes | verb: to slow the movement, action, or progress of | - |
| Plane | noun: a mode of transportation that has wings and an engine and can carry people and things in the air | noun: a flat or level surface that extends outward | noun: a level of though, development, or existence |
| Reservation | noun: an agreement to have something (such as a table, room, or seat) held for use at a later time | noun: a feeling of uncertainty or doubt | noun: an area of land kept separate for Native Americans to live<br><br>an area of land set aside for animals to live for protection |
| Season | noun: one of the four periods in which a year is divided (winter, spring, summer, and fall) | noun: a particular period of time during the year | verb: to add spices to something to give it more flavor |
| Sentence | noun: a group words that expresses a statement, question, command, or wish | noun: the punishment given to someone by a court of law | verb: to officially state the punishment given by a court of law |

From this chart you will notice that words with multiple meanings may have different **parts of speech**. A part of speech is a category of words that have the same grammatical properties. Some of the main parts of speech for words in the English language are: nouns, adjectives, verbs, and adverbs.

| Part of Speech | Definition | Example |
|---|---|---|
| Noun | a person, place, thing, or idea | *Linda, New York City, toaster, happiness* |
| Adjective | a word that describes a noun or pronoun | *adventurous, young, red, intelligent* |
| Verb | an action or state of being | *run, is, sleep, become* |
| Adverb | a word that describes a verb, adjective, or other adverb | *quietly, extremely, carefully, well* |

For example, in the chart above, *season* is can be a **noun** or a **verb**.

# Using Multiple Meaning Words Properly in Context

When you come across a **multiple meaning word** in a text, it is important to discern which meaning of the word is being used so you do not get confused.

You can once again turn to the **context clues** to clarify which meaning of the word is being used.

Let's take a look at the word *coach*. This word has several definitions:

*COACH:*

1. noun: a person who teaches and trains an athlete or performer
2. noun: a large bus with comfortable seating used for long trips
3. noun: the section on an airplane with the least expensive seats
4. verb: to teach or train someone in a specific area
5. verb: to give someone instructions on what to do or say in a certain situation

Since *coach* has so many definitions, you need to look at the **context clues** to figure out which definition of the word is being used:

*The man was not happy that he had to sit in *coach* on the 24-hour flight to Australia.*

In this sentence, the context clues **sit in** and **24-hour flight** help you see that *coach* means the least expensive seat on an airplane.

Let's look at another sentence using the word *coach*:

*The lawyer needed to *coach* her witness so he would answer all the questions properly.*

In this sentence, the context clues **so he would answer all the questions properly** help you see that the lawyer was giving the witness instructions on what to say.

## Let's Review!

- When you come across an unfamiliar word in a text you can use context clues to help you define it.
- Context clues can also help you determine which definition of a multiple meaning word to use.

# MEDICAL TERMINOLOGY

People working in the medical profession must use specific terminology to be able to communicate accurately and consistently with their peers. Understanding and utilizing these domain-specific words will ensure that health care professionals can communicate in the most effective way. This lesson will cover (1) common domain-specific words in the medical industry, (2) how medical words are formed, and (3) determining the meaning of a medical term based on their different word parts.

## Domain-Specific Words in the Medical Industry

**Domain-specific words** are also known as **academic vocabulary**. These are words that are not frequently used in informal conversation or writing. Instead, they are words that pertain to specific academic topics or areas of study.

The medical industry contains many domain-specific vocabulary words that are used by professionals.

Here are just a few examples of medical terms and their definitions:

| MEDICAL TERM | MEANING |
| --- | --- |
| dysentery | abnormal condition of the intestines |
| endoscopy | visual examination of the inside of the body |
| exoskeleton | pertaining to the external skeleton |
| hypertension | high blood pressure |
| hypoglycemia | low blood sugar |
| interarticular | between the joints |
| intravenous | in a vein |
| neoplasm | abnormal new growth of tissue |
| pericardium | tissue surrounding the heart |
| postmortem | after death |
| prenatal | before birth |
| subcutaneous | under the skin |
| unformed | not formed |

## How Medical Words Are Formed

If you look closely at medical terms, you will see that they are made up of certain root words, prefixes, and suffixes. Each of these word parts has a specific meaning.

If you learn what each of these word parts mean, you will be able to define a medical term.

# HESI

Let's take a look at some common root words, prefixes, and suffixes used in medical terminology:

| ROOT WORDS | MEANING |
| --- | --- |
| acoust, ot | ears |
| angi | vessel |
| arteri | arteries |
| arthr | joints |
| capill | capillaries |
| carcin | cancer |
| card, cardi | heart |
| chondr | cartilage |
| col | large intestines |
| cutane, dermat, derm | skin |
| cyto | cell |
| enceph | brain |
| enter | small intestine |
| fasci | fascia |
| gastr | stomach |
| hem, hemat | blood |
| hepat | liver |
| hidr | sweat glands |
| malign | harmful |
| mort | death |
| myel | spinal cord, bone marrow |
| my | muscles |
| nas, rhin | nose |
| nat | birth, born |
| nephr, ren | kidneys |
| neur | nerves |
| ocul, ophthalm | eyes |
| or | mouth |
| oste, oss, ost | bones |
| path | disease |
| phleb, ven | veins |
| pil | hair |
| pneum, pneumon | lungs |

| ROOT WORDS | MEANING |
|---|---|
| ten, tend, tendin | tendons |

| PREFIXES | MEANING |
|---|---|
| a-, an- | without |
| ab- | from, away |
| ad- | toward |
| ana- | up |
| ante- | before |
| anti- | against |
| append- | to hang |
| bi-, bin- | two |
| brady- | slow |
| contra- | against |
| di- | two |
| dis- | undo or free from |
| dys- | difficult |
| ecto-, exo-, extra- | outside |
| epi- | above or surrounding |
| endo- | within |
| erythr- | red |
| glyc- | sweet |
| hypo- | below |
| hyper- | above |
| infra- | under, below |
| inter- | between |
| intra- | inside |
| iso- | equal |
| macro- | large |
| mal- | bad |
| meso- | middle |
| meta- | after |
| micro- | small |
| mono- | one |
| multi- | many |

| PREFIXES | MEANING |
|---|---|
| muti- | change |
| neo- | new |
| para- | beside |
| peri- | surrounding |
| poly- | many |
| post- | after |
| pre- | before |
| re- | back |
| retro- | behind or back |
| semi- | half |
| sub- | under |
| super- | above or over |
| syn- | together, joined |
| tachy- | fast |
| trans- | across, through, beyond |
| tri- | three |
| ultra- | beyond, excess |
| uni- | one |

| SUFFIXES | MEANING |
|---|---|
| -al | pertaining to |
| -algia | pain |
| -ase | enzyme |
| -centesis | surgical puncture |
| -clast | broken |
| -crit | to separate |
| -cyte | cell |
| -ectomy | surgical removal, excision |
| -emia | blood condition |
| -emisi | vomiting |
| -gen, -genesis, -genic | causing, producing |
| -gram | written |
| -ia | condition of, diseased or abnormal state |

| SUFFIXES | MEANING |
|---|---|
| -iac, ic, ior | pertaining to |
| -ism | state of |
| -itis | inflammation of |
| -ist | one who specializes in |
| -logy | study of |
| -lyte | dissolvable |
| -lytic | destroy, reduce |
| -mania | madness |
| -megaly | enlargement |
| -odia | smell |
| -ologist | one who practices or studies |
| -oma | swelling, tumor |
| -opia | vision |
| -opsy | to view |
| -orrhea | flow, excessive discharge |
| -orrhexis | rupture |
| -osis | abnormal increase in production |
| -ostomy | creation of an artificial opening |
| -otomy | incision, cut into |
| -oxia | oxygen |
| -plasty | surgical repair |
| -sclerosis | hardening of |
| -scope | instrument used for visual examination |
| -scopy | visual examination of |
| -sepsis | infection |
| -stasis | stop or control |
| -tomy | cutting |
| -tropic | influencing |
| -toxic | poison |

# Determining the Meaning of a Medical Word Based on its Parts

Now that you know the common root words, prefixes, and suffixes used in medical terminology, you can determine the meaning of a medical term by putting these word parts together.

Let's take a look at a few examples:

| Medical Term | Root | Prefix | Suffix | Meaning |
|---|---|---|---|---|
| pathology | patho = "disease" | - | logy = "study of" | the study of diseases |
| epidermis | derm = "skin" | epi = "above, surrounding" | - | pertaining to the outer parts of the skin |
| rhinorrhoea | Rhino = "nose" | - | orrhea = "flow" | flow form the nose |
| tachycardia | cardi = "heart" | tachy = "fast" | - | rapid heart beat |

## Let's Review!

- People in the health care must have knowledge of medical terminology.
- Medical terms are made up of roots, prefixes, and suffixes, all of which have their own meanings.
- You can decipher what a medical term means by putting together all the word parts.

# CHAPTER 4 VOCABULARY ACQUISITION PRACTICE QUIZ

1. Which suffix would you affix to the word "cardi" to complete the following sentence? The student was studying to become a cardi_____.

   A. -Ology

   B. -Ologist

   C. -Otomy

   D. -Ostomy

2. Select the word from the following sentence that has more than one meaning. Cassandra's voice has a much different pitch than her brother's, so they sound great when they sing together.

   A. Voice

   B. Different

   C. Pitch

   D. Sing

3. An amicable person is one who is

   A. Timid

   B. Friendly

   C. Capable

   D. Uncertain

4. Circumvent most nearly means

   A. To create something

   B. To destroy something

   C. To move across something

   D. To find a way around something

5. Which prefix would you affix to the word "operative" to complete the following sentence? The surgeon wanted to conduct a ____operative exam a week before the patient's surgery.

   A. Pre-

   B. Peri-

   C. Post-

   D. Para-

6. Select the word from the following sentence that has more than one meaning. It was a grave situation, and many people had given up hope.

   A. Hope

   B. Grave

   C. People

   D. Situation

# CHAPTER 4 VOCABULARY ACQUISITION PRACTICE QUIZ – ANSWER KEY

**1. B**. The suffix "ologist" would make the word "cardiologist" to complete the sentence. **See Lesson: Domain-Specific Words: Medical Industry.**

**2. C**. The word "pitch" has more than one meaning. **See Lesson: Context Clues and Multiple Meaning Words.**

**3. B**. The root *ami* means "love," so an amicable person would show love or be friendly. **See Lesson: Root Words, Prefixes, and Suffixes.**

**4. D**. The root *circum* means "around," so circumvent means to find a way around something. **See Lesson: Root Words, Prefixes, and Suffixes.**

**5. A**. The prefix "pre" would make the word "preoperative" to complete the sentence. **See Lesson: Medical Terminology.**

**6. B**. The word "grave" has more than one meaning. **See Lesson: Context Clues and Multiple Meaning Words.**

# SECTION IV
# GRAMMAR

# Grammar: 50 questions, 60 minutes

**Areas assessed:** Conventions of Standard English, Parts of Speech, and Knowledge of Language

*GRAMMAR TIPS*

- Rules of Language Arts and Grammar may be explicitly asked.

- Know the eight parts of a basic sentence: nouns, pronouns, verbs, adjectives, adverbs, conjunctions, prepositions, and interjections.

- Understand dependent and independent clauses of a complex sentence. Know how to join two independent clauses.

- Know subject-verb agreement.

- Study grammar terms. Know what they are and how they work i.e. coordinate conjunctions, subject verb agreement.

- Review basic rules of punctuation; i.e. semi-colon and dash usage.

# Chapter 5 Conventions of Standard English

## Spelling

Spelling correctly is important to accurately convey thoughts to an audience. This lesson will cover (1) vowels and consonants, (2) suffixes and plurals, (3) homophones and homographs.

### Vowels and Consonants

**Vowels** and **consonants** are different speech sounds in English.

The letters A, E, I, O, U and sometimes Y are **vowels** and can create a variety of sounds. The most common are short sounds and long sounds. Long **vowel** sounds sound like the name of the letter such as the *a* in late. Short **vowel** sounds have a unique sound such as the *a* in cat. A rule for **vowels** is that when two vowels are walking, the first does the talking as in pain and meat.

**Consonants** include the other twenty-one letters in the alphabet. **Consonants** are weak letters and only make sounds when paired with **vowels**. That is why words always must have a **vowel**. This also means that **consonants** need to be doubled to make a stronger sound like sitting, grabbed, progress. Understanding general trends and patterns for **vowels** and **consonants** will help with spelling. The table below represents the difference between short and long **vowels** and gives examples for each.

|  | Symbol | Example Words |
|---|---|---|
| Short a | a | Cat, mat, hat, pat |
| Long a | ā | Late, pain, pay, they, weight, straight |
| Short e | e | Met, said, bread |
| Long e | ē | Breeze, cheap, dean, equal |
| Short i | i | Bit, myth, kiss, rip |
| Long i | ī | Cry, pie, high |
| Short o | o | Dog, hot, pop |
| Long o | ō | Snow, nose, elbow |
| Short u | u | Run, cut, club, gum |
| Long u | ū | Duty, rule, new, food |
| Short oo | oo | Book, foot, cookie |
| Long oo | ōō | Mood, bloom, shoot |

# Suffixes and Plurals

A **suffix** is a word part that is added to the ending of a root word. A **suffix** changes the meaning and spelling of words. There are some general patterns to follow with **suffixes**.

- Adding -er, -ist, or -or changes the root to mean *doer* or *performer*
    - Paint -→ Painter
    - Abolition -→ Abolitionist
    - Act -→ Actor
- Adding -ation or -ment changes the root to mean *an action* or *a process*
    - Ador(e) -→ Adoration
    - Develop -→ Development
- Adding -ism changes the root to mean *a theory or ideology*
    - Real -→ Realism
- Adding -ity, -ness, -ship, or -tude changes the root to mean *a condition, quality, or state*
    - Real -→ Reality
    - Sad -→ Sadness
    - Relation -→ Relationship
    - Soli(tary) -→ Solitude

**Plurals** are similar to suffixes as letters are added to the end of the word to signify more than one person, place, thing, or idea. There are also general patterns to follow when creating **plurals**.

- If a word ends in -s,-ss,-z,-zz,-ch, or -sh, add -es.
    - Bus -→ Buses
- If a word ends in a -y, drop the -y and add -ies.
    - Pony -→ Ponies
- If a word ends in an -f, change the f to a v and add -es.
    - Knife -→ Knives
- For all other words, add an -s.
    - Dog -→ Dogs

# Homophones and Homographs

A **homophone** is a word that has the same sound as another word, but does not have the same meaning or spelling.

- To, too, and two
- There, their, and they're
- See and sea

A **homograph** is a word that has the same spelling as another word, but does not have the same sound or meaning.

- Lead (to go in front of) and lead (a metal)
- Bass (deep sound) and bass (a fish)

# Let's Review!

- Vowels include the letters A, E, I, O, U and sometimes Y and have both short and long sounds.

- Consonants are the other twenty-one letters and have weak sounds. They are often doubled to make stronger sounds.

- Suffixes are word parts added to the root of a word and change the meaning and spelling.

- To make a word plural, add -es, -ies, -ves, or -s to the end of a word.

- Homophones are words that have the same sound, but not the same meaning or spelling.

- Homographs are words that have the same spelling, but not the same meaning or sound.

# CAPITALIZATION

Correct capitalization helps readers understand when a new sentence begins and the importance of specific words. This lesson will cover the capitalization rules of (1) geographic locations and event names, (2) organizations and publication titles, (3) individual names and professional titles, and (4) months, days, and holidays.

## Geographic Locations and Event Names

North, east, south, and west are not **capitalized** unless they relate to a **definite region**.

- Go north on I-5 for 200 miles.
- The West Coast has nice weather.

Words like northern, southern, eastern, and western are also not **capitalized** unless they describe **people or the cultural and political activities of people**.

- There is nothing interesting to see in eastern Colorado.
- Midwesterners are known for being extremely nice.
- The Western states almost always vote Democratic.

These words are not **capitalized** when placed before a name or region unless it is part of the **official name**.

- She lives in southern California.
- I loved visiting Northern Ireland.

**Continents, countries, states, cities,** and **towns** need to be **capitalized**.

- Australia has a lot of scary animals.
- Not many people live in Antarctica.
- Albany is the capital of New York.

**Historical events** should be **capitalized** to separate the specific from the general.

- The bubonic plague in the Middle Ages killed a large portion of the population in Europe.
- The Great Depression took place in the early 1930s.
- We are living in the twenty-first century.

## Organizations and Publication Titles

The **names of national organizations** need to be **capitalized.** Short prepositions, articles, and conjunctions within the title are not **capitalized** unless they are the first word.

- The National American Woman Suffrage Association was essential in passing the Nineteenth Amendment.
- The House of Representatives is one part of Congress.
- The National Football League consists of thirty-two teams.

The **titles of books, chapters, articles, poems, newspapers, and other publications** should be **capitalized**.

- Her favorite book is *A Wrinkle in Time*.
- I do the crossword in *The New York Times* every Sunday.
- *The Jabberwocky* by Lewis Carroll has many silly sounding words.

# Individual Names and Professional Titles

**People's names** as well as their **familial relationship title** need to be **capitalized**.

- Barack Obama was our first African American president.
- Uncle Joe brought the steaks for our Memorial Day grill.
- Aunt Sarah lives in California, but my other aunt lives in Florida.

**Professional titles** need to be **capitalized** when they precede a name, or as a direct address. If it is after a name or is used generally, titles do not need to be **capitalized**.

- Governor Cuomo is trying to modernize the subway system in New York.
- Andrew Cuomo is the governor of New York.
- A governor runs the state. A president runs the country.
- Thank you for the recommendation, Mr. President.
- I need to see Doctor Smith.
- I need to see a doctor.

**Capitalize** the **title of high-ranking government officials** when an individual is referred to.

- The Secretary of State travels all over the world.
- The Vice President joined the meeting.

With **compound titles**, the prefixes or suffixes do not need to be **capitalized**.

- George W. Bush is the ex-President of the United States.

# Months, Days, and Holidays

**Capitalize all months of the year** (January, February, March, April, May, June, July, August, September, October, November, December) and **days of the week** (Sunday, Monday, Tuesday, Wednesday, Thursday, Friday, Saturday).

- Her birthday is in November.
- People graduate from college in May or June.
- Saturdays and Sundays are supposed to be fun and relaxing.

**Holidays** are also **capitalized**.

- Most kid's favorite holiday is Christmas.
- The new school year usually starts after Labor Day.
- It is nice to go to the beach over Memorial Day weekend.

The **seasons** are not **capitalized**.

- It gets too hot in the summer and too cold in the winter.
- The flowers and trees bloom so beautifully in the spring.

# Let's Review!

- Only **capitalize** directional words like north, south, east, and, west when they describe **a definite region, people, and their political and cultural activities**, or when it is part of the **official name**.
- **Historical periods and events** are **capitalized** to represent their importance and specificity.
- Every word except short prepositions, conjunctions, and articles in the **names of national organizations** are **capitalized**.
- The **titles of publications** follow the same rules as **organizations**.
- The **names of individual people** need to be **capitalized**.
- **Professional titles** are **capitalized** if they precede a name or are used as a direct address.
- All **months of the year, days of the week**, and **holidays** are **capitalized**.
- **Seasons** are **not capitalized**.

# PUNCTUATION

Punctuation is important in writing to accurately represent ideas. Without correct punctuation, the meaning of a sentence is difficult to understand. This lesson will cover (1) periods, question marks, and exclamation points, (2) commas, semicolons, and colons, and (3) apostrophes, hyphens, and quotation marks.

## Terminal Punctuation Marks: Periods, Question Marks, and Exclamation Points

Terminal punctuation are used at the end of a sentence. Periods, question marks, and exclamation points are the three types of terminal punctuation.

**Periods (.)** mark the end of a declarative sentence, one that states a fact, or an imperative sentence, one that states a command or request). Periods can also be used in abbreviations.

- Doctors save lives.
- She has a B.A. in Psychology.

**Question Marks (?)** signify the end of a sentence that is a question. Where, when, who, whom, what, why, and how are common words that begin question sentences.

- Who is he?
- Where is the restaurant?
- Why is the sky blue?

**Exclamation Points (!)** indicate strong feelings, shouting, or emphasize a feeling.

- Watch out!
- That is incredible!
- I hate you!

## Internal Punctuation: Commas, Semicolons, and Colons

Internal punctuation is used within a sentence to help keep words, phrases, and clauses in order. These punctuation marks can be used to indicate elements such as direct quotations and definitions in a sentence.

A **comma (,)** signifies a small break within a sentence and separates words, clauses, or ideas.

**Commas** are used before conjunctions that connect two independent clauses.

- I ate some cookies, and I drank some milk.

**Commas** are also used to set off an introductory phrase.

- After the test, she grabbed dinner with a friend.

Short phrases that emphasis thoughts or emotions are enclosed by **commas**.

- The school year, thankfully, ends in a week.

**Commas** set off the words yes and no.

- Yes, I am available this weekend.
- No, she has not finished her homework.

**Commas** set off a question tag.

- It is beautiful outside, isn't it?

**Commas** are used to indicate direct address.

- Are you ready, Jack?
- Mom, what is for dinner?

**Commas** separate items in a series.

- We ate eggs, potatoes, and toast for breakfast.
- I need to grab coffee, go to the store, and put gas in my car.

**Semicolons (;)** are used to connect two independent clauses without a coordinating conjunction like *and* or *but*. A **semicolon** creates a bond between two sentences that are related. Do not capitalize the first word after the **semicolon** unless it is a word that is normally capitalized.

- The ice cream man drove down my street; I bought a popsicle.
- My mom cooked dinner; the chicken was delicious.
- It is cloudy today; it will probably rain.

**Colons (:)** introduce a list.

- She teaches three subjects: English, history, and geography.

At the end of a sentence, **colons** can create emphasis of a word or phrase.

- She had one goal: pay the bills.

# More Internal Punctuation: Apostrophes, Hyphens, and Quotation Marks

**Apostrophes (')** are used to indicate possession or to create a contraction.

- Bob has a car -→ Bob's car is blue.
- Steve's cat is beautiful.

For plurals that are also possessive, put the **apostrophe** after the s.

- Soldiers' uniforms are impressive.

Make contractions by combining two words.

- I do not have a dog -→ I don't have a dog
- I can't swim.

Its and it's do not follow the normal possessive rules. Its is possessive while it's means it is.

- It's a beautiful day to be at the park.
- The dog has many toys, but its favorite is the rope.

**Hyphens (-)** are mainly used to create compound words.

- The documentary was a real eye-opener for me.
- We have to check-in to the hotel before midnight.
- The graduate is a twenty-two-year-old woman.

**Quotation Marks (")** are used when directly using another person's words in your own writing. Commas and periods, sometimes question marks and exclamation points, are placed within **quotation marks**. Colons and semicolons are placed outside of the **quotation marks**, unless they are part of the quoted material. If quoting an entire sentence, capitalize the first word. If it is a fragment, do not capitalize the first word.

- Ernest Hemingway once claimed, "There is nothing noble in being superior to your fellow man; true nobility is being superior to your former self."
- Steve said, "I will be there at noon."

An indirect quote which paraphrases what someone else said does not need **quotation marks**.

- Steve said he would be there at noon.

**Quotation marks** are also used for the titles of short works such as poems, articles, and chapters. They are not italicized.

- Robert Frost wrote "The Road Not Taken."

## Let's Review!

- **Periods (.)** signify the end of a sentence or are used in abbreviations.
- **Question Marks (?)** are also used at the end of a sentence and distinguish the sentence as a question.
- **Exclamation Points (!)** indicate strong feelings, shouting, or emphasis and are usually at the end of the sentence.
- **Commas (,)** are small breaks within a sentence that separate clauses, ideas, or words. They are used to set off introductory phrases, the words yes and no, question tags, indicate direct address, and separate items in a series.
- **Semicolons (;)** connect two similar sentences without a coordinating conjunctions such as and or but.
- **Colons (:)** are used to introduce a list or emphasize a word or phrase.
- **Apostrophes (')** indicate possession or a contraction of two words.
- **Hyphens (-)** are used to create compound words.
- **Quotation Marks (")** are used when directly quoting someone else's words and to indicate the title of poems, chapters, and articles.

# CHAPTER 5 CONVENTIONS OF STANDARD ENGLISH PRACTICE QUIZ

1. **Every runner needs a good ____ of shoes.**

   A. Pair

   B. Piar

   C. Pear

   D. Pare

2. **A ____ is sixty seconds.**

   A. Minit

   B. Minute

   C. Muinet

   D. Mionute

3. **Choose the correct sentence.**

   A. They used to live in the pacific northwest.

   B. They used to live in the Pacific northwest.

   C. They used to live in the pacific Northwest.

   D. They used to live in the Pacific Northwest.

4. **What is missing from the following sentence?**

   Classical music helps with studying, I always listen to it before a test.

   A. There needs to be a colon after studying.

   B. There needs to be a semicolon after studying.

   C. There should be an exclamation point at the end.

   D. Nothing is missing.

5. **What is missing from the following sentence?**

   He asked, When is the assignment due?

   A. There should be quotation marks.

   B. There needs to be a semicolon after asked.

   C. There should be a comma after assignment.

   D. Nothing is missing.

6. **Choose the correct sentence.**

   A. The Victorian era is marked by strict modesty.

   B. The Victorian Era is marked by strict modesty.

   C. The victorian era is marked by strict modesty.

   D. the victorian era is marked by strict modesty.

# CHAPTER 5 CONVENTIONS OF STANDARD ENGLISH PRACTICE QUIZ – ANSWER KEY

1. **A.** *Pair* is spelled correctly and has the appropriate meaning for the sentence. **See Lesson: Spelling.**

2. **B.** *Minute* is the only correctly spelled option. **See Lesson: Spelling.**

3. **D.** They used to live in the Pacific Northwest. Specific geographic regions are capitalized. **See Lesson: Capitalization.**

4. **B.** *There needs to be a semicolon after studying.* A semicolon is used to connect two related sentences. **See Lesson: Punctuation.**

5. **A.** *There should be quotation marks.* Direct quotes from someone else should be enclosed in quotation marks. **See Lesson: Punctuation.**

6. **B.** The Victorian Era is marked by strict modesty. All specific historical time periods are capitalized. **See Lesson: Capitalization.**

# CHAPTER 6 PARTS OF SPEECH

# NOUNS

In this lesson, you will learn about nouns. A noun is a word that names a person, place, thing, or idea. This lesson will cover (1) the role of nouns in sentences and (2) different types of nouns.

## Nouns and Their Role in Sentences

A **noun** names a person, place, thing, or idea.

Some examples of nouns are:

- Gandhi
- New Hampshire
- garden
- happiness

A noun's role in a sentence is as **subject** or **object**. A subject is the part of the sentence that does something, whereas the object is the thing that something is done to. In simple terms, the subject acts, and the object is acted upon.

A. Look for the nouns in these sentences.

1. The Louvre is stunning. (subject noun: The Louvre)
2. Marco ate dinner with Sara and Petra. (subject noun: Marco; object nouns: dinner, Sara, Petra)
3. Honesty is the best policy. (subject noun: honesty; object noun: policy)
4. After the election, we celebrated our new governor. (object nouns: governor, election)
5. I slept. (0 nouns)

B. Look for the nouns in these sentences.

> **KEEP IN MIND . . .**
> The subjects *I* and *we* in the two sentences above are pronouns, not nouns.

1. Mrs. Garcia makes a great pumpkin pie. (subject noun: Mrs. Garcia; object noun: pie)
2. We really need to water the garden. (object noun: garden)
3. Love is sweet. (subject noun: love)
4. Sam loves New York in the springtime. (subject noun: Sam; object nouns: New York, springtime)
5. Lin and her mother and father ate soup, fish, potatoes, and fruit for dinner. (subject nouns: Lin, mother, father; object nouns: soup, fish, potatoes, fruit, dinner)

Why isn't the word *pumpkin* a noun in the first sentence? *Pumpkin* is often a noun, but here it is used as an adjective that describes what kind of *pie*.

Why isn't the word *water* a noun in the second sentence? Here, *water* is an **action verb**. To *water the garden* is something we do.

How is the word *love* a noun in the third sentence and not in the fourth sentence? *Love* is a noun (thing) in sentence 3 and a verb (action) in the sentence 4.

How many nouns can a sentence contain? As long as the sentence remains grammatically correct, it can contain an unlimited number of nouns.

**BE CAREFUL!**
Words can change to serve different roles in different sentences. A word that is usually a noun can sometimes be used as an adjective or a verb. Determine a word's function in a sentence to be sure of its part of speech.

# Types of Nouns

## A. Singular and Plural Nouns

Nouns can be **singular** or **plural**. A noun is singular when there is only one. A noun is plural when there are two or more.

- The book has 650 pages.

*Book* is a singular noun. *Pages* is a plural noun.

Often, to make a noun plural, we add -*s* at the end of the word: *cat/cats*. This is a **regular** plural noun. Sometimes we make a word plural in another way: *child/children*. This is an **irregular** plural noun. Some plurals follow rules, while others do not. The most common rules are listed here:

| Singular noun | Plural noun | Rule for making plural |
|---|---|---|
| star | stars | for most words, add -*s* |
| box | boxes | for words that end in -*j*, -*s*, -*x*, -*z*, -*ch* or -*sh*, add -*es* |
| baby | babies | for words that end in -*y*, change -*y* to -*i* and add -*es* |
| woman | women | irregular |
| foot | feet | irregular |

**KEEP IN MIND . . .**
**Some nouns are countable,** and others are not. For example, we eat *three blueberries*, but we **do not** drink *three milks*. Instead, we drink *three glasses of milk* or *some milk*.

## B. Common and Proper Nouns

**Common nouns** are general words, and they are written in lowercase. **Proper nouns** are specific names, and they begin with an uppercase letter.

Examples:

| Common noun | Proper noun |
|---|---|
| ocean | Baltic Sea |
| dentist | Dr. Marx |
| company | Honda |
| park | Yosemite National Park |

## C. Concrete and Abstract Nouns

**Concrete nouns** are people, places, or things that physically exist. We can use our senses to see or hear them. *Turtle, spreadsheet,* and *Australia* are concrete nouns.

**Abstract nouns** are ideas, qualities, or feelings that we cannot see and that might be harder to describe. *Beauty, childhood, energy, envy, generosity, happiness, patience, pride, trust, truth,* and *victory* are abstract nouns.

Some words can be either concrete or abstract nouns. For example, the concept of *art* is abstract, but *art* that we see and touch is concrete.

- We talked about *art.* (abstract)
- She showed me the *art* she had created in class. (concrete)

## Let's Review!

- A noun is a person, place, thing, or idea.
- A noun's function in a sentence is as subject or object.
- Common nouns are general words, while proper nouns are specific names.
- Nouns can be concrete or abstract.

# PRONOUNS

A pronoun is a word that takes the place of or refers to a specific noun. This lesson will cover (1) the role of pronouns in sentences and (2) the purpose of pronouns.

## Pronouns and Their Role in Sentences

A **pronoun** takes the place of a noun or refers to a specific noun.

### A. Subject, Object, and Possessive Pronouns

A pronoun's role in a sentence is as **subject, object,** or **possessive**.

| Subject Pronouns | Object Pronouns | Possessive Pronouns |
|---|---|---|
| I | me | my, mine |
| you | you | your, yours |
| he | her | his |
| she | him | her, hers |
| it | it | its |
| we | us | ours |
| they | them | their, theirs |

In simple sentences, subject pronouns come before the verb, object pronouns come after the verb, and possessive pronouns show ownership.

Look at the pronouns in these examples:

- <u>She</u> forgot <u>her</u> coat. (subject: she; possessive: her)
- <u>I</u> lent <u>her</u> <u>mine</u>. (subject: I; object: her; possessive: mine)
- <u>She</u> left <u>it</u> at school. (subject: she; object: it)
- <u>I</u> had to go and get <u>it</u> the next day. (subject: I; object: it)
- <u>I</u> will never lend <u>her</u> something of <u>mine</u> again! (subject: I; object: her; possessive: mine)

**BE CAREFUL!**

It is easy to make a mistake when you have multiple words in the role of subject or object.

| Correct | Incorrect | Why? |
|---|---|---|
| *John and I* went out. | *John and me* went out. | *John and I* is a subject. *I* is a subject pronoun; *me* is not. |
| Johan took *Sam and me* to the show. | Johan took *Sam and I* to the show. | *Sam and me* is an object. *Me* is an object pronoun; *I* is not. |

115

## B. Relative Pronouns

**Relative pronouns** connect a clause to a noun or pronoun.

These are some relative pronouns:

> who, whom, whoever, whose, that, which

- Steve Jobs, *who founded Apple*, changed the way people use technology.

The pronoun *who* introduces a clause that gives more information about Steve Jobs.

- This is the movie *that Emily told us to see*.

The pronoun *that* introduces a clause that gives more information about the movie.

## C. Other Pronouns

Some other pronouns are:

> this, that, what, anyone, everything, something

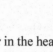

> **DID YOU KNOW?**
>
> Pronouns can sometimes refer to general or unspecified things.

Look for the pronouns in these sentences.

- <u>What</u> is <u>that</u>?
- There is <u>something</u> over there!
- Does <u>anyone</u> have a pen?

# Pronouns and Their Purpose

The purpose of a pronoun is to replace a noun. Note the use of the pronoun *their* in the heading of this section. If we did not have pronouns, we would have to call this section *Pronouns and Pronouns' Purpose*.

## What Is an Antecedent?

A pronoun in a sentence refers to a specific noun, and this noun called the **antecedent**.

> **BE CAREFUL!**
>
> Look out for unclear antecedents, such as in this sentence:
>
> - Take the furniture out of the room and paint *it*.
>
> What needs to be painted, the furniture or the room?

John Hancock signed the Declaration of Independence. <u>He</u> signed <u>it</u> in 1776.

The antecedent for *he* is John Hancock. The antecedent for *it* is the Declaration of Independence.

Find the pronouns in the following sentence. Then identify the antecedent for each pronoun.

Erin had an idea *that she* suggested to Antonio: "*I*'ll help *you* with *your* math homework if *you* help *me* with *my* writing assignment."

| Pronoun | Antecedent |
|---------|------------|
| that | idea |
| she | Erin |
| I | Erin |
| you | Antonio |
| your | Antonio's |
| you | Antonio |
| me | Erin |
| my | Erin's |

## What Is Antecedent Agreement?

A pronoun must agree in **gender** and **number** with the antecedent it refers to. For example:

- Singular pronouns *I, you, he, she*, and *it* replace singular nouns.
- Plural pronouns *you, we*, and *they* replace plural nouns.
- Pronouns *he, she,* and *it* replace masculine, feminine, or neutral nouns.

| Correct | Incorrect | Why? |
|---------|-----------|------|
| <u>Students</u> should do <u>their</u> homework every night. | <u>A student</u> should do <u>their</u> homework every night. | The pronoun *their* is plural, so it must refer to a plural noun such as *students*. |
| When <u>an employee</u> is sick, <u>he or she</u> should call the office. | When <u>an employee</u> is sick, <u>they</u> should call the office. | The pronoun *they* is plural, so it must refer to a plural noun. *Employee* is not a plural noun. |

## Let's Review!

- A pronoun takes the place of or refers to a noun.
- The role of pronouns in sentences is as subject, object, or possessive.
- A pronoun must agree in number and gender with the noun it refers to.

# ADJECTIVES AND ADVERBS

An **adjective** is a word that describes a noun or a pronoun. An **adverb** is a word that describes a verb, an adjective, or another adverb.

## Adjectives

An **adjective** describes, modifies, or tells us more about a **noun** or a **pronoun**. Colors, numbers, and descriptive words such as *healthy, good,* and *sharp* are adjectives.

Look for the adjectives in the following sentences:

|  | Adjective | Noun or pronoun it describes |
|---|---|---|
| I rode the blue bike. | blue | bike |
| It was a long trip. | long | trip |
| Bring two pencils for the exam. | two | pencils |
| The box is brown. | brown | box |
| She looked beautiful. | beautiful | she |
| That's great! | great | that |

> **KEEP IN MIND . . .**
> Adjectives typically come **before the noun** in English, as in the first three examples above. However, with **linking verbs** (non-action verbs such as *be, seem, look*), the adjective may come **after the verb** instead. Think of it like this: a linking verb **links** the adjective to the noun or pronoun.

Multiple adjectives can be used in a sentence, as can multiple nouns. Look at these examples:

|  | Adjectives | Noun or pronoun it describes |
|---|---|---|
| The six girls were happy, healthy, and rested after their long beach vacation. | six, happy, healthy, rested; long, beach | girls; vacation |
| Leo has a good job, but he is applying for a better one. | good; better | job; one |

## Articles: *A, An, The*

**Articles** are a unique part of speech, but they work like adjectives. An article tells more about a noun.

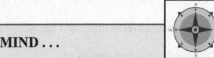

*A* and *an* are **indefinite** articles. Use *a* before a singular **general** noun. Use *an* before a singular general noun that begins with a vowel.

*The* is a **definite** article. Use *the* before a singular or plural **specific** noun.

Look at how articles are used in the following sentences:

- I need *a* pencil to take *the* exam. (any pencil; specific exam)
- Is there *a* zoo in town? (any zoo)
- Let's go to *the* zoo today. (specific zoo)
- Can you get me *a* glass of milk? (any glass)
- Would you bring me *the* glass that's over there? (specific glass)

> **KEEP IN MIND . . .**
> Note comparative and superlative forms of adjectives, such as:
>
> fast, faster, fastest
> far, farther, farthest
> good, better, best
> bad, worse, worst

# Adverbs

An **adverb** describes, modifies, or tells us more about a **verb**, an **adjective**, or another **adverb**. Many adverbs end in *-ly*. Often, adverbs tell when, where, or how something happened. Words such as *slowly, very*, and *yesterday* are adverbs.

## Adverbs that Describe Verbs

Adverbs that describe verbs tell something more about the action.

Look for the adverbs in these sentences:

|  | Adverb | Verb it describes |
|---|---|---|
| They walked quickly. | quickly | walked |
| She disapproved somewhat of his actions, but she completely understood them. | somewhat; completely | disapproved; understood |
| The boys will go inside if it rains heavily. | inside; heavily | go; rains |

## Adverbs that Describe Adjectives

Adverbs that describe adjectives often add intensity to the adjective. Words like *quite, more*, and *always* are adverbs.

Look for the adverbs in these sentences:

|  | Adverb | Adjective it describes |
|---|---|---|
| The giraffe is very tall. | very | tall |
| Do you think that you are more intelligent than them? | more | intelligent |
| If it's really loud, we can make the volume slightly lower. | really; slightly | loud; lower |

## Adverbs that Describe Other Adverbs

Adverbs that describe adverbs often add intensity to the adverb.

Look for the adverbs in these sentences:

|  | Adverb | Adverb it describes |
|---|---|---|
| The mouse moved too quickly for us to catch it. | too | quickly |
| This store is almost never open. | almost | never |
| Those women are quite fashionably dressed. | quite | fashionably |

## Adjectives vs. Adverbs

Not sure whether a word is an adjective or an adverb? Look at these examples.

|  | Adjective | Adverb | Explanation |
|---|---|---|---|
| fast | You're a *fast* driver. | You drove *fast*. | The adjective *fast* describes *driver* (noun); the adverb *fast* describes *drove* (verb). |
| early | I don't like *early* mornings! | Try to arrive *early*. | The adjective *early* describes *mornings* (noun); the adverb *early* describes *arrive* (verb). |
| good/well | They did *good* work together. | They worked *well* together. | The adjective *good* describes *work* (noun); the adverb *well* describes *worked* (verb). |
| bad/badly | The dog is *bad*. | The dog behaves *badly*. | The adjective *bad* describes *dog* (noun); the adverb *badly* describes *behaves* (verb). |

**BE CAREFUL!**

When an adverb ends in *-ly*, add *more* or *most* to make comparisons.

**Correct:** The car moved *more slowly*.

**Incorrect:** The car moved *slower*.

## Let's Review!

- An **adjective** describes, modifies, or tells us more about a **noun** or a **pronoun**.
- An **adverb** describes, modifies, or tells us more about a **verb**, an **adjective**, or another **adverb.**

# CONJUNCTIONS AND PREPOSITIONS

A **conjunction** is a connector word; it connects words, phrases, or clauses in a sentence. A **preposition** is a relationship word; it shows the relationship between two nearby words.

## Conjunctions

A **conjunction** connects words, phrases, or clauses. *And, so,* and *or* are conjunctions.

### Types of Conjunctions

- **Coordinating** conjunctions connect two words, phrases, or independent clauses.

- **Subordinating** conjunctions connect a main (independent) clause and a dependent clause. The conjunction may show a relationship or time order for the two clauses.

- **Correlative** conjunctions are pairs of conjunctions that work together to connect two words or phrases.

**KEEP IN MIND . . .**

A clause is a phrase that has a subject and a verb.

Some clauses are **independent**. An independent clause can stand alone.

Some clauses are **dependent**. A dependent clause relies on another clause in order to make sense.

**DID YOU KNOW?**

The full list of **coordinating conjunctions** is:

> *and, or, but, so, for, nor, yet*

Some **subordinating conjunctions** are:

> *after, as soon as, once, if, even though, unless*

Some **correlative conjunctions** are:

> *either/or, neither/nor, as/as*

| Example | Conjunction | What it is connecting |
|---------|-------------|----------------------|
| *Verdi, Mozart,* **and** *Wagner* are famous opera composers. | and | three nouns |
| Would you like *angel food cake, chocolate lava cake,* **or** *banana cream pie* for dessert? | or | three noun phrases |
| *I took the bus to work,* **but** *I walked home.* | but | two independent clauses |
| *It was noisy at home,* **so** *we went to the library.* | so | two independent clauses |
| *They have to clean the house* **before** *the realtor shows it.* | before | a main clause and a dependent clause |
| Use **either** hers **or** mine. | either/or | two pronouns |
| **After** everyone leaves, make sure you lock up. | after | a main clause and a dependent clause |
| I'd **rather** *fly* **than** *take the train.* | rather/than | two verb phrases |
| **As soon as** they announced the winning number, she looked at her ticket and shouted, "Whoopee!" | as soon as | a main clause and a dependent clause |

**DID YOU KNOW?**

In the last example above, "*Whoopee!*" is an interjection.

An **interjection** is a short phrase or clause that communicates emotion.

Some other interjections are:

- *Way to go!*
- *Oops.*
- *Yuck.*
- *Hooray!*
- *Holy cow!*

# Prepositions

A **preposition** shows the relationship between two nearby words. Prepositions help to tell information such as direction, location, and time. *To, for,* and *with* are prepositions.

| Example | Preposition | What it tells us |
|---------|-------------|-----------------|
| The desk is in the classroom. | in | location |
| We'll meet you at 6:00. | at | time |
| We'll meet you at the museum. | at | place |
| The book is on top of the desk. | on top of | location |

## Prepositional Phrases

A preposition must be followed by an **object of the preposition**. This can be a noun or something that serves as a noun, such as a pronoun or a gerund.

**DID YOU KNOW?**

A gerund is the *-ing* form a verb that serves as a noun. *Hiking* is a gerund in this sentence:

- I wear these shoes for *hiking*.

A **prepositional phrase** is a preposition plus the object that follows it.

Look for the prepositional phrases in the following examples. Note that a sentence can have more than one prepositional phrase.

| Example | Preposition | Object of the preposition |
|---|---|---|
| The tiny country won the war *against all odds*. | against | all odds |
| Look *at us*! | at | us |
| Why don't we go swimming *instead of sweating in this heat*? | instead of; in | sweating; this heat |
| Aunt Tea kept the trophy *on a shelf of the cabinet between the sofas in the living room*. | on; of; between; in | a shelf; the cabinet; the sofas; the living room |

## Let's Review!

- A **conjunction** connects words, phrases, or clauses. *And, so,* and *or* are conjunctions.

- A **preposition** shows the relationship between two nearby words. *To, for,* and *with* are prepositions.

- A **prepositional phrase** includes a preposition plus the object of the preposition.

**BE CAREFUL!**

Sometimes a word looks like a preposition but is actually part of the verb. In this case, the verb is called a phrasal verb, and the preposition-like word is called a particle. Here is an example:

- *Turn on* the light. (*Turn on* has a meaning of its own; it is a phrasal verb. *On* is a particle here, rather than a preposition.)

- *Turn on that street*. (*On that street* shows location; it is a prepositional phrase. *On* is a preposition here.)

# VERBS AND VERB TENSES

A **verb** is a word that describes a **physical or mental action** or a **state of being**. This lesson will cover the role of verbs in sentences, verb forms and tenses, and helping verbs.

## The Role of Verbs in Sentences

A verb describes an action or a state of being. A complete sentence must have at least one verb.

Verbs have different tenses, which show time.

### Verb Forms

Each verb has three primary forms. The **base form** is used for simple present tense, and the **past form** is used for simple past tense. The **participle form** is used for more complicated time situations. Participle form verbs are accompanied by a helping verb.

| Base Form | Past Form | Participle Form |
|---|---|---|
| end | ended | ended |
| jump | jumped | jumped |
| explain | explained | explained |
| eat | ate | eaten |
| take | took | taken |
| go | went | gone |
| come | came | come |

Some verbs are **regular**. To make the **past** or **participle** form of a regular verb, we just add *-ed*. However, many verbs that we commonly use are **irregular**. We need to memorize the forms for these verbs.

In the chart above, *end, jump,* and *explain* are regular verbs. *Eat, take, go*, and *come* are irregular.

### Using Verbs

A simple sentence has a **subject** and a **verb**. The subject tells us who or what, and the verb tells us the action or state.

| Example | Subject | Verb | *Explanation/Time* |
|---|---|---|---|
| They ate breakfast together yesterday. | They | ate | *happened yesterday* |
| I walk to school. | I | walk | *happens regularly* |
| We went to California last year. | We | went | *happened last year* |
| She seems really tired. | She | seems | *how she seems right now* |
| The teacher is sad. | teacher | is | *her state right now* |

You can see from the examples in this chart that **past tense verbs** are used for a time in the past, and **present tense verbs** are used for something that happens regularly or for a state or condition right now.

Often a sentence has more than one verb. If it has a connector word or more than one subject, it can have more than one verb.

- The two cousins <u>live</u>, <u>work</u>, and <u>vacation</u> together.(3 verbs)
- The girls <u>planned</u> by phone, and then they <u>met</u> at the movies. (2 verbs)

> **BE CAREFUL!**
> When you have more than one verb in a sentence, make sure both verb tenses are correct.

# Helping Verbs and Progressive and Perfect Tenses

## Helping Verbs

A **helping verb** is a supporting verb that accompanies a main verb.

Questions, negative sentences, and certain time situations require helping verbs.

| forms of helping verb "to be" | forms of helping verb "to have" | forms of helping verb "to do" | some modals (used like helping verbs) |
|---|---|---|---|
| am, are, is, was, were, be, being, been | have, has, had, having | do, does, did, doing | will, would, can, could, must, might, should |

Here are examples of helping verbs in questions and negatives.

- Where is he going?
- Did they win?
- I don't want that.
- The boys can't go.

## Progressive and Perfect Tenses

Helping verbs accompany main verbs in certain time situations, such as when an action is or was ongoing, or when two actions overlap in time. To form these tenses, we use a **helping verb** with the **base form plus *-ing*** or with the **participle form** of the main verb.

The **progressive tense** is used for an action that is or was ongoing. It takes base form of the main verb plus *-ing*.

| Example sentence | Tense | *Explanation/Time* |
|---|---|---|
| I <u>am taking</u> French this semester. | Present progressive | *happening now, over a continuous period of time* |
| I <u>was working</u> when you stopped by. | Past progressive | *happened over a continuous period of time in the past* |

The **perfect tense** is used to cover two time periods. It takes the *participle* form of the main verb.

| Example sentence | Tense | *Explanation/Time* |
|---|---|---|
| I <u>have lived</u> here for three years. | Present perfect | *started in the past and continues to present* |
| I <u>had finished</u> half of my homework when my computer stopped working. | Past perfect | *started and finished in the past, overlapping in time with another action* |

125

Sometimes we use both the **progressive** and **perfect** tenses together.

| Example sentence | Tense | Explanation/Time |
|---|---|---|
| I <u>have been walking</u> for hours! | Present perfect progressive | *started in the past, took place for a period of time, and continues to present* |
| She <u>had been asking</u> for a raise for months before she finally received one. | Past perfect progressive | *started in the past, took place for a period of time, and ended* |

## Let's Review!

- A verb describes an action or state of being.
- Each verb has three primary forms: base form, past form, and participle form.
- Verbs have different tenses, which are used to show time.
- Helping verbs are used in questions, negative sentences, and to form progressive and perfect tenses.

# CHAPTER 6 PARTS OF SPEECH PRACTICE QUIZ

1. **Select the correct verb form to complete the following sentence.**

   William didn't think he would enjoy the musical, but he ___.

   A. do

   B. did

   C. liked

   D. would

2. **How many pronouns are in the following sentence?**

   I wanted to call you last night, but I couldn't find my phone.

   A. 2

   B. 3

   C. 4

   D. 5

3. **How many prepositional phrases are in the following sentence?**

   Marguerite framed a photograph of her grandfather and gave it to him for his birthday.

   A. 1

   B. 2

   C. 3

   D. 4

4. **Choose the common noun that correctly completes the following sentence.**

   Someone was there to greet the students when they arrived at ___.

   A. School

   B. school

   C. the Elementary School

   D. West Elementary School

5. **Choose a proper noun to complete the following sentence.**

   ____walked to work.

   A. We

   B. Sharon

   C. The girls

   D. My mom and dad

6. **How many adjectives are in the following sentence?**

   The new building is tall and modern.

   A. 1

   B. 2

   C. 3

   D. 4

**7. How many helping verbs are in the following sentence?**

The chipmunks collected food for the winter.

A. 0

B. 1

C. 2

D. 3

**8. Which is _not_ a prepositional phrase?**

A. On the bus

B. Against the wall

C. Oh no

D. To him

**9. How many adjectives are in the following sentence?**

The children love to play with the cute, furry kitten.

A. 0

B. 1

C. 2

D. 3

**10. How many pronouns are in the following sentence?**

I called her, but she didn't return my call.

A. 1

B. 2

C. 3

D. 4

# CHAPTER 6 PARTS OF SPEECH
# PRACTICE QUIZ – ANSWER KEY

**1. B.** *Did* can be used here, for a shortened form of *did enjoy it*. **See Lesson: Verbs and Verb Tenses.**

**2. C.** *I, you, I, and my* are pronouns. **See Lesson: Pronouns.**

**3. C.** *Of her grandfather, to him,* and *for his birthday* are prepositional phrases. **See Lesson: Conjunctions and Prepositions.**

**4. B.** *School* is the only common noun listed with correct capitalization. **See Lesson: Nouns.**

**5. B.** *Sharon* is the only proper noun offered. **See Lesson: Nouns.**

**6. C.** The adjectives *new, tall,* and *modern* describe the noun *building*. **See Lesson: Adjectives and Adverbs.**

**7. A.** *Collected* is the only verb in the sentence. **See Lesson: Verbs and Verb Tenses.**

**8. C.** *Oh no* is an interjection. It does not contain a preposition. **See Lesson: Conjunctions and Prepositions.**

**9. C.** *Cute* and *furry* are adjectives that describe the noun *kitten.* **See Lesson: Adjectives and Adverbs**

**10.    D.** *I, her, she,* and *my* are pronouns. **See Lesson: Pronouns.**

# CHAPTER 7 KNOWLEDGE OF LANGUAGE

## SUBJECT AND VERB AGREEMENT

Every sentence must include a **subject** and a **verb**. The subject tells **who or what**, and the verb describes an **action or condition**. Subject and verb agree in number and person.

## Roles of Subject and Verb

A complete sentence includes a **subject** and a **verb**. The verb is in the part of the sentence called the **predicate**. A predicate can be thought of as a verb phrase.

### A. Simple Sentences

A sentence can be very simple, with just one or two words as **subject** and one or two words as **predicate**.

Sometimes, in a command, a subject is "understood," rather than written or spoken.

Look at these examples of short sentences:

| Sentence | Subject | Predicate, with main verb(s) underlined |
|----------|---------|------------------------------------------|
| I ate. | I | <u>ate</u> |
| They ran away. | They | <u>ran</u> away |
| It's OK. | It | <u>is</u> OK |
| Go and find the cat! | (You) | <u>go</u> and <u>find</u> the cat |

### B. More Complex Sentences

Sometimes a subject or predicate is a long phrase or clause.

Some sentences have more than one subject or predicate, or even a predicate within a predicate.

> **BE CAREFUL!**
>
> *It's* is a contraction of *it is*.
>
> *Its* (without an apostrophe) is the possessive of the pronoun *it*.

| Sentence | Subject(s) | Predicate(s), with main verb(s) underlined |
|----------|-----------|---------------------------------------------|
| My friend from work had a bad car accident. | My friend from work | <u>had</u> a bad car accident |
| John, his sister, and I plan to ride our bikes across the country this summer. | John, his sister, and I | <u>plan</u> to ride our bikes across the country this summer |
| I did so much for them, and they didn't even thank me.* | I;<br>they | <u>did</u> so much for them;<br>didn't even <u>thank</u> me |
| She wrote a letter that explained the problem.** | She | <u>wrote</u> a letter that explained the problem |

*This sentence consists of two clauses, and each clause has its own subject and its own predicate.

**In this sentence, *that explained the problem* is part of the predicate, and it is also a relative clause with own subject and predicate.

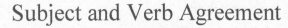

# Subject and Verb Agreement

Subjects and verbs must agree in **number** and **person**. This means that different subjects take different forms of a verb.

**BE CAREFUL!**

The verbs *be, have,* and *do* can be either main verbs or helping verbs.

**KEEP IN MIND . . .**

The third person singular subject takes a different verb form than other subjects.

With **regular** verbs, simply add *-s* to the singular third person verb, as shown below:

|  | Singular | | Plural | |
|---|---|---|---|---|
|  | Subject | Verb | Subject | Verb |
| (first person) | I | play | we | play |
| (second person) | you | play | you | play |
| (third person) | he/she/it | plays | they | play |

Some verbs are **irregular**, so simply adding *-s* doesn't work. For example:

| verb | form for third person singular subject |
|---|---|
| have | has |
| do | does |
| fix | fixes |

**BE CAREFUL!**

The verb *be* is very irregular. Its forms change with several subjects, in both present and past tense.

Look for subject-verb agreement in the following sentences:

- *I* usually <u>eat</u> a banana for breakfast.
- *Marcy* <u>does</u> well in school.
- The *cat* <u>licks</u> its fur.

Subject-Verb Agreement for the Verb *Be*

| Present | | Past | |
|---|---|---|---|
| I am | we are | I was | we were |
| you are | you are | you were | you were |
| he/she/it is | they are | they were | they were |

## Things to Look Out For

Subject-verb agreement can be tricky. Be careful of these situations:

- **Sentences with more than one subject:** If two subjects are connected by *and,* the subject is **plural**. When two singular subjects are connected by *neither/nor,* the subject is **singular**.

  *Sandra and Luiz* <u>shop</u>. (plural)

  *Neither Sandra nor Luiz* <u>has</u> money. (singular)

- **Collective nouns:** Sometimes a noun stands for a group of people or things. If the subject is **one group**, it is considered **singular**.

  *Those students* are still on chapter three. (plural)

  *That class* <u>is</u> still on chapter three. (singular)

- ***There is* and *there are*:** With pronouns such as *there, what,* and *where,* the verb agrees with the noun or pronoun that follows it.

  *There*'s a rabbit! (singular)

  *Where* <u>are</u> my shoes? (plural)

- **Indefinite pronouns:** Subjects such as *everybody, someone,* and *nobody* are **singular**. Subjects such as *all, none,* and *any* can be either **singular or plural**.

  *Everyone* in the band <u>plays</u> well. (singular)

  *All* of the students <u>are</u> there. (plural)

  *All* <u>is</u> well. (singular)

## Let's Review!

- Every sentence has a subject and a verb.
- The predicate is the part of the sentence that contains the verb.
- The subject and verb must agree in number and person.
- The third person singular subject takes a different verb form.

# TYPES OF SENTENCES

Sentences are a combination of words that communicate a complete thought. Sentences can be written in many ways to signal different relationships among ideas. This lesson will cover (1) simple sentences (2) compound sentences (3) complex sentences (4) parallel structure.

## Simple Sentences

A **simple sentence** is a group of words that make up a **complete thought**. To be a complete thought, simple sentences must have one **independent clause.** An independent clause contains a single **subject** (who or what the sentence is about) and a **predicate** (a **verb** and something about the subject.)

Let's take a look at some simple sentences:

| Simple Sentence | Subject | Predicate | Complete Thought? |
|---|---|---|---|
| The car was fast. | car | was fast<br>(verb = was) | Yes |
| Sally waited for the bus. | Sally | waited for the bus<br>(verb = waited) | Yes |
| The pizza smells delicious. | pizza | smells delicious<br>(verb = smells) | Yes |
| Anton loves cycling. | Anton | loves cycling<br>(verb = loves) | Yes |

It is important to be able to recognize what a simple sentence is in order to avoid **run-ons** and **fragments**, two common grammatical errors.

A **run-on** is when two or more independent clauses are combined without proper punctuation:

**FOR EXAMPLE**

*Gregory is a very talented actor he was the lead in the school play.*

If you take a look at this sentence, you can see that it is made up of 2 independent clauses or simple sentences:

1.  *Gregory is a very talented actor*
2.  *he was the lead in the school play*

You <u>cannot</u> have two independent clauses running into each other without proper punctuation.

You can fix this run-on in the following way:

**Gregory is a very talented actor. He was the lead in the school play.**

A **fragment** is a group of words that looks like a sentence. It starts with a capital letter and has end punctuation, but when you examine it closely you will see it is not a complete thought.

---

**FOR EXAMPLE**

*When I woke up.*

If you take a look at this group of words, you can see that it looks like a sentence. It has a capital letter and a period at the end.

But when you read it closely, you can see that it is not a complete thought since you are left wondering: *When I woke up - what happened?*

*When I woke up* is a **dependent clause**. It is a clause that provides information, but it **cannot stand by itself** since it is dependent on other information to make it a complete thought.

You can fix this fragment by adding more information to make it complete:

**When I woke up, I had a terrible headache.**

or

*I had a terrible headache when I woke up.*

---

Let's put this information all together to determine whether a group of words is a simple sentence, a run-on, or a fragment:

| Group of Words | Simple Sentence | Run-On | Fragment |
|---|---|---|---|
| Mondays are the worst they are a drag. | -- | YES! These are two independent clauses running into one another without proper punctuation.<br>FIX: *Mondays are the worst. They are a drag.* | -- |
| Because I wanted soda. | -- | -- | YES! This is a dependent clause and needs more information to make it a complete thought.<br>FIX: *I went to the store because I wanted soda.* |
| Ereni is from Greece. | YES! This is a simple sentence with a subject (*Ereni*) and a predicate (*is from Greece*), so it is a complete thought. | -- | -- |
| While I was apple picking. | -- | -- | YES! This is a dependent clause and needs more information to make it a complete thought.<br>FIX: *While I was apple picking, I spotted a bunny.* |
| New York City is magical it is my favorite place. | -- | YES! These are two independent clauses running into one another without proper punctuation.<br>FIX: New York City is magical. It is my favorite place. | -- |

134

# Compound Sentences

A **compound sentence** is a sentence made up of two independent clauses connected with a **coordinating conjunction**.

Let's take a look at the following sentence:

*Joe waited for the bus, but it never arrived.*

If you take a close look at this compound sentence, you will see that it is made up of two independent clauses:

1. *Joe waited for the bus*
2. *it never arrived*

The word *but* is the coordinating conjunction that connects these two sentences. Notice that the coordinating conjunction has a comma right before it. This is the proper way to punctuate compound sentences.

Here are other examples of compound sentences:

**FOR EXAMPLE**

*I want to try out for the baseball team, and I also want to try out for track.*

*Sally can play the clarinet in the band,* **or** *she can play the violin in the orchestra.*

*Mr. Henry is going to run the half marathon,* **so** *he has a lot of training to do.*

All these sentences are compound sentences since they each have two independent clauses joined by a comma and a coordinating conjunction.

The following is a list of **coordinating conjunctions** that can be used in compound sentences. You can use the mnemonic device "FANBOYS" to help you remember them:

**F**or **A**nd **N**or **B**ut **O**r **Y**et **S**o

Think back to Section 1: Simple Sentences. You learned about run-ons. Another way to fix run-ons is by turning the group of words into a compound sentence:

RUN-ON:     *Gregory is a very talented actor he was the lead in the school play.*

FIX:     *Gregory is a very talented actor,* **so** *he was the lead in the school play.*

# Complex Sentences

A **complex** sentence is a sentence that is made up of an independent clause and one or more dependent clauses connected to it.

Think back to Section 1 when you learned about fragments. You learned about a **dependent clause**, the part of a sentence that cannot stand by itself. These clauses need other information to make them complete.

You can recognize a dependent clause because they always begin with a **subordinating conjunction**. These words are a key ingredient in complex sentences.

135

Here is a list of **subordinating conjunctions:**

| after | although | as | because | before |
|---|---|---|---|---|
| despite | even if | even though | if | in order |
| that | once | provided that | rather than | since |
| so that | than | that | though | unless |
| until | when | whenever | where | whereas |
| wherever | while | why | | |

Let's take a look at a few complex sentences:

**FOR EXAMPLE**

*Since the alarm clock didn't go off, I was late for class.*

This is an example of a complex sentence because it contains:

A dependent clause:                     *Since the alarm clock didn't go off*
An independent clause:                  *I was late for class*
A subordinating conjunction:            *since*

*Sarah studied all night for the exam even though she did not receive an A.*

This is an example of a complex sentence because it contains:

A dependent clause:                     *even though she did not receive an A*
An independent clause:                  *Sarah studied all night*
A subordinating conjunction:            *even though*

*\*NOTE: To make a complex sentence, you can either start with the dependent clause or the independent clause. When beginning with the dependent clause, <u>you need a comma after it</u>. When beginning with an independent clause, <u>you do not need a comma after it</u>.*

# Parallel Structure

**Parallel structure** is the repetition of a grammatical form within a sentence to make the sentence sound more harmonious.

Parallel structure comes into play when you are making a list of items.

Stylistically, you want all the items in the list to line up with each other to make them sound better.

Let's take a look at when to use parallel structure:

1. Use parallel structure with verb forms:

In a sentence listing different verbs, you want all the verbs to use the same form:

*Manuel likes <u>hiking</u>, <u>biking</u>, and mountain <u>climbing</u>.*

In this example, the words *hiking, biking* and *climbing* are all gerunds (having an -ing ending), so the sentence is balanced since the words are all using the gerund form of the verb.

*Manuel likes to <u>hike</u>, <u>bike</u>, and mountain <u>climb</u>.*

In this example, the words *hike, bike* and *climb* are all infinitives (using the basic form of the verb), so the sentence is balanced.

You do not want to mix them up:

*Manuel likes <u>hiking</u>, <u>biking</u>, and <u>to mountain climb</u>.*

This sentence **does not** use parallel structure since *hiking* and *biking* use the gerund form of the verb and *to mountain climb* uses the infinitive form.

2. Use parallel structure with active and passive voice:

In a sentence written in the **active voice**, the subject performs the action:

*Sally kicked the ball.*

Sally, the subject, is the one doing the action, kicking the ball.

In a sentence written in the **passive voice**, the subject is acted on by the verb.

*The ball was kicked by Sally.*

When using parallel structure, you want to make sure your items in a list are either all in **active voice**:

*Raymond baked, frosted, and decorated the cake.*

Or all in **passive voice**:

*The cake was baked, frosted, and decorated by Raymond.*

You do not want to mix them up:

*The cake was baked, frosted, and Raymond decorated it.*

This sentence **does not** use parallel structure because it starts off with passive voice and then switches to active voice.

3. Use parallel structure with the length of terms within a list:

When making a list, you should either have all short individual terms or all long phrases.

Keep these consistent by either choosing short, individual terms:

*Cassandra is <u>bold</u>, <u>courageous</u>, and <u>strong</u>.*

Or longer phrases:

*Cassandra is <u>brave in the face of danger</u>, <u>willing to take risks</u>, and a <u>force to be reckoned with</u>.*

You do not want to mix them up:

*Cassandra is <u>bold</u>, <u>courageous</u>, and <u>a force to be reckoned with</u>.*

This sentence **does not** use parallel structure because the first two terms are short, and the last one is a longer phrase.

## Let's Review!

- A simple sentence consists of a clause, which has a single subject and a predicate.
- A compound sentence is made up of two independent clauses connected by a coordinating conjunction.
- A complex sentence is made up of a subordinating conjunction, an independent clause and one or more dependent clauses connected to it.
- Parallel structure is the repetition of a grammatical form within a sentence to make the sentence sound more harmonious.

# PHRASES AND CLAUSES

There are four types of clauses that are used to create sentences. Sentences with several clauses, and different types of clauses, are considered complex. This lesson will cover (1) independent clauses, (2) dependent clauses and subordinate clauses, and (3) coordinate clauses.

## Independent Clause

An **independent clause** is a simple sentence. It has a subject, a verb, and expresses a complete thought.

- Steve went to the store.
- She will cook dinner tonight.
- The class was very boring.
- The author argues that listening to music helps productivity.

Two **independent clauses** can be connected by a semicolon. There are some common words that indicate the beginning of an **independent clause** such as: moreover, also, nevertheless, however, furthermore, consequently.

- I wanted to go to dinner; however, I had to work late tonight.
- She had a job interview; therefore, she dressed nicely.

## Dependent and Subordinate Clauses

A **dependent clause** is not a complete sentence. It has a subject and a verb but does not express a complete thought. **Dependent clauses** are also called **subordinate clauses**, because they depend on the **independent or main clause** to complete the thought. A sentence that has both at least one **independent clause** and one **subordinate clause** are considered complex.

**Subordinate clauses** can be placed before or after the **independent clause**. When the **subordinate clause** begins the sentence, there should be a comma before the **main clause**. If the **subordinate clause** ends the sentence, there is no need for a comma.

**Dependent clauses** also have common indicator words. These are often called **subordinating conjunctions** because they connect a **dependent clause** to an **independent clause**. Some of these include: although, after, as, because, before, if, once, since, unless, until, when, whether, and while. Relative pronouns also signify the beginning of a **subordinate clause**. These include: that, which, who, whom, whichever, whoever, whomever, and whose.

- When I went to school...
- Since she joined the team...
- After we saw the play...
- *Because she studied hard*, she received an A on her exam.
- *Although the professor was late*, the class was very informative.
- I can't join you unless I finish my homework.

138

# Coordinate Clause

A **coordinate clause** is a sentence or phrase that combines clauses of equal grammatical rank (verbs, nouns, adjectives, phrases, or independent clauses) by using a coordinating conjunction (and, but, for, nor, or so, yet). **Coordinating conjunctions** cannot connect a **dependent or subordinate clause** and an **independent clause.**

- She woke up, and he went to bed.

- We did not have cheese, so I went to the store to get some.

- Ice cream and candy taste great, but they are not good for you.

- Do you want to study, or do you want to go to Disneyland?

## Let's Review!

- An **independent clause** is a simple sentence that has a noun, a verb, and a complete thought. Two **independent clauses** can be connected by a semicolon.

- A **dependent or subordinate clause** depends on the main clause to complete a thought. A **dependent or subordinate clause** can go before or after the **independent clause** and there are indicator words that signify the beginning of the **dependent or subordinate clause.**

- A **coordinate clause** connects two verbs, nouns, adjectives, phrases, or **independent clauses** using a **coordinating conjunction** (and, but, for, nor, or, so, yet).

# MODIFIERS

A modifier is a word, phrase, or clause that adds detail or changes (modifies) another word in the sentence. Descriptive words such as adjectives and adverbs are examples of modifiers.

## The Role of Modifiers in a Sentence

Modifiers make a sentence more descriptive and interesting.

Look at these simple sentences. Notice how much more interesting they are with modifiers added.

| Simple sentence | With modifiers added |
|---|---|
| I drove. | I drove my family along snowy roads to my grandmother's house. |
| They ate. | They ate a fruit salad of blueberries, strawberries, peaches, and apples. |
| The boy looked. | The boy in pajamas looked out the window at the birds eating from the feeder. |
| He climbed. | He climbed the ladder to fix the roof. |

**DID YOU KNOW?**

Adjectives and adverbs are not the only modifiers.

With a participle phrase, **an -ing verb** can act as a modifier. For example, *eating from the feeder* modifies *the birds*.

With an infinitive, **to plus the main form of a verb** can act as a modifier. For example, *to fix the roof* modifies *climbed*.

Look at the modifiers in bold type in the following sentences. Notice how these words add description to the basic idea in the sentence.

|  | Modifier | Word it Modifies | Type |
|---|---|---|---|
| **The hungry** man ate **quickly**. | the; | man | article |
| | hungry; | man; | adjective; |
| | quickly | ate | adverb |
| **The small** child, **who had scraped his knee,** cried **quietly.** | the; | child; | article; |
| | small; | child; | adjective; |
| | who had scraped his knee; | child; | adjective clause; |
| | quietly | cried | adverb |
| **The** horse **standing near the fence** is **beautiful.** | the; | horse; | article; |
| | standing near the fence; | horse; | participle phrase; |
| | beautiful | horse | adjective |
| Hana and Mario stood **by the lake** and watched **a gorgeous** sunset. | by the lake; | stood; | prepositional phrase; |
| | a; | sunset; | article; |
| | gorgeous | sunset | adjective |
| They tried **to duck out of the way as the large spider dangled from the ceiling.** | to duck out of the way; | tried; | infinitive phrase; |
| | as the large spider dangled; | duck; | adverb clause; |
| | from the ceiling | dangled | prepositional phrase |

141

# Misplaced and Dangling Modifiers

A **misplaced modifier** is a modifier that is placed incorrectly in a sentence, so that it modifies the wrong word.

A **dangling modifier** is a modifier that modifies a word that should be included in the sentence but is not.

Look at these examples.

- First, notice the modifier, in bold.
- Next, look for the word it modifies.

> **BE CAREFUL!**
> Sometimes there is a modifier within a modifier. For example, in the clause *as the large spider dangled*, *the* and *large* are words that modify *spider*.

| Incorrect | Problem | How to fix it | Correct |
|---|---|---|---|
| Sam wore his new shirt to school, **which was too big for him**. | Misplaced modifier.<br>Notice the placement of the modifier ***which was too big for him***. It is placed after the word *school*, which makes it seem like *school* is the word it describes. However, this was not the writer's intention. The writer intended for ***which was too big for him*** to describe the word *shirt*. | The modifier needs to be placed after the word *shirt*, rather than after the word *school*. | Sam wore his new shirt, **which was too big for him**, to school. |
| **Running down the hallway,** Maria's bag of groceries fell. | Dangling modifier.<br>The modifier ***running down the hallway*** is placed before the phrase *Maria's bag of groceries*, which makes it seem this is what it describes. However, this was not the writer's intention; the *bag of groceries* cannot run! The correct reference would be the noun *Maria*, which was omitted from the sentence completely. | The modifier must reference *Maria*, rather than *Maria's bag of groceries*. This can be fixed by adding the noun *Maria* as a subject. | **Running down the hallway,** Maria dropped her bag of groceries. |
| **With a leash on,** my sister walked the dog. | Misplaced modifier.<br>The modifier ***with a leash on*** is placed before *my sister*, which makes it seem like she is wearing a leash. | Move the modifier so that it is next to *the dog*, rather than *my sister*. | My sister walked the dog, **who had a leash on**. |

## Let's Review!

- A modifier is a word, phrase, or clause that adds detail by describing or modifying another word in the sentence.

- Adverbs, adjectives, articles, and prepositional phrases are some examples of modifiers.

- Misplaced and dangling modifiers have unclear references, leading to confusion about the meaning of a sentence.

> **BE CAREFUL!**
> A modifier should be placed next to the word it modifies. Misplaced and dangling modifiers lead to confusion about the meaning of a sentence.

# DIRECT OBJECTS AND INDIRECT OBJECTS

A direct or indirect object has a relationship with the action verb that precedes it. A direct object directly receives the action of the verb. An indirect object indirectly receives the action.

## Direct and Indirect Objects in a Sentence

An **object** in grammar is something that is acted on. The **subject** does the action; the **object** receives it.

An object is usually a noun or a pronoun.

There are three types of objects:

- direct object
- indirect object
- object of the preposition

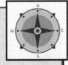

**KEEP IN MIND . . .**

When there is an **indirect object**, it will be placed between the verb and the direct object.

Many sentences have a direct object. Some sentences also have an indirect object.

Look at these examples:

- Kim threw *the ball.*
  *The ball* is the direct object. *Ask yourself:* What did she throw?
- Kim threw *Tommy* the ball.
  *Tommy* is the indirect object. *Ask yourself:* Who did she throw it to?

**BE CAREFUL!**

Some verbs can never take **direct objects**. These are:

- **Linking verbs** such as *is* and *seem*.
- **Intransitive verbs** such as *snore, go, sit,* and *die*.
- *Ask yourself:* Can you *snore* something? No. Therefore, this verb cannot take a direct object.

Look for the objects in the sentences below.

| Sentence | Direct Object | Indirect Object | Be careful! |
|---|---|---|---|
| Her mom poured her a glass of milk. | a glass of milk (*ask:* what did she pour?) | her (*ask:* who did she pour it for? | The indirect object, when there is one, can be found between the verb and the direct object. |
| They work hard. | | | Not all sentences have objects. Here, *hard* is not an object. It is not the recipient of *work*. Instead, it is a modifier; it describes the work. |
| Kazu bought Katrina a present. | a present (*ask:* what did he buy?) | Katrina (*ask:* who did he buy it for?) | |
| Kazu bought a present for Katrina. | a present (*ask:* what did he buy?) | | Don't confuse indirect objects with prepositional phrases. *For* is a preposition, so *Katrina* is the object of the preposition; it is not an indirect object. |

**KEEP IN MIND . . .**

If there is a preposition, the object is the **object of the preposition** rather than an **indirect object**. Compare these two sentences:

- She made *me* dinner. (*Me* is an indirect object.)
- She made dinner *for me*. (*For me* is a prepositional phrase.)

## Let's Review!

- A direct object directly receives the action of the verb.
- An indirect object indirectly receives the action of the verb.
- An indirect object comes between the verb and the direct object.

# CHAPTER 7 KNOWLEDGE OF LANGUAGE PRACTICE QUIZ

1.  **Select the "understood" subject with which the underlined verb must agree.**

    <u>Watch</u> out!

    A.  You

    B.  He

    C.  I

    D.  Out

2.  **How many verbs must agree with the underlined subject in the following sentence?**

    <u>Kareem Abdul-Jabbar</u>, my favorite basketball player, dribbles, shoots, and scores to win the game!

    A.  0

    B.  1

    C.  2

    D.  3

3.  **How many modifiers are in the following sentence?**

    They carried sleeping bags, tents, and backpacks.

    A.  0

    B.  1

    C.  2

    D.  3

4.  **How many modifiers describe the underlined word in the following sentence?**

    Pass that large silver <u>bowl</u>.

    A.  1

    B.  2

    C.  3

    D.  4

5.  **How many indirect objects are in the following sentence?**

    Nigel drove his father's car to their country house.

    A.  0

    B.  1

    C.  2

    D.  3

6.  **How many direct objects are in the following sentence?**

    I read *Gulliver's Travels*, and I loved it!

    A.  0

    B.  1

    C.  2

    D.  3

7. **Which of the following is an example of a compound sentence?**

   A.  The Jankowskis typically go out for Italian food, tonight they tried Thai.

   B.  The Jankowskis typically go out for Italian food and tonight they tried Thai.

   C.  The Jankowskis typically go out for Italian food, but tonight they tried Thai.

   D.  The Jankowskis typically go out for Italian food even though tonight they tried Thai.

8. **Which of the following options would complete this sentence to make it a complex sentence?**

   I enjoy watching the snow fall
   _____.

   A.  the winters are brutally cold.

   B.  but, the winters can be brutally cold.

   C.  however, the winters can be brutally cold.

   D.  even though the winters can be brutally cold.

9. **Identify the type of clause.**

   The reporter stumbled over his words.

   A.  Coordinate clause

   B.  Dependent clause

   C.  Subordinate clause

   D.  Independent clause

10. **Identify the type of clause.**

    I ate, and he drank.

    A.  Coordinate clause

    B.  Dependent clause

    C.  Subordinate clause

    D.  Independent clause

# CHAPTER 7 KNOWLEDGE OF LANGUAGE PRACTICE QUIZ – ANSWER KEY

**1. A.** In a command like this one, the "understood" subject is *you*. **See Lesson: Subject and Verb Agreement.**

**2. D.** The verbs *dribbles, shoots,* and *scores* must agree with the subject *Kareem Abdul-Jabbar*. **See Lesson: Subject and Verb Agreement.**

**3. B.** The only modifier is the word *sleeping*, which is an adjective describing *bags*. **See Lesson: Modifiers.**

**4. C.** *That, large,* and *silver* describe *bowl*. **See Lesson: Modifiers.**

**5. A.** *His father's car* is a direct object of the verb *drove*, but there is no indirect object. **See Lesson: Direct Objects and Indirect Objects.**

**6. C.** *Gulliver's Travels* is a direct object of the verb *read*, and *it* is a direct object of the verb *loved*. **See Lesson: Direct Objects and Indirect Objects.**

**7. C.** This is a compound sentence joining two independent clauses with a comma and the conjunction *but*. **See Lesson: Types of Sentences.**

**8. D.** This option would make the sentence a complex one since it has a subordinating conjunction, *even though*, and a dependent clause. **See Lesson: Types of Sentences.**

**9. D.** Independent clause. The sentence has a subject and a verb and expresses a complete thought. **See Lesson: Types of Clauses.**

**10.   A.** Coordinate clause. A coordinate clause is a sentence or phrase that combines clauses of equal grammatical rank (verbs, nouns, adjectives, phrases, or independent clauses) by using a coordinating conjunction (and, but, for, nor, or so, yet). **See Lesson: Types of Clauses.**

# SECTION V
# BIOLOGY

# Biology: 25 questions, 25 minutes

**Areas assessed:** Life and Physical Sciences

## BIOLOGY TIPS

- Review the periodic table.

- Know quick facts about population growth and decline, and birth and fertility rates.

# CHAPTER 8 LIFE AND PHYSICAL SCIENCES

## AN INTRODUCTION TO BIOLOGY

This lesson introduces the basics of biology, including the process researchers use to study science. It also examines the classes of biomolecules and how substances are broken down for energy.

## Biology and Taxonomy

The study or science of living things is called **biology**. Some characteristics, or traits, are common to all living things. These enable researchers to differentiate living things from nonliving things. Traits include reproduction, growth and development, **homeostasis**, and energy processing. Homeostasis is the body's ability to maintain a constant internal environment despite changes that occur in the external environment. With so many living things in the world, researchers developed a **taxonomy** system, which is used for classification, description, and naming. As shown below, there are seven classification levels in the classical Linnaean system.

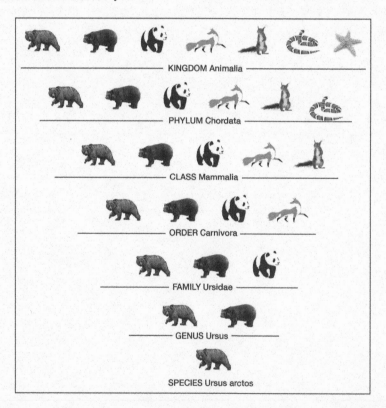

Specificity increases as the levels move from kingdom to species. For example, in the image the genus level contains two types of bears, but the species level shows one type. Additionally, organisms in each level are found in the level above it. For example, organisms in the order level are part of the class level. This classification system is based on physical similarities across living things. It does not account for molecular or genetic similarities.

**DID YOU KNOW?**

Carl Linnaeus only used physical similarities across organisms when he created the Linnaean system because technology was not advanced enough to observe similarities at the molecular level.

## Example

**A researcher classifies a newly discovered organism in the class taxonomy level. What other taxonomic level is this new organism classified in?**

A.  Order

B.  Family

C.  Species

D.  Kingdom

The correct answer is **D.** Each level is found in the level above it. The levels above class are phylum and kingdom. **See Lesson: An Introduction to Biology.**

# Scientific Method

To develop the taxonomic system, researchers had to ask questions. Researchers use seven steps to answer science questions or solve problems. These make up the **scientific method,** described below:

1.  Problem: The question created because of an observation. *Example: Does the size of a plastic object affect how fast it naturally degrades in a lake?*

2.  Research: Reliable information available about what is observed. *Example: Learn how plastics are made and understand the properties of a lake.*

3.  Hypothesis: A predicted solution to the question or problem. *Example: If the plastic material is small, then it will degrade faster than a large particle.*

4.  Experiment: A series of tests used to evaluate the hypothesis. Experiments consist of an **independent variable** that the researcher modifies and a **dependent variable** that changes due to the independent variable. They also include a **control group** used as a standard to make comparisons. *Example: Collect plastic particles both onshore and offshore of the lake over time. Determine the size of the particles and describe the lake conditions during this time period.*

5.  Observe: Analyze data collected during an experiment to observe patterns. *Example: Analyze the differences between the numbers of particles collected in terms of size.*

6.  Conclusion: State whether the hypothesis is rejected or accepted and summarize all results.

7.  Communicate: Report findings so others can replicate and verify the results.

Sometimes, just a few steps of the scientific method are necessary to research a question. At other times, several steps may be repeated as needed. The goal of this method is to find a reliable answer to the scientific question.

**TEST TIP**

Using the first letter in each of the steps, you can create a mnemonic device to remember the steps. For example: "**P**eople **R**eally **H**ave **E**lephants **O**n **C**ompact **C**ars." Try creating your own mnemonic device!

Over the course of many years during which scientists are able to collect sufficient and reliable data, the scientific method can be used to create a law or theory. A **law** is a rule that describes patterns observed in nature. A **scientific theory** explains the how and why of things that happens in nature through observations and experiments. Scientists widely accept both laws and theories, but they can be modified over time.

## Example

**In a study, a researcher describes what happens to a plant following exposure to a dry and hot environment. What step of the scientific method does this most likely describe?**

A.  Forming a hypothesis

B.  Making an observation

C.  Communicating findings

D.  Characterizing the problem

The correct answer is **B.** The researcher is collecting qualitative data by describing what happens to the plant under specific conditions. This data collection corresponds to the observation step of the scientific method. **See Lesson: An Introduction to Biology.**

# Water and Biomolecule Basics

From oceans and streams to a bottle, water is fundamental for life. Without water, life would not exist. Because of water's unique properties, it plays a specific role in living things. The molecular structure of water consists of an oxygen atom bonded to two hydrogen atoms. The structure of water explains some of its properties. For example, water is polar. The oxygen atom is slightly negatively charged, while both hydrogen atoms are slightly positively charged.

As shown below, a single water molecule forms **hydrogen bonds** with nearby water molecules. This type of bonding creates a weak attraction between the water molecules. Hydrogen bonding contributes to water's high boiling point. Water is necessary for biochemical processes like photosynthesis and cellular respiration. It is also a universal solvent, which means water dissolves many different substances.

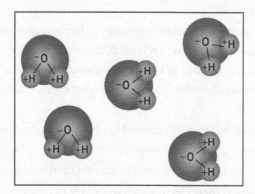

Only two water molecules are needed to show bonding. Remove the partial negative/positive signs and put a − sign next to the oxygen atom and a + sign next to each hydrogen (H) atom. Remove the solid lines between the H and O but keep the dashed line connecting one water molecule to the next.

Biomolecules, or biological molecules, are found in living things. These organic molecules vary in structure and size and perform different functions. Researchers group the wide variety of molecules found in living things into four major classes for organizational purposes: proteins, carbohydrates, lipids, and nucleic acids. Each class of biomolecules has unique **monomers** and **polymers**. Monomers are molecules that covalently bond to form larger molecules or polymers. The table below lists characteristics of each class.

> **KEEP IN MIND**
>
> It takes a lot of heat to create hot water. This is because of water's high specific heat capacity, which is the amount of heat required to raise the temperature of 1 kilogram of water by 1 degree Celsius. This property of water also makes it ideal for living things.

| Biomolecule | Monomer(s) | Function | Example |
|---|---|---|---|
| Protein | Amino acid | A substance that provides the overall basic structure and function for a cell | Enzymes |
| Carbohydrate | Monosaccharides | A form of storage for energy | Glucose Cellulose Starch Disaccharides |
| Lipid | Glycerol and fatty acids | A type of fat that provides a long-term storage for energy | Fats Steroids Oils Hormones |
| Nucleic acid | Nucleotides | A substance that aids in protein synthesis and transmission of genetic information | DNA RNA |

## Example

**During protein synthesis in a cell, the primary structure of the protein consists of a linear chain of monomers. What is another way to describe this structure?**

A.  A linear chain of fatty acids that are hydrogen-bonded together

B.  A linear chain of nucleotides that are hydrogen-bonded together

C.  A linear chain of amino acids that are covalently bonded together

D.  A linear chain of monosaccharides that are covalently bonded together

The correct answer is **C.** The monomers of proteins include amino acids, which are covalently bonded together to form a protein. **See Lesson: An Introduction to Biology.**

# The Metabolic Process

Just like water, energy is essential to life. Food and sunlight are major energy sources. Metabolism is the process of converting food into usable energy. This refers to all biochemical processes or reactions that take place in a living thing to keep it alive.

> **CONNECTIONS**
>
> Energy flows through living things. Energy from the sun is converted to chemical energy via photosynthesis. When living things feed on plants, they obtain this energy for survival.

# HESI

A metabolic pathway is a series of several chemical reactions that take place cyclically to either build or break down molecules. An **anabolic pathway** involves the synthesis of new molecules. These pathways require an input of energy. **Catabolic pathways** involve the breakdown of molecules. Energy is released from a catabolic pathway.

Living things use several metabolic pathways. The most well-studied pathways include glycolysis, the citric acid cycle, and the electron transport chain. These metabolic pathways either release or add energy during a reaction. They also provide a continual flow of energy to living things.

1. **Glycolysis:** This is a catabolic pathway that uses several steps to break down glucose sugar for energy, carbon dioxide, and water. Energy that is released from this reaction is stored in the form of adenosine triphosphate (ATP). Two ATP molecules, two pyruvate molecules, and two NADH molecules are formed during this metabolic pathway.

2. **Citric acid cycle:** The pyruvate molecules made from glycolysis are transported inside the cell's mitochondria. In this catabolic pathway, pyruvate is used to make two ATP molecules, six carbon dioxide molecules, and six NADH molecules.

3. **Electron transport chain and oxidative phosphorylation:** This also takes place in the cell's mitochondria. Many electrons are transferred from one molecule to another in this chain. At the end of the chain, oxygen picks up the electrons to produce roughly 34 molecules of ATP.

The following image provides an overview of **cellular respiration**. Glycolysis, the citric acid cycle, the electron transport chain, and oxidative phosphorylation collectively make up this process. Cellular respiration takes place in a cell and is used to convert energy from nutrients into ATP.

> **BE CAREFUL!**
> Some of these metabolic pathways produce energy in different parts of the cell. Glycolysis takes place in the cytoplasm of the cell. But the citric acid cycle and oxidative phosphorylation occur in the mitochondria.

## Example

**Why are metabolic pathways cyclic?**

A. Metabolic reactions generally take place one at a time.

B. All of the products created in metabolic reactions are used up.

C. The reactions are continuous as long as reactants are available.

D. Energy in the form of ATP is sent to different cells for various uses.

The correct answer is **C**. Metabolic reactions are cyclic, which means they keep occurring as long as enough starting materials are available to allow the reaction to proceed. **See Lesson: An Introduction to Biology.**

# Let's Review!

- This lesson explored how living things are organized, what the scientific method is, and how biomolecules are classified. It also discussed how living things obtain energy via metabolism.

- Biology is the study of living things. Several characteristics distinguish living things from nonliving things.

- All living things are described, classified, and named using a taxonomic system.

- The scientific method uses seven steps to answer a question or solve a problem.

- Biomolecules are organic molecules that are organized into four classes: proteins, carbohydrates, lipids, and nucleic acids

- Living things rely on various metabolic pathways to produce energy and store it in the form of ATP.

# CELL STRUCTURE, FUNCTION, AND TYPE

This lesson describes the cell structure and two different types of cells. The lesson also explores the functions of various cell parts.

## Cell Theory and Types

All living things are made of cells. **Cells** are the smallest structural units and basic building blocks of living things. Cells contain everything necessary to keep living things alive. Varying in size and shape, cells carry out specialized functions. Robert Hooke discovered the first cells in the mid-eighteenth century. Many years later, after advancements in microscopy, the cell theory was formed. This theory, or in-depth explanation, about cells consists of three parts:

1. All living things are composed of one or more cells.
2. Cells are alive and represent the basic unit of life.
3. All cells are produced from preexisting cells.

**DID YOU KNOW?**

More than a trillion cells and at least 200 different types of cells exist in the human body!

Many different types of cells exist. Because of this, cells are classified into two general types: prokaryotic cells and eukaryotic cells. The following comparison table lists key differences between prokaryotes and eukaryotes:

| Characteristic | Prokaryote | Eukaryote |
|---|---|---|
| Cell size | Around 0.2–2.0 mm in diameter | Around 10–100 mm in diameter |
| Nucleus | Absent | True nucleus |
| Organelles | Absent | Several present, ranging from ribosomes to the endoplasmic reticulum |
| Flagella | Simple in structure | Complex in structure |

As shown in the image, prokaryotic cells lack nuclei. Their DNA floats in the **cytoplasm**, which is surrounded by a **plasma membrane**. Very simplistic in structure, these cells lack organelles but do have cell walls. **Organelles** are specialized structures with a specific cellular function. They also may have **ribosomes** that aid in protein synthesis. Also, these cells have a **flagellum** that looks like a tail attached to the cell. Flagella aid in locomotion. The **pili**, or hair-like structures surrounding the cells, aid in cellular adhesion. Bacteria and Archaea are the most common prokaryotes. Most prokaryotes are **unicellular**, or made of a single cell, but there are a few **multicellular organisms**.

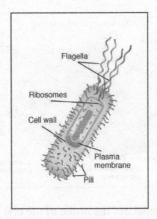

Eukaryotic cells contain a membrane-bound nucleus where DNA is stored. Membrane-bound organelles also exist in eukaryotic cells. Similar to prokaryotic cells, eukaryotic cells have cytoplasm, ribosomes, and a plasma membrane. Eukaryotic organisms can be either unicellular or multicellular. Much larger than prokaryotes, examples of eukaryotic organisms include fungi and even people.

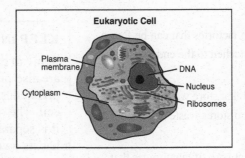

## Example

**What is an organelle?**

A.  The building block of all living things

B.  A substance that is able diffuse inside a cell

C.  The specific receptor found on a cell's surface

D.  A membrane-bound structure with a special function

The correct answer is **D.** Organelles such as ribosomes and the nucleus are membrane-bound structures that have specific functions in a cell. **See Lesson: Cell Structure, Function, and Type**.

# A Peek Inside the Animal Cell

Animal cells are eukaryotic cells. Cheek, nerve, and muscle cells are all examples of animal cells. Because there are many different types, each animal cell has a specialized function. But all animal cells have the same parts, or organelles. Use this image as a guide while going through following list, which describes the organelles found in a eukaryotic (or animal) cell.

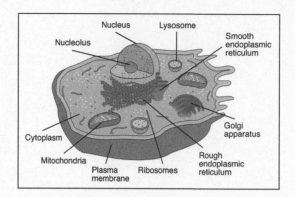

- **Cell membrane:** A double layer that separates the inside of the cell from the outside environment. It is semi-permeable, meaning it only allows certain molecules to enter the cell.

- **Nucleus:** A membrane-bound organelle that contains the genetic material, such as DNA, for a cell. Inside the nucleus is the **nucleolus** that plays a role in assembling subunits required to make ribosomes.

- **Mitochondria:** The cell's powerhouses that provide energy to the cell for it to function. Much of the energy in the form of ATP is produced here.

- **Ribosomes:** The cell's protein factories that can be found floating in the cytoplasm or attached to the endoplasmic reticulum.

- **Vacuoles:** Small sacs in a cell that store water and food for survival. This organelle also stores waste material that is mostly in the form of water.

> **KEEP IN MIND!**
> Some of the organelles in animal cells are also present in plant cells. In addition, all organelles are found in the cytoplasm of the cell. The only exception is the nucleus, which it is separated from the cytoplasm because it has its own membrane.

- **Endoplasmic reticulum:** A network of membranes that functions as a cell's transportation system, shuttling proteins and other materials around the cell. The **smooth endoplasmic reticulum** lacks ribosomes, and the **rough endoplasmic reticulum** has ribosomes.

- **Lysosomes:** Sac-like structures that contain digestive enzymes that are used to break down food and old organelles.

- **Golgi apparatus:** A stack of flattened pouches that plays a role in processing proteins received from the endoplasmic reticulum. It modifies proteins from the endoplasmic reticulum and then packages them into a vesicle that can be sent to other places in the cell.

## Example

**Which two organelles work together to facilitate protein synthesis?**

A. Cytoplasm and lysosome

B. Vacuole and mitochondria

C. Nucleus and cell membrane

D. Ribosome and endoplasmic reticulum

The correct answer is **D.** After a protein is synthesized by ribosomes, it is shuttled to the endoplasmic reticulum, where it is further modified and prepared to be transported by vesicles to other places in the cell. **See Lesson: Cell Structure, Function, and Type**.

# Plant Cells

Recall that plant cells are also eukaryotic cells. Structurally, these cells are similar to animal cells because some of the parts in a plant cell are also found in an animal cell. However, there are some notable differences. The following image shows the structure of a plant cell.

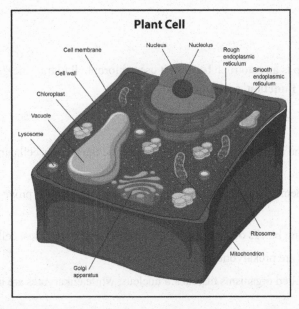

First, only plant cells have a **cell wall**. The purpose of this structure is to provide protection and support to plant cells. The cell wall also enforces the overall structural integrity of the plant cell, and it is found outside the cell membrane. The next organelle is a chloroplast. It is found in the cytoplasm of only plant cells. **Chloroplasts** are photosynthetic compounds used to make food for plant cells by harnessing energy from the sun. These organelles play a role in photosynthesis.

Chloroplasts and mitochondria are both designed to collect, process, and store energy for the cell. Thus, organisms are divided into autotrophs or heterotrophs based on how they obtain energy. **Autotrophs** are organisms that make energy-rich biomolecules from raw material in nature. They do this by using basic energy sources such the sun. This explains why most autotrophs rely on photosynthesis to transform sunlight into usable food that can produce energy necessary for life. Plants and certain species of bacteria are autotrophs.

Animals are **heterotrophs** because they are unable to make their own food. Heterotrophs have to consume and metabolize their food sources to absorb the stored energy. Examples of heterotrophs include all animals and fungi, as well as certain species of bacteria.

**DID YOU KNOW?**
More than 99% of all energy for life on Earth is provided through the process of photosynthesis.

HESI

# Example

**Kelp use chlorophyll to capture sunlight for food. What are these organisms classified as?**

A.  Autotrophs

B.  Chemotrophs

C.  Heterotrophs

D.  Lithotrophs

The correct answer is **A.** Kelp is an autotroph because it uses chlorophyll to trap energy from the sun to make food. **See Lesson: Cell Structure, Function, and Type**.

# Let's Review!

- This lesson focused on the cell theory, different cell types, and the various cell parts found in plant and animal cells.

- The cell theory is an in-depth explanation, supported with scientific data, to prove a cell is a living thing and has unique characteristics.

- Cells are the basic building blocks of life. Coming in various sizes and shapes, cells have specialized functions.

- Two broad types of cells are prokaryotic and eukaryotic cells.

- Prokaryotes are single-celled organisms that lack a nucleus, while eukaryotes are multicellular organisms that contain a nucleus.

- Chloroplasts and cell walls are only found in plant cells.

- Both animal and plant cells have similar organelles such as ribosomes, mitochondria, and an endoplasmic reticulum.

- Living things can be classified as autotrophs or heterotrophs based on how they obtain energy.

# CELLULAR RESPIRATION

This lesson introduces basic processes including cellular reproduction and division, cellular respiration, and photosynthesis. These processes provide ways for cells to make new cells and to convert energy to and from food sources.

## Cell Reproduction

Cells divide primarily for growth, repair, and reproduction. When an organism grows, it normally needs more cells. If damage occurs, more cells must appear to repair the damage and replace any dead cells. During reproduction, this process allows all living things to produce offspring. There are two ways that living things reproduce: asexually and sexually.

**Asexual reproduction** is a process in which only one organism is needed to reproduce itself. A single parent is involved in this type of reproduction, which means all offspring are genetically identical to one another and to the parent. All prokaryotes reproduce this way. Some eukaryotes also reproduce asexually. There are several methods of asexual reproduction.

**Binary fission** is one method. During this process, a prokaryotic cell, such as a bacterium, copies its DNA and splits in half. Binary fission is simple because only one parent cell divides into two daughter cells (or offspring) that are the same size.

**Sexual reproduction** is a process in which two organisms produce offspring that have genetic characteristics from both parents. It provides greater genetic diversity within a population than asexual reproduction. Sexual reproduction results in the production of **gametes**. These are reproductive cells. Gametes unite to create offspring.

### Example

**Binary fission is a method**

A. where one daughter cell is produced.

B. required to produce reproductive cells.

C. that represents a form of asexual reproduction.

D. where two parent cells interact with each other.

The correct answer is **C.** Binary fission is a method organisms use to reproduce asexually. It involves a single parent cell that splits to create two identical daughter cells. **See Lesson: Cellular Reproduction, Cellular Respiration, and Photosynthesis.**

## When the Cell Cycle Begins

For a cell to divide into more cells, it must grow, copy its DNA, and produce new daughter cells. The **cell cycle** regulates cellular division. This process can either prevent a cell from dividing or trigger it to start dividing.

# HESI

The cell cycle is an organized process divided into two phases: **interphase** and the **M (mitotic) phase**. During interphase, the cell grows and copies its DNA. After the cell reaches the M phase, division and of the two new cells can occur. The $G_1$, S, and $G_2$ phases make up interphase.

- **$G_1$:** The first gap phase, during which the cell prepares to copy its DNA

- **S:** The synthesis phase, during which DNA is copied

- **$G_2$:** The second gap phase, during which the cell prepares for cell division

It may appear that little is happening in the cell during the gap phases. Most of the activity occurs at the level of enzymes and macromolecules. The cell produces things like nucleotides for synthesizing new DNA strands, enzymes for copying the DNA, and tubulin proteins for building the mitotic spindle. During the S phase, the DNA in the cell doubles, but few other signs are obvious under the microscope. All the dramatic events that can be seen under a microscope occur during the M phase: the chromosomes move, and the cell splits into two new cells with identical nuclei.

## Example

**For an organism, the cell cycle is needed for**

A. competition.

B. dispersal.

C. growth.

D. parasitism.

The correct answer is **C**. The cell cycle is the process during which a cell grows, copies its own DNA, and physically separates into new cells. With help from the cell cycle, more cells can be provided to help an organism grow. **See Lesson: Cellular Reproduction, Cellular Respiration, and Photosynthesis.**

# Mitosis

**Mitosis** is a form of cell division where two identical nuclei are produced from one nucleus. DNA contains the genetic information of the cell. It is stored in the nucleus. During mitosis, DNA in the nucleus must be copied, or replicated. Recall that this happens during the S phase of the cell cycle. During the M phase, this copied DNA is divided into two complete sets, one of which goes to a daughter cell.

When DNA replicates, it condenses to form **chromosomes** that resemble an X. The DNA forms chromosomes by wrapping around proteins called histones. As shown below, it takes two identical sister chromatids to form a chromosome. A **centromere** holds the sister chromatids together.

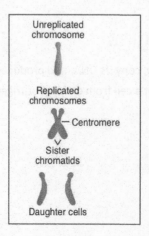

Four phases take place during mitosis to form two identical daughter cells:

1.  **Prophase:** The nuclear membrane disappears, and other organelles move out of the way. The spindle, made of microtubules, begins to form. During **prometaphase**, the microtubules begin to attach to the centromeres at the center of the chromosome.

2.  **Metaphase:** Spindle fibers line the chromosomes at the center of the cell. This is because they are pulled equally by the spindle fibers, which are attached to the opposite poles of the cell.

3.  **Anaphase:** The chromosomes are pulled to the opposite poles of the cell.

4.  **Telophase:** The chromosomes de-condense, the nuclear membrane reappears, and other parts of the cell return to their usual places in the cell.

The cell divides into two daughter cells by way of **cytokinesis**. The illustration below demonstrates the process of mitosis.

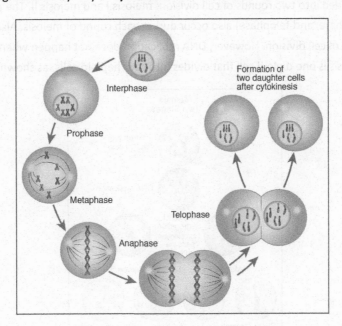

## Example

**Before mitosis occurs**

A.  the spindle fibers must elongate.

B.  DNA must wrap around histones.

C.  chromosomes must split into chromatids.

D.  the cell cycle process must be suspended.

The correct answer is **B.** After DNA replicates, it wraps around proteins called histones to form a chromosome. The chromosome must be formed for mitosis to occur. **See Lesson: Cellular Reproduction, Cellular Respiration, and Photosynthesis.**

# Meiosis

**Meiosis**, sexual cell division in eukaryotes, involves two phases of mitosis that take place one after the other but without a second replication of DNA. This provides the reduction in chromosome number from $2n$ to $n$ needed for fertilization to restore the normal $2n$ state. Diploid multicellular organisms use meiosis, which reduces the number of chromosomes by half. Then, when two haploid ($n$) sex cells (sperm, egg) unite, the normal number of chromosomes is restored. Diploid organisms, such as humans and oak trees, have two copies of every chromosome per cell (2*n*), as opposed to *n*, when one copy of every chromosome is present per cell.

---

**DID YOU KNOW?**

During prophase I of meiosis, **crossing over** occurs to increase genetic diversity. Corresponding chromosomes from the mother and the father of the organism undergoing meiosis are physically bound, and *X*-shaped structures called **chiasmata** form. These are where corresponding DNA from the different parental chromosomes are exchanged, resulting in increased diversity.

---

The process of meiosis is divided into two rounds of cell division: meiosis I and meiosis II. The phases that occur in mitosis (prophase, metaphase, anaphase, and telophase) also occur during each round of meiosis. Also, cytokinesis occurs after telophase during each round of cell division. However, DNA replication does not happen when meiosis I proceeds to meiosis II. The result of meiosis is one diploid cell that divides into four haploid cells, as shown in the following image.

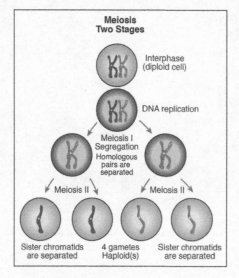

Cytokinesis looks different in plant and animal cells. Plant cells build a new wall, or cell plate, between the two cells, while animal cells split by slowly pinching the membrane toward the center of the cell as the cell divides. Microtubules are more important for cytokinesis in plant cells, while the actin cytoskeleton performs the pinching-off operation during animal cytokinesis.

---

**KEY POINT**

Meiosis and mitosis both require cytokinesis to physically separate a cell into daughter cells. Also, the sequence of events that occur in mitosis are the same in meiosis. However, there are two primary differences between the types of cell division: (1) meiosis has two rounds of cell division, and (2) daughter cells are genetically identical to the parent cell in mitosis but are not genetically identical in meiosis.

---

## Example

**How many rounds of cell division occur during meiosis?**

A. 1          B. 2          C. 3          D. 4

The correct answer is **B.** A difference between mitosis and meiosis is that meiosis requires two rounds of cell division. At the end of both rounds, four haploid daughter cells have been produced. **See Lesson: Cellular Reproduction, Cellular Respiration, and Photosynthesis.**

# Cell Respiration

Once cells have been made, they need to be powered. Plants and some other cells can capture the energy of light and convert it into stored energy in ATP. However, most prokaryotic cells and all eukaryotic cells can perform a metabolic process called **cellular respiration**. Cellular respiration is the process by which the mitochondria of a cell break down glucose to produce energy in the form of ATP. The following is the general equation for cellular respiration:

$$O_2 + C_6H_{12}O_6 \rightarrow CO_2 + H_2O + ATP$$

Reactions during cellular respiration occur in the following sequence:

1. **Glycolysis:** One molecule of glucose breaks down into two smaller sugar molecules called **pyruvate**. This is an anaerobic process, which means it does not need oxygen to be present. Glycolysis takes place in the cell's cytoplasm. End product yield from this reaction per one glucose molecule is

   - two molecules of ATP
   - two molecules of pyruvate
   - two molecules of NADH

2. **Oxidation of pyruvate:** Pyruvate is converted into **acetyl coA** in the mitochondrial matrix. This transition reaction must happen for pyruvate to enter the next phase of cellular respiration. Pyruvate is **oxidized**, which means it loses two electrons and a hydrogen molecule. This results in the formation of NADH and loss of $CO_2$.

> **DID YOU KNOW?**
> The citric acid cycle is not identical for all organisms. Plants have some differences in terms of the enzymes used and energy carriers produced.

3. **Citric acid cycle:** Also called the **Krebs cycle**, during this cycle an acetyl group detaches from the coenzyme A in the acetyl coA molecule. This process is **aerobic,** which means it must occur in the presence of oxygen. The net yield per one glucose molecule is

   - two molecules of ATP
   - six molecules of NADH
   - two molecules of $FADH_2$
   - four molecules of $CO_2$

4. **Electron transport chain:** This process happens in the inner mitochondrial membrane. It consists of a series of enzymatic reactions. Both NADH and FADH$_2$ molecules are passed through a series of enzymes so that electrons and protons can be released from them. During this process, energy is released and used to fuel **chemiosmosis**. During chemiosmosis, protons are transported across the inner mitochondrial membrane to the outer mitochondrial compartment. This flow of protons drives the process of ATP synthesis. This step of cellular respiration creates an approximate net yield of 34 ATP per glucose molecule. Six molecules of water are also formed at the end of the electron transport chain.

## Example

**Before a molecule of glucose can be run through the citric acid cycle, it must experience**

A. ATP production.

B. NADH production.

C. pyruvate oxidation.

D. oxygen deprivation.

The correct answer is **C.** A glucose molecule must first experience pyruvate oxidation because one CO$_2$ molecule must be removed from each pyruvate molecule after glycolysis and before the citric acid cycle. **See Lesson: Cellular Reproduction, Cellular Respiration, and Photosynthesis.**

# Photosynthesis

**Photosynthesis** is the process plants use to make a food source from energy. This process can be thought of as the reverse of cellular respiration. Instead of glucose being broken down into carbon dioxide to create energy-containing molecules, energy is captured from the sun and used to turn carbon dioxide into glucose (and other organic chemicals the plant needs). The energy source is the sun. The reaction for photosynthesis is shown below:

$$CO_2 + H_2O \rightarrow C_6H_{12}O_6 + O_2$$

Energy is captured from the sun and used to turn carbon dioxide into glucose (and other organic chemicals). **Chloroplasts** are **organelles** in plants that contain green chlorophyll, which helps the plants absorb light from the sun.

The photosynthetic reaction involves two distinct phases: light reactions and dark reactions. Light-dependent reactions require light to produce ATP and NADPH. During dark reactions, also known as the **Calvin cycle**, light is not required. These reactions use ATP and NAPDH to produce sugar molecules like glucose.

## Let's Review!

- Cells are needed for growth, repair, and reproduction.
- Mitosis is a form of cell division where one parent cell divides into identical two daughter cells.
- Meiosis involves two rounds of cell division to divide two parent cells into four haploid cells.
- Cells are powered by cellular respiration and photosynthesis, which make ATP and organic chemicals.
- Cellular respiration goes from glycolysis to the citric acid cycle to the electron transport chain.
- Photosynthesis proceeds from the light reactions to the dark reactions, which are known as the Calvin cycle.

# GENETICS AND DNA

The lesson introduces genetics, which is the study of heredity. Heredity is the characteristics offspring inherit from their parents. This lesson also examines Gregor Mendel's theories of heredity and how they have affected the field of genetics.

## Gregor Mendel and Garden Peas

From experiments with garden peas, Mendel developed a simple set of rules that accurately predicted patterns of heredity. He discovered that plants either **self-pollinate** or **cross-pollinate**, when the pollen from one plant fertilizes the pistil of another plant. He also discovered that traits are either **dominant** or **recessive**. Dominant traits are expressed, and recessive traits are hidden.

### Mendel's Theory of Heredity

To explain his results, Mendel proposed a theory that has become the foundation of the science of genetics. The theory has five elements:

1. Parents do not transmit traits directly to their offspring. Rather, they pass on units of information called **genes**.
2. For each trait, an individual has two factors: one from each parent. If the two factors have the same information, the individual is **homozygous** for that trait. If the two factors are different, the individual is **heterozygous** for that trait. Each copy of a factor, or **gene**, is called an **allele**.
3. The alleles determine the physical appearance, or **phenotype**. The set of alleles an individual has is its **genotype**.
4. An individual receives one allele from each parent.
5. The presence of an allele does not guarantee that the trait will be expressed.

### Punnett Squares

Biologists can predict the probable outcomes of a cross by using a diagram called a **Punnett square**. In the Punnett square illustrated at the right, the yellow pea pods are dominant, as designated by a capital Y, and the green pea pods are recessive, as designated with a lowercase y. In a cross between one homozygous recessive (yy) parent and a heterozygous dominant parent (Yy), the outcome is two heterozygous dominant offspring (Yy) and two homozygous recessive offspring (yy), which gives a ratio of 2:2.

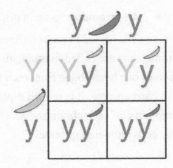

## Example

**In the Punnett square below, homozygous green pea pods are crossed with dominant yellow pea pods. What is the probability of a homozygous green pea pod?**

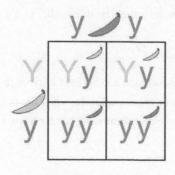

A.  25%          B.  50%          C.  75%          D.  100%

The correct answer is **B.** There is a 2 out of 4, or 50%, chance of a homozygous green pea pod.
**See Lesson: Genetics and DNA.**

# Chromosomes

A **gene** is a segment of DNA, deoxyribonucleic acid, which transmits information from parent to offspring. A single molecule of DNA has thousands of genes. A **chromosome** is a rod-shaped structure that forms when a single DNA molecule and its associated proteins coil tightly before cell division.

Chromosomes have two components:

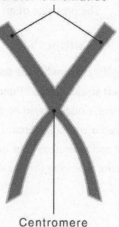

- **Chromatids:** two copies of each chromosome
- **Centromeres:** protein discs that attach the chromatids together

Human cells have 23 sets of different chromosomes. The two copies of each chromosome are called **homologous** chromosomes, or homologues. An offspring receives one homologue from each parent. When a cell contains two homologues of each chromosome, it is termed **diploid (2n)**. A **haploid (n)** cell contains only one homologue of each chromosome. The only haploid cells humans are the sperm and eggs cells known as **gametes**.

## Example

**What is the difference between a diploid cell and a haploid cell?**

A.  A haploid cell is only found in skin cells.

B.  A diploid cell is only found in heart cells.

C.  A diploid cell has a full number of chromosomes, and a haploid cell does not.

D.  A haploid cell has a full number of chromosomes, and a diploid cell does not.

The correct answer is **C.** Diploid cells have a full number of chromosomes, and haploid cells have half the number of chromosomes. **See Lesson: Genetics and DNA.**

# Deoxyribonucleic Acid

The **DNA molecule** is a long, thin molecule made of subunits called **nucleotides** that are linked together in a **nucleic acid** chain. Each nucleotide is constructed of three parts: a **phosphate group**, **five-carbon sugar**, and **nitrogen base**.

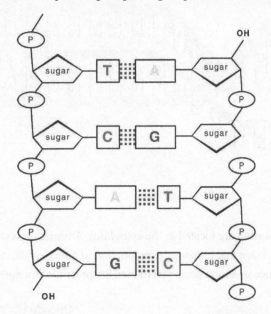

The four nitrogenous bases are

- adenine (A);
- guanine (G);
- thymine (T); and
- cytosine (C).

Adenine and guanine belong to a class of large, organic molecules called **purines**. Thymine and cytosine are **pyrimidines**, which have a single ring of carbon and nitrogen atoms. Base pairs are formed as adenine pairs with thymine and guanine pairs with cytosine. These are the only possible combinations.

## DNA Replication

The process of synthesizing a new strand of DNA is called **replication**. A DNA molecule replicates by separating into two strands, building a complementary strand, and twisting to form a double helix.

## Transcription

The first step in using DNA to direct the making of a protein is **transcription**, the process that "rewrites" the information in a gene in DNA into a molecule of messenger RNA. Transcription manufactures three types of RNA:

- Messenger RNA (mRNA)
- Transfer RNA (tRNA)
- Ribosomal RNA (rRNA)

**Messenger RNA** is an RNA copy of a gene used as a blueprint for a protein. In eukaryotes, transcription does not produce mRNA directly; it produces a pre-mRNA molecule. **Transfer RNA** translates mRNA sequences into amino acid sequences. **Ribosomal RNA** plays a structural role in ribosomes.

Transcription proceeds at a rate of about 60 nucleotides per second until the **RNA polymerase** (an enzyme) reaches a **stop codon** on the DNA called a **terminator** and releases the RNA molecule.

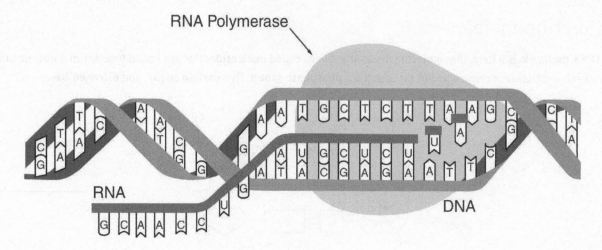

## Translation

The components necessary for **translation** are located in the cytoplasm. Translation is the making of proteins by mRNA binding to a ribosome with the start codon that initiates the production of amino acids. A **peptide bond** forms and connects the amino acids together. The sequence of amino acids determines the protein's structure, which determines its function.

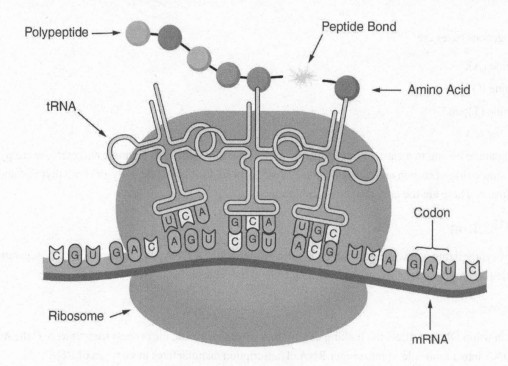

## Example

**Which type of RNA acts as an interpreter molecule?**

A.  mRNA

B.  pre-mRNA

C.  rRNA

D.  tRNA

The correct answer is **D.** Transfer RNA (tRNA) acts as an interpreter molecule, translating mRNA sequences into amino acid sequences. **See Lesson: Genetics and DNA.**

## Let's Review!

- Gregor Mendel developed a simple set of rules that accurately predicts patterns of heredity.
- Mendel proposed a theory that has become the foundation of the science of genetics.
- Biologists can predict the probable outcomes of a cross by using a diagram called a Punnett square.
- A gene is a segment of DNA that transmits information from parent to offspring
- A chromosome is a rod-shaped structure that forms when a single DNA molecule and its associated proteins coil tightly before cell division.
- Deoxyribonucleic acid is a long, thin molecule made of subunits called nucleotides that are linked together in a nucleic acid chain.
- Replication is the process of synthesizing a new strand of DNA.
- Transcription is the first step in using DNA to direct the making of a protein.
- Translation is the process of making proteins.

# CHAPTER 8 LIFE AND PHYSICAL SCIENCES PRACTICE QUIZ

1. **Fats and steroids belong to what biomolecule class?**

   A. Lipids

   B. Proteins

   C. Nucleic acids

   D. Carbohydrates

2. **How many hydrogen atoms are bonded to oxygen in water?**

   A. 1

   B. 2

   C. 3

   D. 4

3. **A protein is synthesized in the ribosome. Where does it travel next?**

   A. Vacuole

   B. Lysosome

   C. Golgi apparatus

   D. Endoplasmic reticulum

4. **Chromosomes contain all of the information necessary to run a cell and pass on a cell's hereditary traits to new cells. Where are these structures found in a cell?**

   A. Nucleus

   B. Ribosome

   C. Cytoplasm

   D. Golgi apparatus

5. **A chemist decides to study reactions occurring in a cell's cytoplasm. Which of the following reactions does she observe?**

   A. Mitosis

   B. Cell cycle

   C. Glycolysis

   D. Carbon cycle

6. **A scientist is watching a colony of bacteria on a plate, and the colony is growing. Which process is most likely responsible for this growth?**

   A. Mitosis

   B. Binary fission

   C. Photosynthesis

   D. Sexual reproduction

7. **Adenine and guanine belong to a class of organic molecules called ____.**

   A. enzymes

   B. nucleotides

   C. purines

   D. pyrimidines

8. **A ____ is a rod-shaped structure that forms when a single DNA molecule and its associated proteins coil tightly before cell division.**

   A. centromere

   B. chromatid

   C. chromosome

   D. gene

# CHAPTER 8 LIFE AND PHYSICAL SCIENCES PRACTICE QUIZ – ANSWER KEY

**1. A.** Lipids are a class of biomolecules that provide a long-term storage solution for energy in living things. Examples of lipids include fats, steroids, and oils. See **Lesson: An Introduction to Biology.**

**2. B.** In the molecular structure of water, a partially negative oxygen atom is bonded to two partially positive hydrogen atoms. See **Lesson: An Introduction to Biology.**

**3. C.** After a protein is synthesized, it goes to the Golgi apparatus where the protein is further modified and then packaged for transport in the cell. See **Lesson: Cell Structure, Function, and Type**.

**4. A.** The nucleus is where genetic information is found in a cell. This genetic information, or DNA, is packaged into chromosomes. See **Lesson: Cell Structure, Function, and Type**.

**5. C.** The first step of cellular respiration is glycolysis. This process happens in the cell's cytoplasm, where glucose is broken down to pyruvate, yielding two molecules of ATP. See **Lesson: Cellular Reproduction, Cellular Respiration, and Photosynthesis.**

**6. B.** Bacteria are able to reproduce asexually using binary fission. See **Lesson: Cellular Reproduction, Cellular Respiration, and Photosynthesis.**

**7. C.** Adenine and guanine belong to a class of organic molecules called purines, which are large molecules. See **Lesson: Genetics and DNA.**

**8. C.** A chromosome is a rod-shaped structure that forms when a single DNA molecule and its associated proteins coil tightly before cell division. **See Lesson: Genetics and DNA.**

# SECTION VI
# CHEMISTRY

# Chemistry: 25 questions, 25 minutes

**Areas assessed:** Chemistry and Scientific Reasoning

## *CHEMISTRY TIPS*

- Know how to balance an equation in chemistry (atomic mass, protons, neutrons, etc.)

- Review atomic structure, chemical bonding, chemical equations, chemical reactions, nuclear chemistry and the periodic table

# CHAPTER 9 SCIENTIFIC REASONING

## DESIGNING AN EXPERIMENT

This lesson introduces the idea of experimental design and the factors one must consider to build a successful experiment.

## Scientific Reasoning

When conducting scientific research, two types of scientific reasoning can be used to address scientific problems: inductive reasoning and deductive reasoning. Both forms of reasoning are also used to generate a hypothesis. **Inductive reasoning** involves drawing a general conclusion from specific observations. This form of reasoning is referred to as the "from the bottom up" approach. Information gathered from specific observations can be used to make a general conclusion about the topic under investigation. In other words, conclusions are based on observed patterns in data.

**Deductive reasoning** is the logical approach of making a prediction about a general principle to draw a specific conclusion. It is recognized as the "from the top down" approach. For example, deductive reasoning is used to test a theory by collecting data that challenges the theory.

> **FOR EXAMPLE**
>
> Use your inductive reasoning to determine the next item in the sequence of events:
>
> 1. fall, winter, spring . . .
> 2. 4, 8, 12 . . .

> **DID YOU KNOW?**
> While Francis Bacon was developing the scientific method, he advocated for the use of inductive reasoning. This is why inductive reasoning is considered to be at the heart of the scientific method.

## Example

**Which is an example of deductive reasoning?**

A. A scientist concludes that a plant species is drought resistant after watching it survive a hot summer.

B. After a boy observes where the sun rises, he tells his mom that the sun will rise in the east in the morning.

C. Since it is well established that noble gases are stable, scientists can safely say that the noble gas neon is stable.

D. A state transportation department decides to use sodium road salt after studies show that calcium road salt is ineffective.

The correct answer is **C.** The statement that noble gases are stable is a general principle or well-accepted theory. Thus, the specific conclusion that the noble gas neon is stable can be drawn from this general principle. **See Lesson: Designing an Experiment.**

# Designing an Experiment

According to the scientific method, the following steps are followed after making an observation or asking a question: (1) conduct background research on the topic, (2) formulate a hypothesis, (3) test the hypothesis with an experiment, (5) analyze results, and (6) report conclusions that explain whether the results support the hypothesis. This means after using logical reasoning to formulate a hypothesis, it is time to design a way to test this hypothesis. This is where **experimental design** becomes a factor.

Experimental design is the process of creating a reliable experiment to test a hypothesis. It involves organizing an experiment that produces the amount of data and right type of data to answer the question. A study's validity is directly affected by the construction and design of an experiment. This is why it is important to carefully consider the following components that are used to build an experiment:

- **Independent variable:** This factor does not depend on what happens in the experiment. The independent variable has values that can be changed or manipulated in an experiment. Data from the independent variable is graphed on the $x$-axis.

- **Dependent variable:** This factor depends on the independent variable. Recognized as the outcome of interest, its value cannot change. It can only be observed during an experiment. Data from the dependent variable is graphed on the $y$-axis.

- **Treatment group:** This is the group that receives treatment in an experiment. It is the item or subject in an experiment that the researcher manipulates. During an experiment, treatment is directly imposed on a group and the response is observed.

- **Control group:** This is a baseline measure that remains constant. Used for comparison purposes, it is the group that neither receives treatment nor is experimentally manipulated. One type of control is a **placebo**. This false treatment is administered to a control group to account for the placebo effect. This is a psychological effect where the brain convinces the body that a fake treatment is the real thing. Often, experimental drug studies use placebos.

---

**TEST TIP**

It can be hard to remember the differences between an independent and a dependent variable. Use the following mnemonic to help keep those differences clear:

| | | |
|---|---|---|
| **D** = dependent | **M** = manipulated variable | **Y** = $y$-axis |
| **R** = responding variable | **I** = independent variable | **X** = $x$-axis |

---

## Example

**A control group**

A. modifies the desired outcome of an experiment.

B. fluctuates in value if an experimental factor is manipulated.

C. establishes a baseline measure to compare dependent variables to.

D. depends on the type of independent variable chosen for an experiment.

The correct answer is **C.** A control group functions as a baseline measure or constant that is not influenced by experimental manipulations. It does not receive treatment in a study. **See Lesson: Designing an Experiment.**

# Data Analysis and Interpretation

When researchers test their hypotheses, the next step in the scientific method is to analyze the data and collect empirical evidence. **Empirical evidence** is acquired from observations and through experiments. It is a repeatable form of evidence that other researchers, including the researcher overseeing the study, can verify. Thus, when analyzing data, empirical evidence must be used to make valid conclusions.

While analyzing data, scientists tend to observe cause-and-effect relationships. These relationships can be quantified using correlations. **Correlations** measure the amount of linear association between two variables. There are three types of correlations:

- **Positive correlation:** As one variable increases, the other variable also increases. This is also known as a direct correlation.

- **Negative correlation:** As one variable increases, the other decreases. The opposite is true if one variable decreases. A negative correlation is also known as an inverse correlation or an indirect correlation.

- **No correlation:** There is no connection or relationship between two variables.

From graphs to tables, there are many ways to visually display data. Typically, graphs are a powerful way to visually demonstrate the relationships between two or more variables. This is the case for correlations. A positive correlation is indicated as a positive slope in a graph, as shown below. Negative correlations are indicated as a negative slope in a graph. If there is no correlation between two variables, data points will not show a pattern.

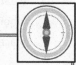

**FOR EXAMPLE**

Studies have shown there is a positive correlation between smoking and lung cancer development. The more you smoke, the greater your risk of developing lung cancer. An example of a negative correlation is the relationship between speed and time when distance is kept constant. The faster a car travels, the amount of time to reach the destination decreases.

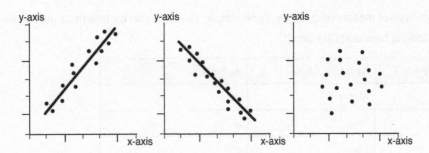

## Examples

1. **What is another term used to describe a direct correlation?**

    A. Positive slope

    B. Negative slope

    C. Inverse correlation

    D. Indirect correlation

    The correct answer is **A.** A direct correlation occurs when one variable increases as another increases. Graphically, this is shown as a positive slope. **See Lesson: Designing an Experiment.**

2. **If a researcher notices a negative slope while analyzing his data, what can he conclude?**

    A. The variables exhibit no correlation.

    B. A different control group should be used.

    C. The variables exhibit a direct correlation.

    D. The variables exhibit an indirect correlation.

    The correct answer is **D.** A negative slope is indicative of an indirect, negative, or inverse correlation. **See Lesson: Designing an Experiment.**

# Scientific Tools and Measurement

Researchers use a wide variety of tools to collect data. The most common types of measuring tools are outlined below:

| Barometer | Used to determines the air pressure in a space. |
|---|---|
| Clock or stopwatch | Used to record time. |
| Graduated cylinder | Used to measure the volume of liquid. |
| Ruler | Used to measure the length of an object. |
| Thermometer | Used to measure temperature. Measurement values may be expressed in degrees Celsius or Fahrenheit. |
| Triple beam balance | Used to measure the mass of an object or to determine the unit of mass. Electronic balances are used to measure very small masses. |

Measured values are often associated with scientific units. Typically, the metric system is preferred when reporting scientific results. This is because nearly all countries use the metric system. Additionally, there is a single base unit of measurement for each type of measured quantity. For example, the base unit for length cannot be the same as the base unit for mass. The following base units are used:

| Unit of Measurement | Base Unit Name | Abbreviation |
|---|---|---|
| Length | Meter | m |
| Mass | Gram | g |
| Volume | Liter | L |

Another benefit of the metric system is that units are expressed in multiples of 10. This allows a researcher to express reported values that may be very large or small. This expression is facilitated by using the following metric prefixes, which are added to the base unit name:

| Prefix | Abbreviation | Value | Description |
|---|---|---|---|
| kilo | k | 1,000 | thousand |
| hecto | h | 100 | hundred |
| deka | da | 10 | ten |
| BASE | N/A | 1 | one |
| deci | d | 0.1 | tenth |
| centi | c | 0.01 | hundredth |
| milli | m | 0.001 | thousandth |

## Example

**What base measurement unit is associated with reported values measured by a graduated cylinder?**

A. Celsius          B. Gram          C. Liter          D. Meter

The correct answer is **C.** Liter is a base unit for volume. Volume is measured using a graduated cylinder. **See Lesson: Designing an Experiment.**

## Let's Review!

- Formulating a hypothesis requires using either inductive or deductive reasoning.
- A good experimental design properly defines all variables and considers how data will be analyzed.
- Correlations illustrate the cause-and-effect relationships between two variables.
- Positive and negative correlations can be displayed graphically by analyzing the slope of a line.
- Different devices are used to measure objects in an experimental study.
- The metric system is usually used when expressing the units of measured values.

# SCIENTIFIC NOTATION

This lesson begins by explaining how to convert measurements with very large or very small values into more manageable numbers using scientific notation. It then explores the structure of the atom and describes how to determine the number of protons, neutrons, and electrons in an atom of a specific element. Finally, it describes the relationship between isotopes of the same element and the effects that these isotopes have on the average atomic mass of an element.

## Scientific Notation

Scientists often work with very large and very small numbers. For example, the radius of Earth's orbit around the sun is very large: 15,000,000,000,000 centimeters. On the other extreme, the radius of a hydrogen atom is very small: 0.00000000529 centimeters. To make these numbers more manageable, scientists write them using **scientific notation**. Scientific notation is a way to represent numbers and contains three components, which are shown in the diagram below.

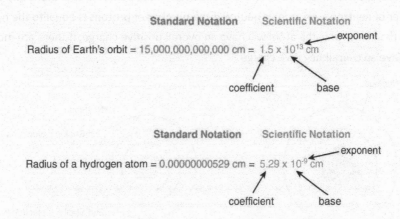

Understanding how these components relate to one another makes it possible to convert between standard notation and scientific notation. The coefficient is a number that has a value of at least 1 but less than 10 and includes all significant digits in the given value. Another way to think about this is that there should always be one non-zero digit before the decimal point.

In scientific notation, the base is always 10.

The exponent indicates the number of places the decimal point needs to move. Notice that when the exponent is positive, the decimal place moves to the right; this is how larger numbers are represented. When the exponent is negative, the decimal place moves to the left; this is how smaller numbers are represented. When the decimal must move beyond the digits that are in the measurement, the "empty" spaces are filled in with zeros.

> **KEY POINT**
> When converting from scientific notation to standard notation, a negative exponent requires the decimal point to move to the left, and a positive exponent requires the decimal point to move to the right.

## Example

**The length of a year is 31,560,000 seconds. What is this value in scientific notation?**

A. $0.3156 \times 10^{-6}$ s          B. $3.156 \times 10^{-7}$ s          C. $3.156 \times 10^{7}$ s          D. $31.56 \times 10^{6}$ s

The correct answer is **C.** The coefficient is a value between 1 and 10 and includes all digits, which is 3.156. Starting with that coefficient, the decimal must be moved seven places to the right to get the value in standard notation, which means that the exponent is a positive seven. **See Lesson: Scientific Notation.**

# The Atom

All matter is made of atoms. Every atom contains a dense core in the center called a **nucleus**. The nucleus is composed of subatomic particles called **protons** and **neutrons**. Surrounding this core is an area known as the **electron cloud**, in which smaller subatomic particles known as **electrons** are moving.

The Bohr model below shows these components of the atom. In the model, each subatomic particle is marked with a charge. Protons have a positive (+) charge, electrons have a negative (–) charge, and neutrons do not carry any charge; they are neutral. Therefore, the overall charge of an atom depends on the numbers of protons and electrons and is not influenced by the number of neutrons. An atom is neutral if the number of protons is equal to the number of electrons. If there are more protons than electrons, the atom will have an overall positive charge; if there are more electrons than protons, the atom will have an overall negative charge.

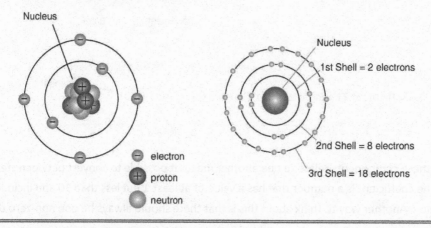

---

### COMPARE THE BOHR MODEL TO A REAL ATOM.

Note that this model is not to scale. The nucleus should be much smaller because it is about 10,000 times smaller than the electron cloud in a real atom. Also, the space between the electrons a real atom is much greater than in the model. In a real atom, the electron cloud is mostly empty space.

---

To further compare these three subatomic particles, their locations, charges, and masses are shown in the table below. The unit used for mass is the **atomic mass unit (amu)**. The masses of a proton or neutron are considerably larger than the mass of an electron. This difference in mass has important implications. First, because the nucleus is so small relative to the overall size of the atom and contains the more massive protons and neutrons, it is extremely dense. Second, because the electrons are almost 2,000 times less massive than the other subatomic particles, they do not significantly influence the atom's mass.

| Subatomic Particle | Symbol | Location | Charge | Mass (amu) |
|---|---|---|---|---|
| Proton | $p^+$ | Nucleus | +1 | 1.0 |
| Neutron | $n^0$ | Nucleus | 0 | 1.0 |
| Electron | $e^-$ | Electron cloud | −1 | 0.00054 |

One final note about the Bohr model of the atom is that the electrons lie on rings. These rings represent energy levels, sometimes referred to as electron "shells." Electrons that occupy energy levels that are closest to the nucleus have the least energy. Electrons found farther from the nucleus have more energy. A limited number of electrons can occupy each energy level. The first energy level can fit up to 2 electrons. The second energy level can fit up to 8 electrons. The third energy level can fit up to 18 electrons. An atom in its normal state will have electrons lying in the lowest possible energy levels.

While the Bohr model provides a good way to visualize the atom, its representation of the electron cloud is not completely accurate. Electrons move around the nucleus in different energy levels, but this movement is not restricted to specific circular orbits as the Bohr model indicates. The **quantum mechanical model** (also known as the electron cloud model) describes the probable locations of electrons because their exact pathways, locations, and speeds cannot be determined simultaneously.

## Example

**Which subatomic particles affect the overall charge of the atom?**

A.  Only protons

B.  Protons and neutrons

C.  Protons and electrons

D.  Protons, neutrons, and electrons

The correct answer is **C**. Because protons are positively charged and electrons are negatively charged, they affect the overall charge of the atom. Neutrons do not affect the charge because they are uncharged. **See Lesson: Scientific Notation.**

# The Periodic Table of the Elements

The atom is not only the basic building block of matter, but also the smallest unit of an element that can be defined as that element. All known elements are listed in the periodic table.

## Periodic Table of Elements

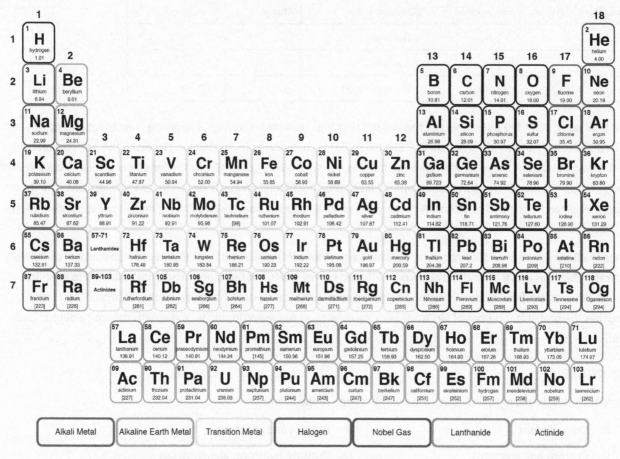

In the periodic table, elements are arranged in rows, also known as **periods**, and columns, also known as **groups**. Both the periods and the groups can be referred to by number. For example, argon is in period 3 and group 18.

Elements with similar properties are put into families that are outlined in different colors in the periodic table above. Note that these families generally correspond to the groups in the periodic table. For example, the elements in group 18 are in a family called the noble gases, while the elements in group 2 are all alkaline earth metals.

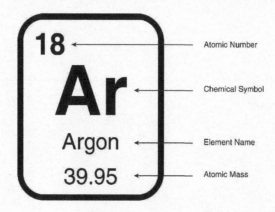

Periodic tables differ in the information they provide, and an example of a block is shown above. This block shows the name of the element and its **chemical symbol**, which is an abbreviation for the name. The chemical symbol is one, two, or three letters with the first letter capitalized and all subsequent letters letter lowercase. The symbol for the element argon is Ar.

Each element is assigned an **atomic number**. The atomic number is equal to the number of protons in a single atom of that element and is how an element is identified. Argon, for example, has an atomic number of 18. Therefore, every atom of argon has 18 protons, regardless of how many neutrons or electrons it has.

## Example

**Which of the following statements is true?**

A.  A tin atom has 22 protons.

B.  An iron atom has 26 protons.

C.  A sodium atom has 16 protons.

D.  A potassium atom has 15 protons.

The correct answer is **B.** In the periodic table, iron has an atomic number of 26, which means it has 26 protons. **See Lesson: Scientific Notation.**

# Average Atomic Mass and Mass Number

Some periodic tables also provide the **average atomic mass** of an element in atomic mass units (amu). Because not all atoms of argon have the same mass, the periodic table shows the average mass of all argon atoms. These forms of argon are differentiated based on their **mass numbers**, which are determined by adding the number of protons and neutrons. Argon has three stable forms, called isotopes, which are shown in the table below.

| Name | Abundance | Mass (amu) | Mass Number | Number of protons | Number of neutrons |
|------|-----------|------------|-------------|-------------------|--------------------|
| Argon-36 | 0.337% | 35.97 | 36 | 18 | 18 |
| Argon-38 | 0.063% | 37.96 | 38 | 18 | 20 |
| Argon-40 | 99.6% | 39.96 | 40 | 18 | 22 |

The mass number can be used to determine the number of neutrons, as shown by the equation below. Argon-40 is the most abundant and has a mass number of 40. Its 18 protons contribute 18 to the mass number of the atom. The remaining mass is from the neutrons.

mass number = number of protons + number of neutrons

40 = 18 + number of neutrons

number of neutrons = 40 − 18 = 22 neutrons

To determine the number of electrons, the charge of the atom must be considered. If a charge is not indicated, it can be assumed that the atom in question is neutral. A neutral atom has an equal number of positively charged protons and negatively charged electrons. Therefore, a neutral atom of argon has 18 electrons that balance the charge of its 18 protons, given by the atomic number.

**CHECKLIST**

Here are reminders for how to determine the numbers of subatomic particles using information found in the periodic table:

❑ Number of protons = atomic number
❑ Number of neutrons = mass number – number of protons (atomic number)
❑ Number of electrons = number of protons (atomic number) in a neutral atom

## Example

**Using the periodic table, determine how many protons and electrons a neutral atom of potassium has.**

A.  19 protons, 19 electrons

B.  19 protons, 20 electrons

C.  19 protons, 39 electrons

D.  39 protons, 39 electrons

The correct answer is **A.** The atomic number of potassium is 19, which means it has 19 protons. Because the atom is neutral, the number of electrons must equal the number of protons. **See Lesson: Scientific Notation.**

# Isotopes

All atoms of an element have the same number of protons, but the number of neutrons may be different. Atoms that have the same number of protons but different numbers of neutrons are called **isotopes**. Because they have the same number of protons, they are the same element. However, because they contain different numbers of neutrons, their masses and mass numbers are different. The Bohr models for three isotopes of carbon are shown below.

**Isotopes of Carbon**

| Carbon-12 | Carbon-13 | Carbon-14 |
|---|---|---|
| 6 protons | 6 protons | 6 protons |
| 6 neutrons | 7 neutrons | 8 neutrons |

$$^{12}_{6}\text{C} \qquad ^{13}_{6}\text{C} \qquad ^{14}_{6}\text{C}$$

Different mass numbers

Same atomic number

All three isotopes have 6 protons because they are all different forms of carbon. They all have 6 electrons because these are neutral atoms of carbon, which means that the positive and negative charges balance each other. The different numbers of neutrons and the different masses differentiate these isotopes.

The isotopes can be named according to their masses. Carbon-12 has a mass number of 12, with 6 protons and 6 neutrons. Carbon-13 has a mass number of 13, with 6 protons and 7 neutrons. Carbon-14 has a mass number of 14, with 6 protons and 8 neutrons. The figure above shows how isotopes can be represented using the element symbols.

Isotopes are present in varying amounts. Carbon-12 makes up 98.93% of all carbon on Earth, and carbon-13 makes up 1.07%. Although carbon-14 exists, its amount is negligible. When calculating the average atomic mass, all isotopes are taken into account. In the periodic table, carbon has an atomic mass of 12.01 amu, which is extremely close to the mass of the most abundant isotope, carbon-12. Though not always true, the average atomic mass of an element is often closest to the mass of the most common isotope.

## Example

**Atom X has 7 protons and 8 neutrons, and Atom Y has 7 protons and 7 neutrons. Which of the following statements describes the relationship between Atom X and Atom Y?**

A. They are different elements because they have different masses.

B. They are different elements because they have different numbers of neutrons.

C. They are isotopes because they have different atomic numbers but the same masses.

D. They are isotopes because they have the same number of protons but different numbers of neutrons.

The correct answer is **D.** Atom X and Y are different isotopes of nitrogen. They both have 7 protons, but the different numbers of neutrons give them different masses. **See Lesson: Scientific Notation.**

## Let's Review!

- Scientific notation is used to make very large numbers and very small numbers easier to use.
- An atom is composed of protons, neutrons, and electrons. Protons and neutrons are found in the nucleus, and electrons are found in the electron cloud that surrounds the nucleus.
- The number of protons in an atom determines its identity (which element it is).
- The mass number of an atom is determined by adding the number of protons and the number of neutrons.
- The charge of an atom is determined by the numbers of protons and electrons.
- Isotopes are atoms of the same element that have different numbers of neutrons and, therefore, different masses.

# TEMPERATURE AND THE METRIC SYSTEM

This lesson introduces the metric system, including how to do metric conversions and use prefixes. It also explores the three different types of temperature systems.

## The English and Metric System

A universal language is used in science and research. This scientific language is called the **metric system**. Also known as the International System of Units (SI), the metric system is easy to use, and its design is simple. Prior to the metric system, several different units were used in scientific measurement, which led to confusion. The metric system was created to standardize units and simplify how they are used. By using a universally accepted measurement standard, scientists around the world can easily communicate with one another.

There are two principles of the metric system to keep in mind:

- Only one unit is assigned to a given quantity that is measured. This unit is called the **SI base unit**. The three most common base units are gram (for mass), meter (for length), and liter (for volume).

- The base unit can be expressed in multiples of 10 to account for measured objects that are very large or very small. This means when performing a metric conversion, the base units can either be multiplied or be divided by 10.

When performing metric conversions, it is important to understand the **metric prefixes**. These are used to distinguish among the base units according to size. The following table provides a list of the most commonly used metric prefixes, including the multiplying factor. Metric prefixes are attached to the beginning of a base unit term. The prefixes can be added to any of the base units.

> **FOR EXAMPLE**
>
> A large container that holds 250,000 grams of sand can be said to hold 250 kilograms of sand.

| Metric Prefix | Symbol | Multiplying Factor | Equivalent Value |
|---|---|---|---|
| tera | T | $10^{12}$ | 1,000,000,000,000 |
| giga | G | $10^{9}$ | 1,000,000,000 |
| mega | M | $10^{6}$ | 1,000,000 |
| kilo | k | $10^{3}$ | 1,000 |
| hecto | h | $10^{2}$ | 100 |
| deca | da | $10^{1}$ | 10 |
| deci | d | $10^{-1}$ | 0.1 |
| centi | c | $10^{-2}$ | 0.01 |
| milli | m | $10^{-3}$ | 0.001 |
| micro | $\mu$ | $10^{-6}$ | 0.000001 |
| nano | n | $10^{-9}$ | 0.000000001 |
| pico | p | $10^{-12}$ | 0.000000000001 |
| femto | f | $10^{-15}$ | 0.000000000000001 |

The **English system** is another recognized system of measurement. It is not universally accepted, and it consists of several units of measurements that are not functionally related to one another. This means the multiple of 10 cannot be used to convert one English unit to another. The following list provides the equivalent values of commonly used English measurements for length, weight, and volume. These values can be used when performing conversions from one English unit to another.

*Length*

- 12 inches = 1 foot (ft)
- 3 feet = 1 yard (yd)
- 5,280 feet = 1 mile (mi)

*Weight*

- 16 ounces (oz) = 1 pound (lb)
- 1 ton = 2,000 pounds

*Volume*

- 8 ounces = 1 cup (c)
- 2 cups = 1 pint (pt)
- 2 pints = 1 quart (qt)
- 4 quarts = 1 gallon (gal)

**DID YOU KNOW?**

The English system was created because people needed a way to describe measurements. Many of the measurements were based on the size of body parts and familiar objects. Eventually, this system was standardized into the system used today.

## Example

**Thalia wants to measure the distance a solar-powered toy car travels over time. What SI base unit should she use?**

A. Feet          B. Inches          C. Liter          D. Meter

The correct answer is **D.** Meter is an SI base unit that is used to measure length or distance. When recording the distance the car travels, Thalia would use meters as the unit. **See Lesson: Temperature and the Metric System.**

# Metric Conversions

Recall that the metric system involves the use of prefixes and base units. The prefixes help a person identify how big or small the measured object is. What happens if one base unit needs to be converted to a different base unit? This is where the concept of using multiples of 10 is important.

When making metric conversions, it is helpful to create a metric staircase, as shown below.

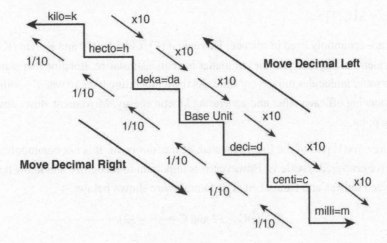

Look at each step on the staircase. It represents a ten-fold change in the metric system. In other words, each step indicates that the decimal place of the measured unit value moves to the left or to the right. Moving to the right (or down the staircase) requires multiplication, which involves using multiples of 10 to convert the larger unit to a smaller unit. When moving to the left (or up the staircase), a smaller unit is converted to a larger unit by dividing using a multiple of 10.

Sometimes, it is necessary to do conversions between the metric and English systems. The following list provides commonly used English measurements and their respective (approximate) metric equivalent values.

*Length*

- 1 inch = 2.54 centimeters
- 1 yard = 0.91 meters

*Weight*

- 1 ounce = 28.3 grams
- 2.20 pounds = 1 kilogram

*Volume*

- 1.06 quart = 1 liter
- 3.79 liters = 1 gallon

**KEEP IN MIND**

It is helpful to use the following mnemonic to remember the order of the metric prefixes to ensure proper movement of the decimal between units from largest to smallest.

*King Henry Doesn't [Usually] Drink Chocolate Milk*

Where *king* means "kilo," *Henry* means "hecto," *doesn't* means "deca," *usually* represents the base unit, *drink* means "deci," *chocolate* means "centi," and *milk* means "milli."

**FOR EXAMPLE**

*How many grams are in 2.52 kilograms?*

The metric staircase indicates that kilogram is a larger unit than gram. Going down the staircase means the decimal must move to the right to give a value of 2,520 grams. If 2.52 is multiplied by the multiplying factor of $10^3$, this will give the same value.

## Example

**A patient needs a dose of 0.3 g of medicine. How much medicine is this in milligrams?**

A. 3          B. 30          C. 300          D. 3,000

The correct answer is **C**. Gram is a larger unit than milligram. Thus, this value must be divided by a factor of 0.001 to get 300 milligrams. If using the metric staircase, the decimal in 0.3 g would move three units to the right to give 300 milligrams. **See Lesson: Temperature and the Metric System.**

# Temperature Systems

Three temperature scales are commonly used in science: Fahrenheit (F), Celsius (C), and Kelvin (K). **Temperature** measures the amount of kinetic energy that particles of matter have in a substance. Imagine that someone wants to boil a pot of water. Initially, the water molecules move very little. As the temperature rises to water's boiling point, these molecules move faster, bouncing off each other and generating kinetic energy. Movement slows down as the temperature lowers to water's freezing point.

The Fahrenheit temperature scale is part of the English system of measurement. It is not commonly used for scientific purposes like the Celsius (or centigrade) scale is. However, it is important to recognize and know how to use the conversion formulas between Celsius and Fahrenheit. The formulas are shown below:

$$F = (\frac{9}{5})C + 32 \text{ and } C = \frac{5}{9}(F - 32).$$

The Fahrenheit scale is based on 32°F for the freezing point of water and 212°F for the boiling point of water. This corresponds to 0°C and 100°C, respectively, on the Celsius scale. The Celsius scale is part of the metric system, which means it is universally accepted when reporting temperature measurements. A thermometer is used to measure temperature. The following thermometers show common temperature values.

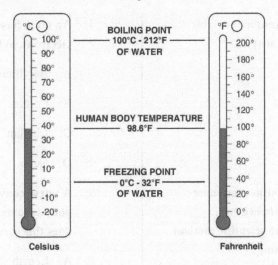

Kelvin is another temperature scale that is used. Its degrees are similar in size to degrees Celsius, but its zero is set to an absolute zero, or 0 K. This is the point where all molecular motion ends. On the Kelvin scale, the freezing point of water is 273.15 K. The boiling point is 373.15 K. The following equation is used to convert a Celsius reading to Kelvin: K = °C + 273

**BE CAREFUL!**

A degree sign is not used in the temperature designation for Kelvin. This symbol is only used with Fahrenheit and Celsius measurements.

## Example

**On which molecule's boiling and freezing points are the Celsius and Fahrenheit scales based?**

A. Alcohol      B. Chloride      C. Glucose      D. Water

The correct answer is **D.** Both the Fahrenheit and Celsius scales are based on the boiling and freezing point of water. The boiling point of water is 212°F (100°C), and the freezing point is 32°F (0°C). **See Lesson: Temperature and the Metric System.**

## Let's Review!

- The metric system is a universally accepted standard method that is used to determine the units of a given measurement.
- The English system is not universally accepted but provides a collection of measurements whose units are functionally unrelated.
- Meter (length), gram (weight), and liter (volume) are the most common types of SI base units.
- Metric prefixes are added to base units to describe the measurement of an object according to size.
- The metric staircase can be used for metric-metric conversions, and specific equivalent values are used for English-metric conversions.
- Three temperature scales, Celsius, Fahrenheit, and Kelvin, are used in science.
- Formulas are used to convert Celsius values to Fahrenheit or to Kelvin.

# CHAPTER 9 SCIENTIFIC REASONING PRACTICE QUIZ

1. As a variable increases, another variable increases. This describes a(n)

   A. positive variation.

   B. negative variation.

   C. inverse correlation.

   D. indirect correlation.

2. When a researcher determines the cause-and-effect relationship between two variables, what part of the scientific method is the researcher performing?

   A. Analysis

   B. Conclusion

   C. Experiment

   D. Hypothesis

3. An atom has 17 protons, 20 neutrons, and 17 electrons. What is its mass, in amu?

   A. 17

   B. 20

   C. 37

   D. 54

4. An atom has 3 protons, 4 neutrons, and 3 electrons. Which element is it?

   A. Beryllium

   B. Carbon

   C. Lithium

   D. Neon

5. A nurse converts a recorded value of 180 pounds to ounces. What unit of measurement does this correspond to?

   A. Length

   B. Temperature

   C. Weight

   D. Volume

6. An equivalency factor of 0.001 corresponds to which of the following metric prefixes?

   A. Deca-

   B. Hecto-

   C. Milli-

   D. Pico-

# CHAPTER 9 SCIENTIFIC REASONING
# PRACTICE QUIZ – ANSWER KEY

**1. A.** When a variable increases as another variable increases, this relationship is described as a positive correlation, direct correlation, or positive variation. **See Lesson: Designing an Experiment.**

**2. A.** During experimental analysis, results from data collection are analyzed for cause-and-effect relationships. **See Lesson: Designing an Experiment.**

**3. C.** The mass is determined by adding the numbers of protons and neutrons (17 + 20 = 37). **See Lesson: Scientific Notation.**

**4. C.** The atomic number of an element is determined by its number of protons. Lithium has an atomic number of 3, which means that if an atom has 3 protons, it is an atom of lithium. **See Lesson: Scientific Notation.**

**5. C.** Ounces and pounds are units in the English system that are used to describe weight measurements. **See Lesson: Temperature and the Metric System.**

**6. C.** The equivalency factor of 0.001 corresponds to the *milli-* prefix. When looking at the metric staircase, this unit is smaller than the base unit. **See Lesson: Temperature and the Metric System**

# CHAPTER 10 CHEMISTRY

## STATES OF MATTER

This lesson explains the differences between solids, liquids, gases, and plasmas. It also describes how a sample can change from one state of matter to another.

## States of Matter

On Earth, substances are found in four states of matter: solid, liquid, gas, and plasma. Many properties of these states of matter are familiar. For example, solids are rigid and hard, liquids can flow inside their containers, and gases can spread throughout an entire room. But what happens at the molecular level may not be as familiar. The differences among them can be explained by the amount of energy that the particles have and the strength of the cohesive forces that hold the particles together. **Cohesion** is the tendency of particles of the same kind to stick to each other and is an important property to consider when looking at states of matter. The motion and density of particles in a substance and the tendency of a substance to take the shape and volume of its container differentiate states of matter.

**Solids** have the lowest energy. The particles are packed close together, and their structure is relatively rigid. Strong cohesive forces prevent particles from moving very far or very fast. Therefore, both the shape and volume of a solid are fixed.

**DID YOU KNOW?**
While particles are generally more tightly packed in solids than in other states, water is an exception. When liquid water freezes, it expands. The molecules are pushed apart as strong intermolecular forces, known as hydrogen bonds, allow the particles to form crystals. This property of water is important in many processes on Earth.

In **liquids**, particles have more energy than in solids and can overcome the cohesive forces to some degree. Since particles can move more freely, they flow and take the shape of their container. However, cohesive forces are strong enough to somewhat restrict the movement of particles. While the shape of the liquid is not fixed, the volume is.

**Gases** have more energy than solids or liquids. In a gas, the cohesive forces are very weak because the particles move very quickly. Gas particles move more freely than liquids, which means that gas particles can not only take the shape of the container, but also spread to occupy the entire volume of the container.

**CONNECTIONS**
Gases and liquids are considered fluids because of their ability to "flow" and take the shape of their containers.

In **plasma**, the particles have so much energy that the electrons separate from their nuclei. The result is a substance composed of moving positively and negatively charged particles. Although plasmas are less common in everyday life than the other states of matter, there are a few familiar examples. First, the hottest parts of the sun are made of plasma because of the high temperature (up to 15,000,000 K). Also, neon signs glow when plasma is produced by passing an electric current through a gas.

## Example

**In which state of matter are particles moving slowest?**

A. Solid          B. Liquid          C. Gas          D. Plasma

The correct answer is **A.** Because solid particles have less energy than particles in other states of matter, they have the most restricted movement. **See Lesson: States of Matter.**

# Phase Changes

Whenever a substance transforms from one state of matter to another, it undergoes a phase change. These processes are physical changes because the chemical composition of the substance remains the same; only its appearance is different. The six most common phase changes are summarized in the diagram and chart below. Note that the states of matter are arranged in order of increasing energy from left to right.

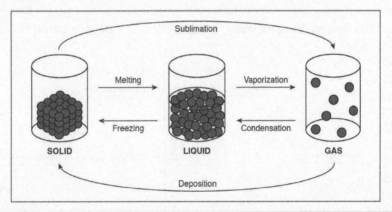

| Phase Change | Name | Absorb or Release Energy |
|---|---|---|
| solid to liquid | melting | absorb |
| liquid to gas | vaporization | absorb |
| solid to gas | sublimation | absorb |
| liquid to solid | freezing | release |
| gas to liquid | condensation | release |
| gas to solid | deposition | release |

All phase changes require the system to either absorb or release energy. Any phase change that moves to the right in the diagram above requires energy to be added to the system because the substance has more energy at the end of the phase change. The phase changes are **melting**, **vaporization (boiling)**, and **sublimation**. When energy is added, particles move faster and can break away from each other more easily as they move to a state of matter with a higher amount of energy. This is most commonly done by heating the substance.

Any phase change that moves to the left in the diagram requires energy to be removed from the system because the substance has less energy at the end of the phase change. These phase changes are **freezing**, **condensation**, and **deposition**.

195

When the particles release energy, they move more slowly. The cohesive forces bring these particles closer together as they move to a state of matter with a lower amount of energy. This is most commonly done by cooling the substance.

The temperatures at which phase changes occur depends the strength of the cohesive forces between particles. For substances like metals that have high melting and boiling points, it takes a relatively large amount of energy to overcome the intermolecular forces enough to change states of matter. Similarly, substances with low melting and boiling points, like the gases that make up Earth's atmosphere, do not require as much energy to overcome their intermolecular forces.

## Example

**Which of the following phase changes requires a substance to release energy?**

A. Boiling             B. Condensation

C. Melting            D. Sublimation

The correct answer is **B.** During condensation, a gas turns to a liquid. For this to occur, high-energy particles in the gas must release some energy for the cohesive forces to bring the particles closer together. **See Lesson: States of Matter.**

# Heating and Cooling Curves

When studying phase changes, one can examine the heating or cooling curve of a substance. Heating and cooling curves are plots of temperature versus time that occur as energy is added to or removed from the system at a constant rate.

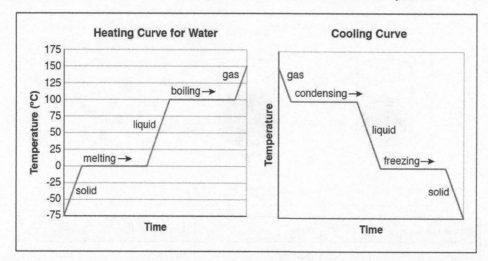

The heating curve for water is shown above. Notice that at the beginning of the experiment, the substance is a solid. As heat is added, the temperature of the solid increases until it reaches its melting point, 0°C. The temperature remains constant at the melting point until the entire sample has changed to a liquid. Note that even though heat is still being added, the temperature is not increasing. This is because the added energy is used to disrupt the cohesive forces in the solid, allowing the particles to move more freely as the substance changes to a liquid.

Once the sample is completely melted, the temperature increases again. It increases until the boiling point, 100°C, is reached. Heat is still being added, but the temperature remains constant as the substance boils. This time, the added energy is being used to break the intermolecular bonds in the liquid as the particles transform into a gas and move farther away from each other. It is not until the phase change is complete and the sample is entirely gas that the temperature starts increasing again.

**KEEP IN MIND**

The temperature of a substance is a measure of the kinetic energy of the particles that make up a substance. In other words, temperature is related to how fast the particles are moving.

A cooling curve has the opposite shape of a heating curve, as seen in the graph above. In these experiments, the sample starts as a high-temperature gas. As heat is removed, the temperature of the gas decreases to its boiling point. At this point, the temperature remains constant until the entire sample is liquid. The liquid then cools to a lower temperature until it reaches the freezing point. The temperature remains constant as the substance freezes, and once it is completely solid, the temperature decreases again.

**KEY POINT!**

As a substance undergoes a phase change, its temperature remains constant. The only time a substance experiences an increase or decrease in temperature is when it is entirely in one state of matter.

## Example

**If a sample of water is losing energy but its temperature is not changing, what may be happening?**

A. Freezing          B. Melting          C. Sublimation          D. Vaporization

The correct answer is **A.** When a substance is freezing, the liquid particles lose enough energy to become a solid. The temperature will not change until the phase change is complete. **See Lesson: States of Matter.**

## Let's Review!

- Solids, liquids, gases, and plasmas differ from one another in the amount of energy that the particles have and the strength of the cohesive forces that hold the particles together.

- A substance can undergo a phase change if it either absorbs or releases enough energy.

- Heating and cooling curves show the temperature of a substance as heat is consistently added or removed.

- As a substance changes states, its temperature remains constant. Any energy that is absorbed or released is used to change the way in which the particles interact with one another.

# PROPERTIES OF MATTER

This lesson introduces the properties of matter, which are fundamental to the understanding of chemistry.

## Matter and its Properties

Aluminum, clothing, water, air, and glass are all different kinds of matter. **Matter** is anything that takes up space and has mass. A golf ball contains more matter than a table-tennis ball. The golf ball has more mass. The amount of matter that an object contains is its **mass**.

Table sugar is 100 percent sugar. Table sugar (sucrose) is an example of a substance. A **substance** is matter that has a uniform and definite composition. Lemonade is not a substance because not all pitchers of lemonade are identical. Different pitchers of lemonade may have different amounts of sugar, lemon juice, or water and may taste different.

All crystals of sucrose taste sweet and dissolve completely in water. All samples of a substance have identical physical properties. A **physical property** is a quality or condition of a substance that can be observed or measured without changing the substance's composition. Some physical properties of matter are color, solubility, mass, odor, hardness, density, and boiling point.

Just as every substance has physical properties, every substance has chemical properties. For example, when iron is exposed to water and oxygen, it corrodes and produces a new substance called iron (III) oxide (rust). The chemical properties of a substance are its ability to undergo chemical reactions and to form new substances. Rusting is a chemical property of iron. **Chemical properties** are observed only when a substance undergoes a change in composition, which is a chemical change.

### Physical vs. Chemical Properties

| Physical Properties | Chemical Properties |
|---|---|
| ● Color | ● Flammability |
| ● Shape | ● Rusting |
| ● Size | ● Burning |
| ● Density | ● Corrosion |
| ● Amount | ● Reactivity |
| ● Volume | |

### Intensive and Extensive Properties

**Intensive** properties do not depend on the amount of matter that is present. Intensive properties do not change according to the conditions. They are used to identify samples because their characteristics do not depend on the size of the sample. In contrast, **extensive** properties do depend on the amount of a sample that is present. A good example of the difference between the two types of properties is that mass and volume are extensive properties, but their ratio (density) is an intensive property. Notice that mass and volume deal with amounts, whereas density is a physical property.

198

Intensive Properties
versus
Extensive Properties

| Intensive properties are physical properties that do not depend on the amount of matter | Extensive properties are physical properties that depend on the amount of matter |
|---|---|
| Independant of the amount of matter | Depend of the amount of matter |
| Some examples include melting point, boiling point, density, etc. | Some examples include volume, mass, energy, etc. |

## Example

**Which of the following explains the difference between chemical and physical properties?**

A.  Physical properties can easily change, while chemical properties are constant.

B.  Chemical properties always involve a source of heat, and physical properties always involve light.

C.  Chemical properties involve a change in the chemical composition of a substance, while physical properties can easily be observed.

D.  Physical properties involve a change in the chemical composition of a substance, while chemical properties can easily be observed.

The correct answer is **C.** A physical property is a quality or condition of a substance that can be observed or measured without changing the substance's composition, while a chemical property is one where a change in chemical composition has occurred. **See Lesson: Properties of Matter.**

# Phase Changes

There are six phase changes: condensation, evaporation, freezing, melting, sublimation, and deposition.

**Condensation** is the change of a gas or vapor to a liquid. A change in the pressure and the temperature of a substance causes this change. The condensation point is the same as the boiling point of a substance. It is most noticeable when there is a large temperature difference between an object and the atmosphere. Condensation is also the opposite of evaporation.

**Evaporation** is the change of a liquid to a gas on the surface of a substance. This is not to be confused with boiling, which is a phase transition of an entire substance from a liquid to a gas. The evaporation point is the same as the freezing point of a substance. As the temperature increases, the rate of evaporation also increases. Evaporation depends not only on the temperature, but also on the amount of substance available.

**Freezing** is the change of a liquid to a solid. It occurs when the temperature drops below the freezing point. The amount of heat that has been removed from the substance allows the particles of the substance to draw closer together, and the material changes from a liquid to a solid. It is the opposite of melting.

**Melting** is the change of a solid into a liquid. For melting to occur, enough heat must be added to the substance. When this is done, the molecules move around more, and the particles are unable to hold together as tightly as they can in a solid. They break apart, and the solid becomes a liquid.

**Sublimation** is a solid changing into a gas. As a material sublimates, it does not pass through the liquid state. An example of sublimation is carbon dioxide, a gas, changing into dry ice, a solid. It is the reverse of deposition.

**Deposition** is a gas changing into a solid without going through the liquid phase. It is an uncommon phase change. An example is when it is extremely cold outside and the cold air comes in contact with a window. Ice will form on the window without going through the liquid state.

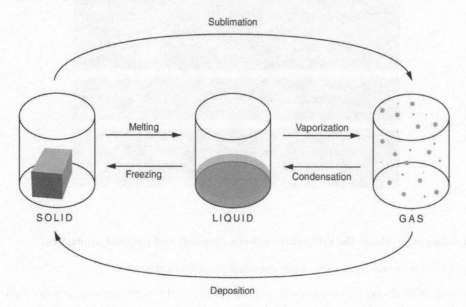

## Example

**Which of the six types of phase changes is the opposite of sublimation?**

A.  Condensation

B.  Deposition

C.  Evaporation

D.  Freezing

The correct answer is **B**. Sublimation is the changing of a solid to a gas, and deposition is the changing of a gas to a solid. **See Lesson: Properties of Matter.**

# Adhesiveness and Cohesiveness

Because of polarity, water is attracted to water, a property called **cohesion**. The typical water molecule has a polar configuration, as seen below.

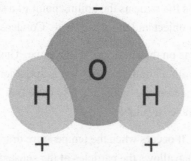

Notice that there is a negative end and a positive end. This means it is a polar molecule. In a **polar molecule**, one end of the molecule is slightly negative and one end is slightly positive.

Inside a plant, water has to travel up, against gravity, to reach all the leaves. Because the water molecules are attracted to each other, or demonstrate **cohesion**, they also adhere to the sides of the xylem vessels that transport water up to where it is needed in the plant. This is possible because of **adhesion**. Adhesion is water's ability to be attracted to other substances.

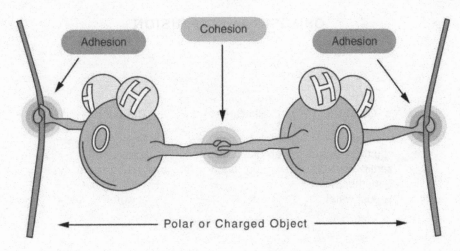

Polar or Charged Object

## Example

**What property allows water to flow against the force of gravity?**

A. Adhesion          B. Cohesion          C. Polarity          D. Xylem

The correct answer is **A.** Adhesion is water's ability to be attracted to other substances. Because of adhesion, water is able to move upward. **See Lesson: Properties of Matter.**

# Diffusion and Osmosis

When a bottle of perfume is opened, perfume molecules diffuse throughout a room. **Diffusion** is the tendency of molecules and ions to move toward areas of lower concentrations until the concentration is uniform throughout the room (that is, it reaches equilibrium). This random movement of individual particles has an important consequence. Because the movement is random, a particle is more likely to move from an area where there are a lot of molecules (area of high concentration) to an area where there are fewer molecules (an area of lower concentration). In the human lungs, oxygen diffuses into the bloodstream because there is a higher concentration of oxygen molecules in the lungs' air sacs than there is in the blood.

Solute and solvent particles tend to diffuse from areas where their concentration is high to areas where their concentration is lower. Imagine that a membrane separates two regions of liquid. As long as solute particles and solvent (water) molecules can pass freely through the membrane, diffusion will equalize the amount of solute and solvent on the two sides. The sides will reach equilibrium.

But what if a polar solute that cannot pass through the membrane is added to one side? This situation is common in cells. An amino acid cannot cross a lipid bilayer, and neither can an ion or a sugar molecule. Unable to cross the membrane, the polar solute particles form hydrogen bonds with the water molecules surrounding them. These "bound" water molecules are no longer free to diffuse through the membrane. The polar solute has reduced the number of free water molecules on that side of the membrane. This means the opposite side of the membrane (without solute) has more free water molecules than the side with the polar solute. As a result, water molecules move by diffusion from the side without the polar solute to the side with the polar solute.

Eventually, the concentration of free water molecules will equalize on the sides of the membrane. At this point, however, there are more water molecules (bound and unbound) on the side of the membrane with the polar solute. Net water movement through a membrane in response to the concentration of a solute is called **osmosis**. Stated another way, osmosis is the diffusion of water molecules through a membrane in the direction of higher solute concentration.

## OSMOSIS and DIFFUSION

**Osmosis**

Molecules
go through a
semipermeable
membrane.
Just water

Similarities

Molecules move
around to create
equilibrium

**Diffusion**

Molecules
spread out
over a large area.
Everything but
water

## Example

**What is the goal of osmosis?**

A. The water will equalize on both side of the semipermeable membrane.

B. The concentration of solutes will diffuse through the semipermeable membrane.

C. The concentration of free water molecules will equalize on both sides of the membrane

D. The solute particles will flow from an area of high concentration to an area of lower concentration.

The correct answer is **C**. As a result of osmosis, the concentration of free water molecules will equalize on both sides of the membrane. **See Lesson: Properties of Matter.**

## Let's Review!

- Matter is anything that takes up space and has mass.
- The difference between physical and chemical properties is that chemical properties involve a change in a substance's chemical composition and physical properties do not.
- The difference between extensive and intensive properties is based on whether the properties depend on the amount of substance that is present.
- Cohesiveness is the attraction of water to itself, and adhesiveness is the attraction of water to other substances.
- Osmosis is the diffusion of water and the movement of molecules from an area of high concentration to an area of lower concentration.

# CHEMICAL BONDS

This lesson introduces bonding and explains the three ways in which atoms can become stable. The rest of the lesson examines different types of bonds in more detail.

## Introduction to Bonding

Chemical elements found in the periodic table have different levels of reactivity. The number of **valence electrons** in an atom is the most important factor in determining how an element will react. Valence electrons, which are found in an atom's outermost energy level, are involved in forming chemical bonds. The periodic table below shows the Bohr models of select elements. The valence electrons appear in red.

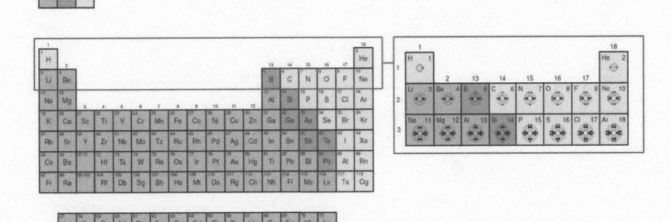

The **octet rule** states that atoms will lose, gain, or share electrons to obtain a stable electron configuration of eight valence electrons. In other words, if an atom needs to become stable, it will react with another atom, which can result in the formation of a chemical compound. Note that the elements in group 18, the noble gases, have eight valence electrons. Helium is an exception and is stable with two valence electrons. Because they have a stable electron configuration, the noble gases do not need to react with other elements to become stable. As a result, they are found in nature as single elements rather than in compounds.

> ### KEY POINT!
> The goal of forming chemical bonds is to become stable by having eight electrons in the outer shell. This is easy to remember because it is described in the *octet* rule. The prefix *octa-* means "eight," and it can be seen in other words, such as *octopus* and *octagon*.

Elements in other groups will react to become stable in predictable ways, depending on how many valence electrons they have. In the periodic table above, elements are classified as metals, nonmetals, or metalloids. Compared to other elements, metals have fewer valence electrons and tend to lose them to become stable. Notice that removing the red valence electrons from the outermost energy level exposes another energy level. This becomes the valence shell, and the atom is stable because it has eight valence electrons.

Nonmetals and metalloids have a relatively high number of valence electrons. Except for the noble gasses, these elements tend to gain or share electrons to become stable.

**Ionic compounds** are formed when electrons are transferred from a metal (which loses one or more electrons) to a nonmetal (which gains one or more electrons). **Covalent compounds** are formed when two nonmetals or metalloids share electrons.

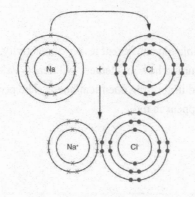

Ionic Bond

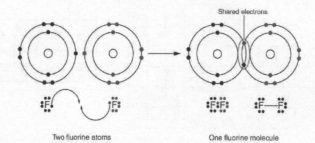

Shared electrons

Two fluorine atoms                One fluorine molecule

Covalent Bond

**TEST TIP**

A quick way to determine if atoms are held together by ionic or covalent bonds is to examine the types of elements involved. If a metal and a nonmetal bond, an ionic bond forms. If two nonmetals or metalloids bond, a covalent bond forms.

## Example

**In the compound sodium bromide (NaBr), electrons are _____. In the compound carbon tetrabromide (CBr₄), electrons are _____.**

A.  shared, shared          B.  shared, transferred

C.  transferred, shared         D.  transferred, transferred

The correct answer is **C**. Electrons are transferred when an ionic compound like sodium bromide forms. Electrons are shared when a covalent compound like carbon tetrabromide forms. **See Lesson: Chemical Bonds.**

# Ion Formation

If an atom has an equal number of positively charged protons and negatively charged electrons, it is neutral and has no **net charge**. When electrons are transferred, atoms end up with either more protons than electrons or more electrons than protons. The atoms are considered **ions** because they have a net positive or negative charge.

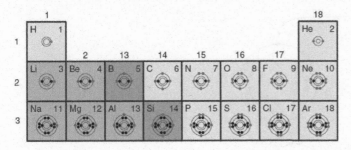

When a metal such as sodium reacts to become stable, it loses its valence electrons. At first, it is a neutral atom with 11 protons and 11 electrons. When it loses an electron, the number of protons does not change, and the atom has 11 protons and 10 electrons. Because there is one more positively charged proton, a **cation** forms. A cation is an ion with a net positive charge.

When a nonmetal such as chlorine reacts to become stable, it gains a valence electron. At first, it is a neutral atom with 17 protons and 17 electrons. When it gains an electron, the number of protons does not change, and the atom has 17 protons and 18 electrons. Because there is one more negatively charged electron, an **anion** forms. An anion is an ion with a net negative charge.

**BE CAREFUL!**

When an atom *gains* electrons, it has a net *negative* charge because it gains negatively charged particles. When an atom *loses* electrons, it has a net *positive* charge. After the loss, there are more protons than electrons, which means there are more positively charged particles.

The way in which an element reacts can be predicted based on that element's position in the periodic table. The table below summarizes the reactivity of elements according to their group number. Elements in each group have a specific number of valence electrons, which dictates what the atoms need to do to obtain a valence shell with eight electrons. Some will lose electrons, and others will gain electrons. This, along with the number of electrons that must be transferred, determines the charge of the stable ion that forms.

| Group | 1 | 2 | 13 | 14 | 15 | 16 | 17 | 18 |
|---|---|---|---|---|---|---|---|---|
| Valence $e^-$ | 1 | 2 | 3 | 4 | 5 | 6 | 7 | 8 |
| Lose/Gain $e^-$ | Lose 1 | Lose 2 | Lose 3 | Lose/Gain 4 | Gain 3 | Gain 2 | Gain 1 | N/A |
| Charge | +1 | +2 | +3 | +/-4 | -3 | -2 | -1 | N/A |

## Example

**What will strontium do to form a stable ion with a +2 charge?**

A. Gain two protons
B. Lose two protons
C. Gain two electrons
D. Lose two electrons

The correct answer is **D**. Atoms gain or lose electrons, not protons, to form ions. Like other metals in group 2, strontium will lose its two valence electrons to become stable. **See Lesson: Chemical Bonds.**

# Ionic Bonding

An ionic compound is composed of a cation and an anion. An ionic bond is formed from the cation's attraction to the oppositely charged anion. The figure below shows how transferring an electron from sodium to chlorine results in the formation of an ionic bond.

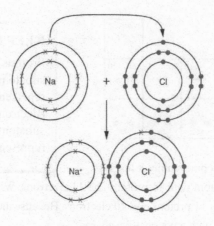

Ionic Bond

Notice that the charges on sodium ($Na^+$) and chlorine ($Cl^-$) ions have the same magnitude (they both have a value of 1). Therefore, the charge of one sodium ion balances the charge of one chlorine ion. When an ionic compound is formed from ions that have equal but opposite charges, the elements will be present in a 1:1 ratio. Examples are shown in the table below.

| Compound Name | Cation | Anion | Compound Formula |
|---|---|---|---|
| Potassium fluoride | $K^+$ | $F^-$ | KF |
| Magnesium oxide | $Mg^{2+}$ | $O^{2-}$ | MgO |
| Aluminum nitride | $Al^{3+}$ | $N^{3-}$ | AlN |

In some cases, atoms need to lose or gain two, three, or, in rare cases, four electrons to become stable. For example, magnesium must give up two electrons to become stable. Because chlorine only needs one electron, magnesium can give an electron to two different chlorine atoms. Then, one magnesium cation with a +2 charge ($Mg^{2+}$) bonds with two chloride anions ($Cl^-$) to form magnesium chloride, ($MgCl_2$). The subscript 2 indicates that there are two chloride ions in this compound.

| Compound Name | Cation | Anion | Compound Formula |
|---|---|---|---|
| Calcium bromide | $Ca^{2+}$ | $Br^-$ | $CaBr_2$ |
| Aluminum fluoride | $Al^{3+}$ | $F^-$ | $AlF_3$ |
| Rubidium oxide | $Rb^+$ | $O^{2-}$ | $Rb_2O$ |
| Sodium phosphide | $Na^+$ | $P^{3-}$ | $Na_3P$ |
| Aluminum oxide | $Al^{3+}$ | $O^{2-}$ | $Al_2O_3$ |
| Calcium phosphide | $Ca^{2+}$ | $P^{3-}$ | $Ca_3P_2$ |

Similarly, when oxygen and lithium react, the oxygen atom receives an electron from each of two lithium atoms. This transfer results in two lithium cations ($Li^+$) and an oxygen anion ($O^{2-}$). They attract each other to form the compound lithium oxide with a formula of $Li_2O$. Other examples are shown in the table below. Notice that in all ionic compounds, the total positive charge balances out the total negative charge, resulting in a neutral compound.

---

**KEY POINT!**

Regardless of how many electrons are transferred, ionic compounds have net charges of zero. They are all neutral because the positive cations attract as many anions as they need to balance their charges, and vice versa.

---

## Example

**What is the formula for the compound formed between calcium and oxygen?**

A.  CaO        B.  $CaO_2$        C.  $Ca_2O$        D.  $Ca_3O_2$

The correct answer is **A.** Calcium is in group 2 and will lose its two valence electrons to become stable. Oxygen is in group 16 and, because it has six valence electrons, will gain two electrons to complete its octet. Therefore, one calcium ion requires one oxide ion to balance its charge to form a neutral ionic compound. **See Lesson: Chemical Bonds.**

## Covalent Bonding

When a nonmetal atom reacts with a nonmetal or metalloid, the atoms share electrons to obtain eight valence electrons each. An example can be seen in the model below. Both the Bohr models and the electron dot structures of the fluorine atoms show their seven valence electrons. After each atom shares an electron with the other, shown by the arrows, a covalent bond forms. In the newly formed fluorine molecule, both fluorine atoms have the stable electron configuration of eight valence electrons. The shared electrons can be represented by two dots or by a line in between the fluorine atoms.

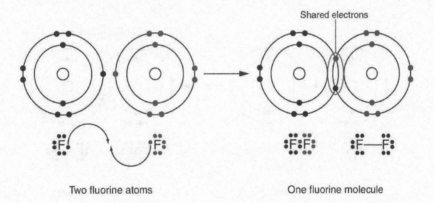

Covalent Bond

Covalent compounds can be modeled in **Lewis structures**. Lewis structures for methane, ammonia, and water are shown below. In a Lewis structure, covalent bonds, also called shared electrons, are represented by lines between two atoms. Valence electrons that are not involved in bonding, also called **lone-pair electrons**, are represented by dots.

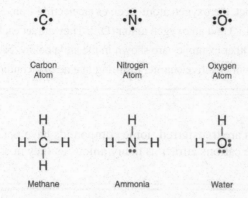

Carbon Atom · Nitrogen Atom · Oxygen Atom

Methane · Ammonia · Water

**KEEP IN MIND**

Each line (bond) in a Lewis structure represents two electrons, one from each atom involved in the bond.

The number of bonds that an atom forms depends on the number of valence electrons that the atom has as a single atom. In a molecule of methane ($CH_4$), one carbon atom bonds to four hydrogen atoms. A single neutral carbon atom has four valence electrons and can share each one with a different hydrogen atom. In the end, it has four covalent bonds. Because each covalent bond involves two electrons, carbon has a total of eight valence electrons and is stable.

Similarly, in a molecule of ammonia ($NH_3$), one nitrogen atom bonds to three hydrogen atoms. Nitrogen shares six electrons total and has two remaining lone-pair electrons that are not involved in bonding for a total of eight. In a water molecule, an oxygen atom bonds to two hydrogen atoms. Oxygen has four shared electrons and four lone-pair electrons for a total of eight.

## Example

**In the Lewis structure of a fluorine molecule shown below, how are the eight valence electrons of each fluorine atom arranged?**

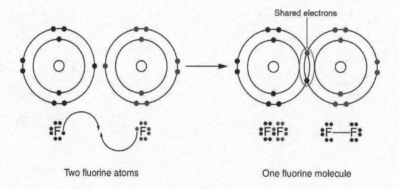

Two fluorine atoms · One fluorine molecule

Covalent Bond

A.  2 are shared, 6 are lone-pair.

B.  4 are shared, 4 are lone-pair.

C.  6 are shared, 2 are lone-pair.

D.  8 are shared, none are lone-pair.

The correct answer is **A.** A fluorine atom forms a single covalent bond with another fluorine atom, which means that two electrons are being shared. The other six valence electrons are lone-pair electrons and are represented by dots around the atom. **See Lesson: Chemical Bonds.**

# Types of Covalent Bonds

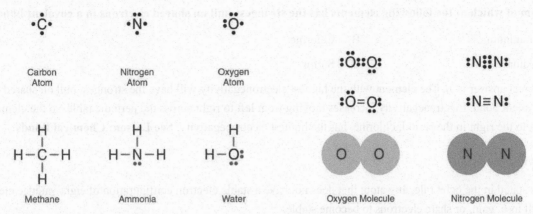

Carbon Atom   Nitrogen Atom   Oxygen Atom

Methane   Ammonia   Water   Oxygen Molecule   Nitrogen Molecule

In methane, ammonia, and water, atoms are joined by **single covalent bonds** in which the atoms share two electrons. However, two atoms may need to share more than one pair of electrons to be stable. For example, two oxygen atoms form a **double bond**, in which two pairs of electrons (four electrons total) are shared. Similarly, two nitrogen atoms form a molecule with a **triple bond**, in which three pairs of electrons (six electrons total) are shared.

As more pairs of electrons are shared, the length of the bond decreases, and the bond strength increases. Single bonds are the longest and weakest bonds. They require the least energy to break because there is not as much energy stored in them.

## CONNECTION

A pair of shared electrons between two atoms can be compared to a rubber band stretching between two objects. Having two or three rubber bands, rather than one, increases the strength of the "bond" that holds them together, making it harder to separate the objects.

Regardless of how many electrons are shared, the strength of a covalent bond comes from the positively charged nuclei of both atoms attracting the negatively charged electrons that are being shared. However, not all atoms attract shared electrons equally. This property is known as **electronegativity**, the tendency of an atom to attract shared electrons in a covalent bond. It is a measure of how hard an atom is pulling on shared electrons. Electronegativity increases going from left to right in the periodic table. Nonmetal atoms pull harder on electrons and do not tend to give them up. Therefore, the halogens in group 17 have the highest electronegativity of all elements.

If the two atoms share electrons equally, the bond is classified as **nonpolar covalent**. This occurs if the two atoms have similar electronegativities, which means that neither atom pulls significantly harder on the shared electrons than the other. If the two atoms share electrons unequally, the bond is **polar covalent**. This occurs if the electronegativity of one atom is significantly higher than the other, causing it to pull significantly harder on the shared electrons.

## CONNECTION

The sharing of electrons is like a game of tug-of-war in which two opposing teams are pulling on a rope in opposite directions. In a nonpolar bond, the opposing teams are pulling with the same force, and the rope is not moving toward one team or the other. In a polar bond, one team is winning by pulling the rope closer to its side.

## Example

**An atom of which of the following elements has the strongest pull on shared electrons in a covalent bond?**

A. Aluminum

B. Chlorine

C. Sodium

D. Sulfur

The correct answer is **B.** The element with the highest electronegativity will have the strongest pull on shared electrons in a covalent bond. Electronegativity increases moving from left to right across the periodic table, so the element farthest to the right in the period, chlorine, has the highest electronegativity. **See Lesson: Chemical Bonds.**

## Let's Review!

- As stated in the octet rule, any atom that does not have a stable electron configuration of eight valence electrons will lose, gain, or share electrons to become stable.

- Exceptions to the octet rule include hydrogen and helium, which are stable when they have two valence electrons.

- Ionic bonds are formed when electrons are transferred from a metal atom to a nonmetal atom.

- Covalent bonds are formed when two atoms share electrons. When two atoms need to share more than one pair of electrons, multiple bonds form. If two pairs are shared, a double bond forms. If three pairs are shared, a triple bond forms.

- The difference in the electronegativities of the two atoms determines if electrons are shared equally, forming a nonpolar covalent bond, or shared unequally, forming a polar covalent bond.

# CHEMICAL SOLUTIONS

This lesson discusses the properties of different types of mixtures, focusing on solutions. Then, it examines aspects of chemical reactions, including the components of the reactions and the types of changes that occur.

## Solutions

When elements and compounds are physically (not chemically) combined, they form a **mixture**. When the substances mix evenly and it is impossible to see the individual components, the mixture is described as **homogeneous**. When the substances mix unevenly and it is possible to see the individual components, the mixture is described as **heterogeneous**.

**Solubility** is the ability of a substance to dissolve in another substance. For example, salt and sugar are both substances that can dissolve in water. They are **soluble**. In contrast, sand does not dissolve in water. It is **insoluble**. Individual particles of sand can be seen in water, but individual particles of salt are completely mixed in.

When one substance dissolves in the other, a type of homogeneous mixture called a **solution** forms. The substance that is being dissolved is the **solute**. The substance in which the solute is dissolved is the **solvent**, which makes up a greater percentage of the mixture than the solute. When salt dissolves in water, salt is the solute, and water is the solvent. Saltwater is an example of an **aqueous solution**, which forms when any substance dissolves in water.

The **concentration** of a solution is the amount of solute in a given volume of solution and can be expressed in several ways:

- **Molarity** (number of moles of a substance in one liter of solution)
- **Molality** (number of moles of a substance per kilogram of solvent)
- **Percent composition by mass** (mass of a solute per unit mass of the solution)
- **Mole fraction** (moles of a solute divided by the total number of moles in the solution)

Solubility can also refer to the *amount* of a substance that can dissolve. Even for soluble substances, there is a limit to how much of it can dissolve. The lines in the graph below show these limits for different substances at different temperatures in 100 grams of water. The area below a line represents masses of solute that dissolve in 100 grams of water. This type of solution is **unsaturated** because more solute can be dissolved. At the line, the solution is **saturated** because the limit has been reached. Any solute added above that mass will remain undissolved.

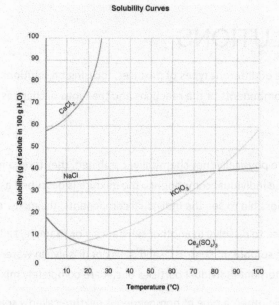

Solubility Curves

## Example

**A beaker contains 50 mL of oil and 50 mL of water. No matter how much the mixture is stirred, the oil and the water still separate into two layers. Which statement accurately describes this mixture?**

A. Oil is insoluble in water.

B. It is an unsaturated solution.

C. It is a homogeneous mixture.

D. Water is a good solvent for oil.

The correct answer is **A.** Because the oil will not mix into the water, it is insoluble. **See Lesson: Chemical Solutions.**

# Chemical Reactions

A chemical reaction involves elements and compounds that combine, break apart, rearrange, or change form in some way. **Reactants** are the substances that are present at the beginning of the reaction and undergo a change. **Products** are the substances that are formed from the reactants. Chemical reactions can be described by chemical equations, an example of which is shown below.

Coefficient

$CH_4(g) + 2O_2(g)$     ⟶     Coefficient   $CO_2(g) + 2H_2O(g)$

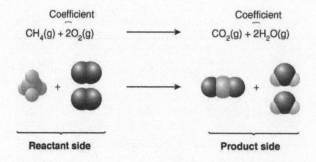

Reactant side      Product side

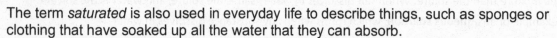

In this reaction, methane ($CH_4$) is burned in the presence of oxygen ($O_2$) to form carbon dioxide ($CO_2$) and water ($H_2O$). In the chemical equation, the formulas of the reactants ($CH_4$ and $O_2$) and products ($CO_2$ and $H_2O$) are used. If there is more than one reactant or more than one product, their formulas are separated by a plus sign (+). The reactants and products are separated by an arrow.

The state of matter may also be shown in the chemical equation in parentheses after the substance formula. Substances can be solid, liquid, or gas, indicated by (s), (l), or (g), respectively. If a substance is dissolved in water, forming an aqueous solution, that state is indicated by (aq) in a chemical equation.

**KEEP IN MIND**

Reactants will always be on the left side of the arrow, and products will always be on the right side.

Finally, coefficients may appear in chemical equations. These coefficients indicate how many particles (atoms or molecules) of each substance react or form. When there is no coefficient present, only one particle is involved. In the example above, one molecule of methane ($CH_4$) reacts with two molecules of oxygen ($O_2$). One molecule of carbon dioxide ($CO_2$) is produced, along with two molecules of water ($H_2O$).

## Example

**The equation describing the formation of ammonia ($NH_3$) from nitrogen and hydrogen is shown below. Which of the following statements is true?**

$$3H_2(g) + N_2(g) \rightarrow 2NH_3(g)$$

A.  $NH_3$ is the reactant, and $H_2$ and $N_2$ are products.

B.  $H_2$ and $N_2$ are the reactants, and $NH_3$ is the product.

C.  N and $H_3$ are the reactants, and $H_2$ and $N_2$ are products.

D.  $H_2$ and $N_2$ are the reactants, and N and $H_3$ are the products.

The correct answer is **B.** Two reactants, $H_2$ and $N_2$, are found on the left side of the arrow. One product, $NH_3$, is found on the right side of the arrow. **See Lesson: Chemical Solutions.**

# Types of Reactions

Chemical reactions can be classified according to the reactants and products involved. This lesson will cover five types of reactions: synthesis, decomposition, single-replacement, double-replacement, and combustion. The first four types are outlined in the table below.

| Type of Reaction | Model | Example |
|---|---|---|
| Synthesis | A + B → AB | $2H_2(g) + O_2(g) \rightarrow 2H_2O(g)$ |
| Decomposition | AB → A + B | $2H_2O_2(aq) \rightarrow 2H_2O(l) + O_2(g)$ |
| Single-Replacement | AB + C → AC + B | $2HCl(aq) + Zn(s) \rightarrow ZnCl_2(aq) + H_2(g)$ |
| Double-Replacement | AB + CD → AD + CB | $AgNO_3(aq) + NaCl(aq) \rightarrow AgCl(s) + NaNO_3(aq)$ |

**Synthesis** reactions involve two or more reactants (A and B) combining to form one product (AB). In the example provided, hydrogen ($H_2$) and oxygen ($O_2$) begin as separate elements. At the end of the reaction, the hydrogen and oxygen atoms are bonded in a molecule of water ($H_2O$).

**Decomposition** reactions have only one reactant (AB) that breaks apart into two or more products (A and B). In the example above, hydrogen peroxide ($H_2O_2$) breaks apart into two smaller molecules: water ($H_2O$) and oxygen ($O_2$).

**Single-replacement** reactions involve two reactants, one compound (AB) and one element (C). In this type of reaction, one element replaces another to form a new compound (AC), leaving one element by itself (B). In the example, zinc replaces hydrogen in hydrochloric acid (HCl). As a result, zinc forms a compound with chlorine, zinc chloride ($ZnCl_2$), and hydrogen ($H_2$) is left by itself.

**Double-replacement** reactions involve two reactants, both of which are compounds made of two components (AB and CD). In the example, silver nitrate, composed of silver ($Ag^{1+}$) and nitrate ($NO_3^{1-}$) ions, reacts with sodium chloride, composed of sodium ($Na^{1+}$) and chloride ($Cl^{1-}$) ions. The nitrate and chloride ions switch places to produce two compounds that are different from those in the reactants.

**Combustion** reactions occur when fuels burn, and they involve specific reactants and products, as seen in the examples below. Some form of fuel that contains carbon and hydrogen is required. Examples of such fuels are methane, propane in a gas grill, butane in a lighter, and octane in gasoline. Notice that these fuels all react with oxygen, which is necessary for anything to burn. In all combustion reactions, carbon dioxide, water, and energy are produced. When something burns, energy is released, which can be felt as heat and seen as light.

| Fuel | Reaction |
|---|---|
| Methane ($CH_4$) | $CH_4 + 2O_2 \rightarrow CO_2 + 2H_2O + energy$ |
| Propane ($C_3H_8$) | $C_3H_8 + 5O_2 \rightarrow 3CO_2 + 4H_2O + energy$ |
| Butane ($C_4H_{10}$) | $2C_4H_{10} + 13O_2 \rightarrow 8CO_2 + 10H_2O + energy$ |
| Octane ($C_8H_{18}$) | $2C_8H_{18} + 25O_2 \rightarrow 16CO_2 + 18H_2O + energy$ |

## Example

**Which of the following equations shows a decomposition reaction?**

A.   $3H_2 + N_2 \rightarrow 2NH_3$

B.   $2KClO_3 \rightarrow 2KCl + 3O_2$

C.   $2C_2H_2 + 5O_2 \rightarrow 4CO_2 + 2H_2O$

D.   $2Na + ZnCl_2 \rightarrow Zn + 2NaCl$

The correct answer is **B.** This reaction starts with a single compound as a reactant that breaks down into two smaller products. **See Lesson: Chemical Solutions.**

# Energy Diagrams

Energy diagrams can be used to show how the energy of the species in a reaction changes over time. The reactants have a certain amount of energy stored in their bonds, and the products usually have a different amount of energy. If energy is released, the products have less energy than the reactants, and the reaction is **exothermic**. If energy is absorbed, the products have more energy than the reactants, and the reaction is **endothermic**. The shapes of the energy diagrams are shown below.

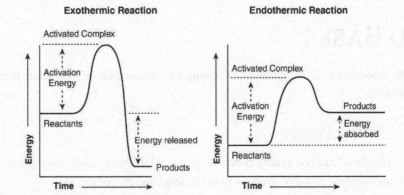

In every reaction, an **activated complex** must form between reactants. This complex can also be referred to as a transition state because it is required to convert, or provide a transition between, the reactants and products. In energy diagrams like the ones above, the activated complex has more energy than both the reactants and the products. The **activation energy** is the amount of energy required to transform the reactants into the activated complex, which then breaks apart to form the products.

The components of an energy diagram are as follows:

- Energy of reactants - energy of substances at the beginning of the reaction
- Energy of products - energy of substances at the end of the reaction
- Energy of the activated complex - energy of the substance represented by the maximum in the energy diagram
- Activation energy - difference in energy between the reactants and the activated complex
- Amount of energy released/absorbed - difference in energy between the reactants and products

## Example

**When iron reacts with oxygen, iron (III) oxide ($Fe_2O_3$), also known as rust, forms according to the equation below. The iron (III) oxide has less energy than the iron and oxygen. How is reaction classified, and why?**

$$4Fe(s) + 3O_2(g) \rightarrow 2Fe_2O_3(s)$$

A. It is exothermic because energy is released.

B. It is exothermic because energy is absorbed.

C. It is endothermic because energy is released.

D. It is endothermic because energy is absorbed.

The correct answer is **A.** It is exothermic because the reactants must release energy to form a product that has less energy. **See Lesson: Chemical Solutions.**

## Let's Review!

- A solution is a type of homogeneous mixture that is formed when a solute dissolves in a solvent.
- The concentration of a solution is the amount of a substance in a given amount of solution.
- Chemical reactions occur when reactants combine, break apart, or rearrange to form products.
- Chemical equations represent chemical reactions using formulas and symbols.
- Chemical reactions can be classified as synthesis, decomposition, single-replacement, double-replacement, or combustion based on the reactants and products.

# ACIDS AND BASES

This lesson introduces the properties of acids and bases, including the various theories that define them. It also covers acid-base reactions and the pH scale.

## Nature of Acids and Bases

**Acids** are compounds that contain at least one hydrogen atom or proton ($H^+$), which, when dissolved in water, can form a hydronium ion ($H_3O^+$). Acids dissolved in water generally have the following properties:

- Taste sour
- Turn litmus red
- Act corrosive

Acids are found in a variety of substances, from vinegar to apple juice. The following table provides a list of common acids and their sources or applications.

| Name of Acid | Chemical Formula | Sources or Applications |
|---|---|---|
| Citric acid | $C_6H_8O_7$ | Citrus fruits such as oranges and lemons |
| Lactic acid | $C_3H_6O_3$ | Yogurt and buttermilk |
| Acetic acid | $C_2H_4O_2$ or $CH_3COOH$ | Nail polish remover and vinegar |
| Hydrochloric acid | HCl | Stomach |
| Phosphoric acid | $H_3PO_4$ | Detergents and soft drinks |
| Nitric acid | $HNO_3$ | Fertilizers |

**Bases** are compounds that form hydroxide ions ($OH^-$) in a water solution. They also accept hydronium ions from acids. Bases dissolved in water generally have the following properties:

- Slippery in solution
- Very corrosive
- Turn litmus blue
- Taste bitter

Like acids, bases have many applications. The following table provides examples of common bases and how they are used.

| Name of Base | Chemical Formula | Applications |
|---|---|---|
| Sodium hydroxide | NaOH | Soap, oven cleaners, and textiles |
| Potassium hydroxide | KOH | Soap and textiles |
| Ammonia | $NH_3$ | Cleaning agents and fertilizers |
| Magnesium hydroxide | $Mg(OH)_2$ | Laxatives and antacids |

Acidic solutions have more hydrogen ions than hydroxide ions, whereas basic solutions have more hydroxide ions than hydrogen ions. All water solutions have both ion types, but the relative numbers dictate whether an aqueous solution is acidic, basic, or neutral. Anything that is dissolved in water is an **aqueous solution**. Neutral solutions are neither acidic nor basic, meaning that an equal number of hydrogen and hydroxide ions are present. Pure water is an example of a neutral solution.

216

Water is the primary solvent used to create an aqueous solution. Thus, it is important to understand how pure water behaves in solution. A small fraction of water molecules breaks down to form hydronium and hydroxide ions. When two water molecules interact, one water molecule gives up a positively charged hydrogen ion to form a hydroxide ion. A hydronium ion forms when a water molecule accepts a hydrogen ion. The following equation illustrates this reaction: $2H_2O \rightarrow H_3O^+ + OH^-$

> **KEEP IN MIND**
>
> Substances that form ions in aqueous solutions are called **electrolytes**. As electrolytes, acids and bases are conductors of electricity in solution. This is because they contain dissolved ions.

## Examples

1.  **Which of the following is an acid?**

    A.  $KNO_3$

    B.  $BaCl_2$

    C.  NaOH

    D.  $H_3PO_4$

    The correct answer is **D**. Phosphoric acid ($H_3PO_4$) is a common acid that is capable of donating one of its hydrogen atoms to form a hydronium ion. **See Lesson: Acids and Bases.**

2.  **Which is a characteristic of a basic solution?**

    A.  Tastes sour

    B.  Accepts $OH^-$ ions

    C.  Turns litmus blue

    D.  Contains a lot of $H_3O^+$ ions

    The correct answer is **C**. A basic solution is made using water as a solvent. Basic solutions turn litmus paper from red to blue. **See Lesson: Acids and Bases.**

# Acid and Base Classification

Recall that an acid produces hydrogen ions, and a base produces hydroxide ions. These compounds are defined as **Arrhenius** acids and bases. The Arrhenius theory explains how acids and bases form ions when dissolved in water. Take, for example, the acid HCl, shown in the equation below. When forming an aqueous solution of HCl, this acid dissociates, or splits, into hydrogen ions and chloride ions in water.

$$HCl\ (g) \rightarrow H^+\ (aq) + Cl^-\ (aq)$$

An Arrhenius base dissociates into hydroxide ions (OH-) in an aqueous solution. This is the case for sodium hydroxide, NaOH, as shown in the following equation:

$$NaOH\ (s) \rightarrow Na^+\ (aq) + OH^-(aq)$$

One limitation of this theory is that it does not account for acids and bases that lack a hydrogen or hydroxide ion in their molecular structure. Another way to define acids and bases is by using the Brønsted-Lowry theory. A Brønsted-Lowry **acid** is a hydrogen ion donor that increases the concentration of hydronium ions in solution. A Brønsted-Lowry **base** is a hydrogen ion acceptor that increases hydroxide ion concentration in solution. The term *proton* is used interchangeably with the term *hydrogen ion*.

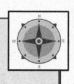

**BE CAREFUL!**

Free H+ ions do not float in an aqueous solution. Rather, they bind with water to form $H_3O^+$. However, it is not uncommon to see the two formulas, H+ and $H_3O^+$, used interchangeably in chemical reactions.

When a base accepts a hydrogen ion, it produces a conjugate acid. When an acid donates a hydrogen ion, it produces a conjugate base. In the following example, ammonia is the base, but its conjugate acid is ammonium ion. What is the conjugate base for the acid?

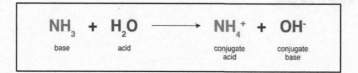

The last theory about acids and bases is called the Lewis theory. This theory is based on electron movement during an acid-base reaction. A **Lewis acid** accepts a pair of electrons, while a **Lewis base** donates an electron pair.

**KEEP IN MIND**

When substances such as pure water act as an acid or a base, they are **amphoteric**.

## Example

**What is the conjugate acid in the following equation?**

$$CH_3COOH + H_2O \rightleftharpoons H_3O^+ + CH_3COO^-$$

A. $H_3O^+$

B. $H_2O$

C. $CH_3COO^-$

D. $CH_3COOH$

The correct answer is **A**. A conjugate acid is a substance that accepts a proton from a base. In this case, the base $H_2O$ accepts a proton to form the conjugate acid, hydronium ion ($H_3O^+$). **See Lesson: Acids and Bases.**

# Acid-Base Reactions

In an aqueous solution, a base increases the hydroxide concentration (OH⁻), while an acid increases the hydrogen ion (H⁺) concentration. Sometimes, **neutralization reactions** also occur. This type of reaction happens when an acid and a base react with each other to form water and salt. Salt is typically defined as an **ionic compound** that includes any cation except H⁺ and any anion except OH⁻. Consider the following example of a neutralization reaction between hydrobromic acid (HBr) and potassium hydroxide (KOH).

$$HBr + KOH \longrightarrow KBr + H_2O$$

In the above equation, one molecule of water forms in addition to the salt potassium bromide (KBr). There are instances where acid-base reactions must be balanced because more than one molecule of an acid or a base react to form products. This is the case for the reaction between hydrochloric acid and magnesium hydroxide, as shown below.

$$2HCl + Mg(OH)_2 \longrightarrow MgCl_2 + 2H_2O$$

When two molecules of hydrochloric acid react with magnesium hydroxide, two water molecules and one molecule of salt, $MgCl_2$, form.

## Example

**Which is a product of a neutralization reaction?**

A.  Acid

B.  Base

C.  Proton

D.  Salt

The correct answer is **D**. When an acid and a base react, they form a salt and water. This type of reaction is called a neutralization reaction. See **Lesson: Acids and Bases.**

# Acid Base Strength and pH

Acids and bases can be classified according to their strength. This strength refers to how readily an acid donates a hydrogen ion. The strength of a base is determined by how readily it removes a hydrogen ion from a molecule, or **deprotonates**. Strong acids are also known as strong electrolytes, which means that they completely ionize in solution. Weak acids are weak electrolytes because they partially ionize in solution. The following diagram shows what happens to a strong or weak acid in an aqueous solution.

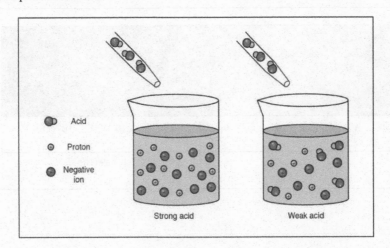

219

The maximum number of ions is produced when strong acids ionize. As shown in the following equations, the weak acid reaction is reversible (and incomplete) in aqueous solutions. This explains why weak acids produce fewer ions than strong acids.

Strong acid in solution

$$HNO_3 \longrightarrow H^+ + NO_3^-$$

Weak base in solution

$$NH_3 + H_2O \rightleftharpoons NH_4^+ + OH^-$$

Like strong acids, strong bases fully dissociate in solution. They produce metal ions and hydroxide ions. Like weak acids, weak bases partially dissociate and participate in reversible reactions. The following table provides a list of common strong acids and bases and common weak acids and bases.

> **BE CAREFUL!**
> Ammonia is a weak base even though it does not have a hydroxide ion ($OH^-$) in its chemical formula. It will accept a proton and form hydroxide ions in aqueous solutions.

| Strong Acid | Weak Acid | Strong Base | Weak Base |
|---|---|---|---|
| Hydrochloric acid (HCl) | Hydrofluoric acid (HF) | Sodium hydroxide (NaOH) | Ammonia ($NH_3$) |
| Nitric acid ($HNO_3$) | Carbonic acid ($H_2CO_3$) | Potassium hydroxide (KOH) | Methylamine ($CH_3NH_2$) |
| Perchloric acid ($HClO_4$) | Phosphoric acid ($H_3PO_4$) | Calcium hydroxide ($Ca(OH)_2$) | Hydrazine ($N_2H_4$) |
| Sulfuric acid ($H_2SO_4$) | Acetic acid ($C_2H_4O_2$ or $CH_3COOH$) | Lithium hydroxide (LiOH) | Pyridine ($C_5H_5N$) |

Researchers can determine the strength of an acid or a base by measuring the **pH** of a solution. The pH value describes how acidic or basic a solution is. On pH scale, shown below, if the number is less than 7 the solution is acidic. A pH greater than 7 means the solution is basic. When the pH is exactly 7, the solution is neutral.

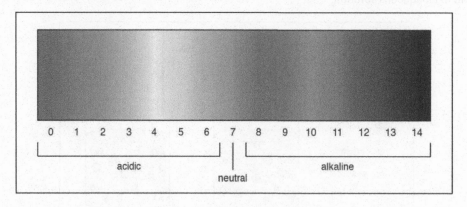

## Example

**Which of the following measured pH values means a solution is basic?**

A. 2

B. 5

C. 7

D. 9

The correct answer is **D.** When the pH of an aqueous solution is greater than 7, which is the case for a solution that has a pH of 9, the solution is basic. **See Lesson: Acids and Bases.**

## Let's Review!

- Acids and bases exhibit unique properties when dissolved in water.

- Arrhenius acids donate hydrogen ions, and Arrhenius bases accept hydrogen ions in solution.

- Brønsted-Lowry acids donate protons (or hydrogen ions), and Brønsted-Lowry bases accept protons (or hydrogen ions).

- Lewis acids are electron pair acceptors, and Lewis bases are electron pair donors.

- A neutralization reaction occurs when an acid and a base react to form a salt and water.

- Strong acids completely ionize in solution, and strong bases fully dissociate in solution.

- Weak acids and weak bases only partially dissociate in solution.

- The pH of a solution determines how acidic or basic it is.

# CHAPTER 10 CHEMISTRY PRACTICE QUIZ

1. _____ is dependent not only on the temperature, but also on the amount of substance available.

   A. Condensation

   B. Deposition

   C. Evaporation

   D. Melting

2. Compare the melting points of three metals: gold (1063°C), lead (328°C), and mercury (–38.9°C). Which of the following statements is true regarding the states of matter of these elements at room temperature (around 23°C)?

   A. All three metals are solid at room temperature.

   B. All three metals are liquid at room temperature.

   C. Gold is solid at room temperature; lead and mercury are liquid at room temperature.

   D. Gold and lead are solid at room temperature; mercury is liquid at room temperature.

3. _____ is the ability of water to be attracted to other substances.

   A. Adhesion

   B. Cohesion

   C. Density

   D. Polar

4. What states of matter are found in a sample that is in the process of freezing?

   A. Only solid

   B. Only liquid

   C. Liquid and gas

   D. Solid and liquid

5. Which of the following elements will gain three electrons to become stable?

   A. Aluminum

   B. Boron

   C. Oxygen

   D. Phosphorus

6. Which of the following type of bond forms between two atoms that have similar electronegativities?

   A. Ionic bond

   B. Polar covalent bond

   C. Nonpolar covalent bond

   D. Any of the bond types listed above could form.

7. Which of the following is an example of a homogeneous mixture?

   A. A bowl of cereal with milk

   B. A glass of lemonade with ice

   C. A mixture of silver and gold coins

   D. A pitcher of cherry-flavored beverage

8.  **Sugar is dissolved in water. Which of the following statements best describes the components of this solution?**

    A.  Sugar and water are both solutes.

    B.  Sugar and water are both solvents.

    C.  Sugar is the solute, and water is the solvent.

    D.  Sugar is the solvent, and water is the solute.

9.  **Which of the following is a weak base?**

    A.  Vinegar

    B.  Ammonia

    C.  Pure water

    D.  Sodium hydroxide

10. **Which of the following is a characteristic of citrus substances?**

    A.  Taste sour

    B.  Have a pH of 7

    C.  Turn litmus blue

    D.  Slippery to touch

# CHAPTER 10 CHEMISTRY
# PRACTICE QUIZ – ANSWER KEY

**1. C.** Unlike condensation, deposition, and melting, evaporation is dependent not only on the temperature, but also on the amount of a substance available. **See Lesson: Properties of Matter.**

**2. D.** Because their melting points are higher than room temperature, gold and lead are solid. Because its melting point is lower than room temperature, mercury is liquid. **See Lesson: States of Matter.**

**3. A.** Adhesion is the ability of water to be attracted to other substances. **See Lesson: Properties of Matter.**

**4. D.** Freezing is the process of changing from a liquid to a solid. Therefore, these two states of matter will be present as that change occurs. **See Lesson: States of Matter.**

**5. D.** Phosphorus is in group 15, which means it has five valence electrons. Gaining three would give it eight valence electrons, making the atom stable. **See Lesson: Chemical Bonds.**

**6. C.** In a nonpolar covalent bond, electrons are shared equally because neither atom pulls significantly harder on them. **See Lesson: Chemical Bonds.**

**7. D.** The cherry-flavored beverage is the only mixture described in which the components are mixed evenly. In the other mixtures, the individual components of the mixture can be seen because substances did not mix completely. **See Lesson: Chemical Solutions.**

**8. C.** Generally, the solute dissolves in the solvent to form a solution. To make sugar water, the sugar dissolves in water. **See Lesson: Chemical Solutions.**

**9. B.** A weak base is a substance that partially dissociates in solution. Ammonia is an example of a weak base because it weakly dissociates to ammonium ions in solution. **See Lesson: Acids and Bases.**

**10. A.** Because citrus substances are acidic, they taste sour, which is a property of acidic substances dissolved in water. **See Lesson: Acids and Bases.**

# SECTION VII
# ANATOMY AND
# PHYSIOLOGY

# Anatomy and Physiology: 25 questions, 25 minutes

**Areas assessed:** Life and Physical Sciences

## *ANATOMY AND PHYSIOLOGY TIPS*

- Know your Anatomy and Physiology.

- Review anatomical systems, structures and general terminology.

- Know basics of the 11 systems of the body, organelles, basic biology.

# CHAPTER 11 HUMAN ANATOMY AND PHYSIOLOGY: ORGANIZATION OF SYSTEMS

## ORGANIZATION OF THE HUMAN BODY

Human anatomy and physiology is the study of the structures and functions of the human body.

## Levels of Organization and Body Cavities

The body can be studied at seven structural levels: **chemical**, **organelle**, **cell**, **tissue**, **organ**, **organ system**, and **organism**.

- **Chemical:** The chemical level involves interactions among atoms and their combination into molecules.

- **Organelle:** An organelle is a small structure contained within a cell that performs one or more specific functions.

- **Cell:** Cells are the basic functional units of life. All cells share many characteristics, but they differ in structure and function.

- **Tissue:** A tissue is a group of cells with similar structures and functions.

- **Organ:** An organ is composed of two or more tissue types that together perform one or more common function.

- **Organ system:** An organ system is a group of organs classified as a unit because of a common function or set of functions.

- **Organism:** An organism is any living thing considered as a whole. Organisms can have anywhere from a single cell to trillions of cells.

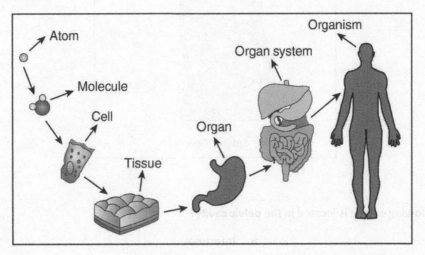

## Body Cavities

The human body has many cavities, some of which open to the exterior. A **cavity** is a fluid-filled space in the body that holds and protects internal organs. The **ventral cavity** (front of the body) contains three major cavities:

- The **thoracic cavity** is surrounded by the rib cage and separated from the abdominal cavity by the diaphragm. It is divided into right and left halves by a structure called the mediastinum. It contains the esophagus, trachea, thymus gland, heart, and both lungs, along with other structures.

- The **abdominal cavity** is bounded by the abdominal muscles below the thoracic cavity and contains the stomach, intestines, liver, spleen, pancreas, and kidneys.

- The **pelvic cavity** is enclosed by the bones of the pelvis and contains the urinary bladder, part of the intestines, and the internal reproductive organs. The abdominal and pelvic cavities are sometimes referred to as the abdominopelvic cavity.

The **dorsal cavity** is the back of the human body, and it is subdivided into two cavities: cranial and spinal.

- The **cranial cavity** contains the brain.
- The **spinal cavity** contains the spinal cord.

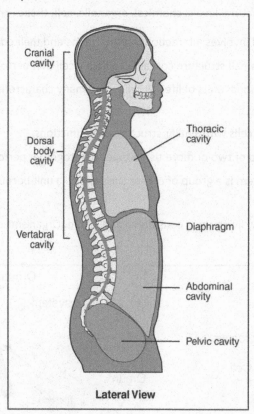

**Lateral View**

## Example

**Which of the following organs is located in the pelvic cavity?**

A.  Heart

B.  Intestines

C.  Liver

D.  Pancreas

The correct answer is **B.** The intestines are located in both the abdominal and pelvic cavities.

**See Lesson: Organization of the Human Body.**

228

# Terminology and the Body Planes and Regions

Directional terms refer to the body in the **anatomical position**, regardless of its actual position. The term *anatomical position* refers to a person standing erect with the feet forward, arms hanging to the sides, and the palms of the hands facing forward.

## Terminology

| Term | Definition |
|---|---|
| Inferior | A structure below another |
| Superior | A structure above another |
| Anterior | Toward the front of the body |
| Posterior | Toward the back of the body |
| Dorsal | Toward the back |
| Ventral | Toward the front |
| Proximal | Closer to the point of attachment to the body than another structure |
| Distal | Farther from the point of attachment to the body |
| Lateral | Away from the midline of the body |
| Medial | Toward the middle or midline of the body |
| Superficial | Toward or on the surface |
| Deep | Away from the surface |
| Anterosuperior | In front or above |
| Midline | A median line |
| Supine position | Lying flat with face and torso facing upward |
| Prone position | Lying face down |

## Body Planes

Sectioning the body is a way to look inside and observe the body's structures. The following are the major planes of the body:

- The **sagittal plane** runs vertically through the body and separates the body into right and left parts.
- The **midsagittal plane** divides the body into two equal halves.
- The **transverse plane** runs parallel to the surface of the ground and divides the body into superior and inferior planes.
- The **coronal plane**, sometimes called the frontal plane, runs vertically from left to right and divides the body into anterior and posterior parts.

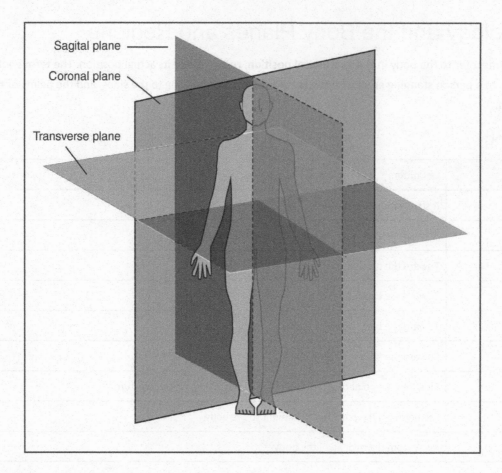

## Body Regions

The body is divided into the following four regions:

- **Upper limb:** The upper limb includes the arm, forearm, wrist, and hand.
- **Lower limb:** The lower limb is divided into the thigh, leg, ankle, and foot.
- **Central region:** The central region includes the neck and trunk.
- **Head region:** The head region includes the entire head.

## Example

**The wrist is _____ to the shoulder.**

A.  distal

B.  lateral

C.  median

D.  superior

The correct answer is **A.** The wrist is farther from the point of attachment than the shoulder is, so it is distal to the shoulder. **See Lesson: Organization of the Human Body.**

# Human Tissues

A **tissue** is a group of cells with similar structure and function and similar extracellular substances located between the cells. The table below describes the four primary tissues found in the human body.

| Tissue | Structure | Function | Example |
|---|---|---|---|
| Connective | characterized by extracellular material that separate cells from one another | 1. enclosing and separating<br>2. connecting tissues to one another<br>3. supportive and moving<br>4. storing<br>5. cushioning and insulating<br>6. transporting<br>7. protecting | cells of the immune system and blood |
| Epithelial | classified according to the number of cell layers and shapes | 1. protecting underlying structures<br>2. acting as barriers<br>3. permitting the passage of substances<br>4. secreting substances | skin, linings of internal organs |
| Muscle | cells of muscles resemble long threads and are called *fibers* | 1. providing movement | heart, organs of digestive system |
| Neural | cells are composed of dendrites, cell bodies, and axons | 1. coordinating and controlling many body activities | brain, spinal cord |

**Four Types of Tissue**

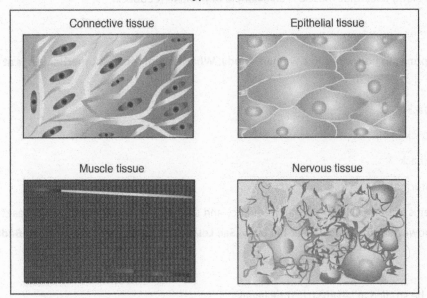

Connective tissue

Epithelial tissue

Muscle tissue

Nervous tissue

# Example

**Which type of tissue controls when the heart beats?**

A. Connective          B. Epithelial          C. Muscle          D. Nervous

The correct answer is **D.** Although the muscle tissue is responsible for the actual movement of the heart, the neural tissue "tells" the heart when to beat. **See Lesson: Organization of the Human Body.**

# Homeostasis and Feedback Mechanisms

**Homeostasis** is the existence and maintenance of a relatively constant environment within the body. Each cell of the body is surrounded by a small amount of fluid, and the normal functions of each cell depend on the maintenance of its fluid environment within a narrow range of conditions, including temperature, volume, and chemical content. These conditions are known as **variables**. For example, body temperature is a variable that can increase in a hot environment or decrease in a cold environment.

There are two types of feedback mechanisms in the human body: negative and positive.

## Negative Feedback

Most systems of the body are regulated by **negative feedback mechanisms**, which maintain homeostasis. *Negative* means that any deviation from the set point is made smaller or is resisted. The maintenance of normal blood pressure is a negative-feedback mechanism. Normal blood pressure is important because it is responsible for moving blood from the heart to tissues.

## Positive Feedback

Positive-feedback mechanisms are not homeostatic and are rare in healthy individuals. *Positive* means that when a deviation from a normal value occurs, the response of the system is to make the deviation even greater. Positive feedback therefore usually creates a cycle leading away from homeostasis and, in some cases, results in death. Inadequate delivery of blood to cardiac muscle is an example of positive feedback.

## Example

**Childbirth is a response to hormones in a woman's body. What type of feedback mechanism is at work during childbirth?**

A. Neutral feedback

B. Positive feedback

C. Negative feedback

D. Need more information

The correct answer is **B.** During childbirth, the frequency and strength of the contractions increases until the contractions are powerful enough to deliver the baby. **See Lesson: Organization of the Human Body.**

## Let's Review!

- The body can be studied at seven structural levels.
- The human body has multiple body cavities.
- Directional terms refer to the body in the anatomical position.
- Sectioning the body is a way to look inside and observe the body's structures.
- The four primary tissues found in the human body are connective, epithelial, muscular and nervous.
- Homeostasis is the existence and maintenance of a relatively constant environment within the body.
- The two types of feedback mechanisms in the human body are negative and positive feedback mechanisms.

# THE CARDIOVASCULAR SYSTEM

This lesson introduces the anatomy of blood and its connection to the cardiovascular system. Explore the parts that make up the cardiovascular system and how this system functions.

## Anatomy of Blood

**Blood** is a type of fluid connective tissue that circulates throughout the body, carrying substances to and away from bodily tissues. It has a pH of about 7.4 and is more viscous than water. Blood consists of three types of formed elements, an extracellular matrix called **plasma,** molecules, cell fragments, and debris. The formed elements consist of red blood cells, white blood cells, and platelets. They are also referred to as **erythrocytes**, **leukocytes**, and **thrombocytes**, respectively. The following table details key characteristics of these elements.

| Characteristic | Red Blood Cells | White Blood Cells | Platelets |
|---|---|---|---|
| Scientific Name | Erythrocytes | Leukocytes | Thrombocytes |
| Size (Diameter) | 0.0008 mm | 0.02 mm | 0.03 mm |
| Function | Participate in gas exchange, primarily with oxygen and carbon dioxide | Protect the body from foreign substances by eliciting an immune response | Aid in blood clotting and wound healing |

Plasma is different from other types of connective tissue because it is a fluid. Consisting of about 92% water, formed elements remain suspended in the matrix where they are circulated throughout the body.

## DID YOU KNOW?

The average volume of blood in the human body, for a 70-kilogram person, is 5 liters. Blood accounts for roughly 8% of a person's body weight.

Consider the following image, which illustrates the composition of blood in a person's blood sample. When a blood sample is spun in a centrifuge, less-dense plasma floats on top of a reddish mass that consists of red blood cells. There is also a thin white layer called the **buffy coat** that consists of white blood cells and platelets. This layer is found between the reddish mass and plasma layers.

## KEEP IN MIND

Blood viscosity is indirectly proportional to blood flow throughout the body. If the viscosity of blood is high, blood flow decreases. When blood viscosity is low, or blood is thin, blood flow increases.

## Example

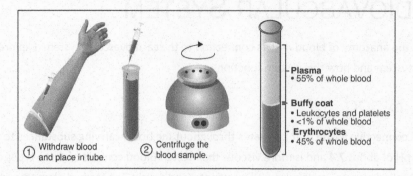

① Withdraw blood and place in tube.
② Centrifuge the blood sample.

**Plasma**
• 55% of whole blood

**Buffy coat**
• Leukocytes and platelets
• <1% of whole blood

**Erythrocytes**
• 45% of whole blood

**A laboratory technician needs to determine the leukocyte count in a patient. From which part of a blood sample are these cells extracted?**

A.  Water

B.  Buffy coat

C.  Liquid plasma

D.  Reddish mass

The correct answer is **B.** Buffy coat contains white blood cells (or leukocytes) and platelets in blood. **See Lesson: Cardiovascular System.**

# Functions of Blood

Transportation, regulation, and protection are three primary functions of blood. Blood transports the following substances throughout the body:

- Gases: Blood delivers oxygen from the lungs to all cells in the body. It also transports carbon dioxide to the lungs for elimination from the body.

- Nutrients: Blood transports nutrients from the digestive tract and storage sites in the body to various places in the body.

- Wastes: Blood transports waste products to the liver, where they are excreted as bile. Waste products also travel by blood to the kidneys when they need to be excreted as urine.

- Hormones: Blood transports hormones from the glands where they are produced to their target organs.

Although blood's primary function is to distribute substances throughout the body, it also has regulatory functions. These functions include the regulation of body temperature, chemical balance, and water balance. Blood ensures the right body temperature is maintained with help from plasma and the speed of blood flow. Plasma is able to absorb or give off heat. As shown in the following image, when blood vessels expand, or **vasodilate**, blood flows slowly, causing heat loss. This occurs when the temperature of the external environment is high. If external environmental temperatures are low, blood vessels contract, or **vasoconstrict**, causing less heat to be released.

> **KEEP IN MIND**
> Albumin is the main protein in blood, accounting for roughly 60% of the plasma proteins in blood. It plays a role in water balance and functions as a carrier protein, shuttling certain molecules throughout the body.

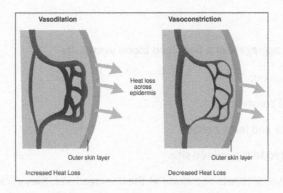

Blood also functions as a form of protection, defending the body against foreign invaders or **pathogens** that harm the body. As blood circulates through the body, it carries white blood cells and **antibodies** that destroy any pathogens they encounter. With the help of platelets and plasma proteins, blood also protects the body from extensive blood loss if a blood vessel is damaged.

## Example

**Platelets are important because they**

A. give blood its natural color.

B. repair broken blood vessels.

C. transport nutrients to the cells.

D. protect the body against infection.

The correct answer is **B**. At the site of injury or damage to a blood vessel, platelets help repair the damaged area.

# Hemostasis

Recall that a function of platelets and plasma proteins is to repair damaged blood vessels. When blood vessels are damaged, a physiological process called hemostasis is activated. **Hemostasis** helps maintain blood in its fluid state and stops blood from leaking out of a damaged blood vessel through clot formation. As shown in the image below, there are three steps of hemostasis.

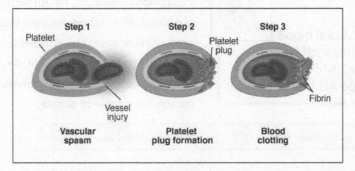

The first step is **vascular spasm**, or vasoconstriction, where the blood vessels constrict to reduce blood loss. Reducing blood loss for several hours, this process works best with small blood vessels. The second step is platelet plug formation. Platelets adhere to the epithelial wall of the blood vessel and aggregate by sticking together. This creates a temporary seal over the damaged site. In the third step, **blood coagulation** occurs. Also known as **blood clotting**, this process is a series of events that strengthen the platelet plug by using fibrin threads to form a mesh around the plug. The protein mesh functions as a molecular glue, securing the plug to the damaged site. Red blood cells and platelets remain trapped at the damaged site, forming a clot that facilitates wound healing.

## Example

**What happens after platelets aggregate at a damaged blood vessel site?**

A. The site of the wound is healed.

B. The damaged blood vessel constricts.

C. The platelets stick together and form a plug.

D. Red blood cells are recruited to the injured site.

The correct answer is **C.** After the platelets aggregate at the damaged site, they stick together to form a plug. Next, blood coagulation occurs when a fibrin mesh forms around the platelet aggregate. **See Lesson: Cardiovascular System.**

# Blood Grouping and Agglutination

There are several different types or groups of blood, and the major groups are A, B, AB, and O. Blood group is a way to classify blood according to inherited differences of red blood cell **antigens** found on the surface of a red blood cell. The type of antibody in blood also identifies a particular blood group. **Antibodies** are proteins found in the plasma. They function as part of the body's natural defense to recognize foreign substances and alert the immune system. Depending on which antigen is inherited, parental offspring will have one of the four major blood groups. Collectively, the following major blood groups comprise the ABO system:

- Blood group A: Displays type A antigens on the surface of a red blood cell and contains B antibodies in the plasma.

- Blood group B: Displays type B antigens on the red blood cell's surface and contains A antibodies in the plasma.

- Blood group O: Does not display A or B antigens on the surface of a red blood cell. Both A and B antibodies are in the plasma.

- Blood group AB: Displays type A and B antigens on the red blood cell's surface, but neither A nor B antibodies are in the plasma.

**KEEP IN MIND**

A person can be a universal blood donor or acceptor. A universal blood donor has type O blood, while a universal blood acceptor has type AB blood.

In addition to antigens, the **Rh factor** protein may exist on a red blood cell's surface. Because this protein can be either present (+) or absent (-), it increases the number of major blood groups from four to eight: A+, A-, B+, B-, O+, O-, AB+, and AB-. The following table summarizes what blood types a person can receive or donate.

| Blood Group | Can accept blood from | Can donate blood to |
| --- | --- | --- |
| A | A, O | A, AB |
| B | B, O | B, AB |
| AB | AB, A, B, O | AB |
| O | O | AB, A, B, O |

When determining an individual's blood type, a sample of blood is mixed with an antiserum. If **agglutination**, or clumping, occurs during this process, the antibody has found an antigen with which to interact. This means there are antigens on the surface of the red blood cell to which the antibodies can bind. Evidence of agglutination is used to interpret the final blood type result from a sample.

## Example

**People with type O blood can accept blood from people with _____ blood.**

A. type O

B. type B

C. type AB

D. type A

The correct answer is **A.** People with type O blood are universal donors but can accept blood only from people with type O blood. **See Lesson: Cardiovascular System.**

# Cardiovascular Anatomy

The **cardiovascular system** circulates substances throughout the body using blood as a transporting mechanism. The organs of the cardiovascular system work together to supply cells and tissues with oxygen and nutrients and remove cellular wastes such as carbon dioxide. Blood, heart, and blood vessels form this system.

Because blood circulation is a closed loop system, blood is contained within the heart or blood vessels at all times. There are three types of blood vessels: arteries, veins, and capillaries. **Arteries** carry blood away from the heart, toward organs and tissues. **Veins** carry blood toward the heart, away from organs and tissues. Arteries branch into smaller blood vessels called **arterioles**, which further divide into capillaries. As shown in the following image, **capillaries** are tiny vessels that form a network around tissues. Veins branch into venules before further dividing into capillaries.

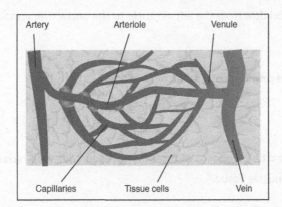

The heart is found between the lungs in the middle of the chest. It rests behind and slightly to the left of the sternum, or breastbone. The human heart is a muscular organ composed primarily of cardiac muscle. It consists of four chambers: two upper chambers called the **atria** and two lower chambers called the **ventricles**. The atria are separated from the ventricles by a muscular structure called the **septum**. Three layers make up the heart wall. These are the **pericardium** or outer layer, the **myocardium** or middle layer, and the **endocardium** or innermost layer. Most cardiac muscle tissue is found in the myocardium.

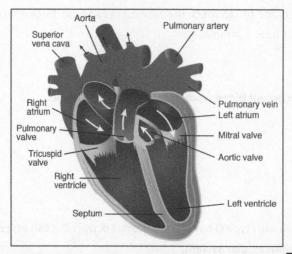

**DID YOU KNOW?**

Capillaries have thin walls and a very large surface area. Because of the capillaries' thin walls, blood flow slows to facilitate exchanges between blood and the body's tissues.

In addition to the four chambers, the heart has four valves that regulate blood flow into and out of the heart:

- **Tricuspid valve** regulates blood flow between the right atrium and right ventricle.
- **Pulmonary valve** regulates blood flow from the right ventricle into the pulmonary artery.
- **Mitral valve** regulates blood flow from the left atrium into the left ventricle.
- **Aortic valve** regulates blood flow from the left ventricle to the **aorta**. The aorta is the largest artery in the body.

## Example

**Which heart layer is composed primarily of cardiac muscle?**

A. Myocardium

B. Pericardium

C. Septum

D. Sternum

The correct answer is **A**. The heart is composed of three layers, the middle of which is the myocardium. The myocardium contains cardiac muscle tissue.

# Circulation and the Cardiac Cycle

Blood continually flows in one direction, beginning in the heart and proceeding to the arteries, arterioles, and capillaries. When blood reaches the capillaries, exchanges occur between blood and tissues. After this exchange happens, blood is collected into venules, which feed into veins and eventually flow back to the heart's atrium. The heart must relax between two heartbeats for blood circulation to begin. Two types of circulatory processes occur in the body:

*Systemic circulation*

1. The pulmonary vein pushes oxygenated blood into the left atrium.
2. As the atrium relaxes, oxygenated blood drains into the left ventricle through the mitral valve.
3. The left ventricle pumps oxygenated blood to the aorta.
4. Blood travels through the arteries and arterioles before reaching the capillaries that surround the tissues.

*Pulmonary circulation*

1. Deoxygenated blood is sent back to the heart via the veins and pooled into the right atrium.

2. Blood travels through the superior vena cava and drains into the right ventricle.

3. The right ventricle contracts, causing the blood to be pushed through the pulmonary valve into the pulmonary artery.

4. Deoxygenated blood becomes oxygenated in the lungs.

5. Oxygenated blood returns from the lungs to the left atrium through the pulmonary veins.

The following image shows the heart's role in systemic and pulmonary circulation.

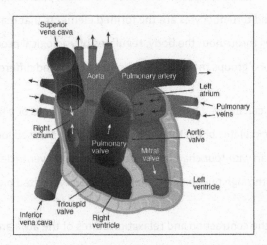

The complete cycle beginning with atrial contraction and ending with ventricular contraction is called the **cardiac cycle**. When the heart contracts and pumps blood into systemic circulation, this is called **systole**. **Diastole** refers to the period of relaxation when the heart chambers fill with blood.

**KEEP IN MIND**

Blood flow is regulated by many mechanisms in the body. This regulated variable is also directly proportional to blood pressure. If blood volume increases, blood pressure increases. The opposite occurs if blood pressure decreases.

Because the heart is a muscle, it transmits electrical impulses that cause the heart to contract. This electrical activity can be recorded using an **electrocardiogram**, or EKG. An EKG is a graph that shows the heart's rate and rhythm over a period of time. As shown in the following image of an EKG, waves in the graph have different meanings.

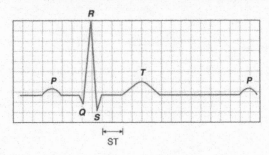

The first wave on an EKG is the P wave. This indicates atrial contraction or systole. The QRS complex represents the combination of Q, R, and S waves. This indicates ventricular systole or contraction. The T wave indicates ventricular diastole. The flat line between the S and T wave is the ST segment.

HESI

# Example

**What segment of the electrocardiogram is associated with atrial systole?**

A.  P wave          B.  S wave          C.  ST segment          D.  QRS complex

The correct answer is **A.** Atrial systole occurs when the atrium contracts. On an EKG, atrial systole is indicated by a P wave. **See Lesson: Cardiovascular System.**

# Let's Review!

- Blood is a type of connective tissue composed of formed elements, plasma, and other substances.

- Erythrocytes, leukocytes, and thrombocytes are the formed elements that make up blood.

- Blood transports substances throughout the body, regulates physiological processes, and protects the body.

- There are four common blood groups that are determined by inherited differences in antigens on red blood cells.

- Agglutination, or clumping, can be used to help interpret the blood type of a blood sample.

- The cardiovascular system circulates blood throughout the body in a closed loop structure.

- The heart is a muscular organ with four chambers: two atria and two ventricles.

- Deoxygenated blood flows through pulmonary circulation, and oxygenated blood flows through systemic circulation.

- The cardiac cycle refers to the contraction and relaxation states of the atria and ventricles.

- An electrocardiogram, or EKG, is used to record heart beat and rhythm.

# THE RESPIRATORY SYSTEM

This lesson introduces the anatomy of the respiratory system and how each organ within this system functions. It also discusses the mechanics of breathing and respiration.

## Anatomy of the Respiratory System

Every living thing requires oxygen for survival. Humans can live for days without water and for weeks without food. But they can only survive a few minutes without air. The respiratory system's primary function is to bring oxygen into the body, in exchange for carbon dioxide. As shown in the following image, organs of the respiratory system include the nose, nasal cavity, mouth, larynx, pharynx, lungs, and diaphragm.

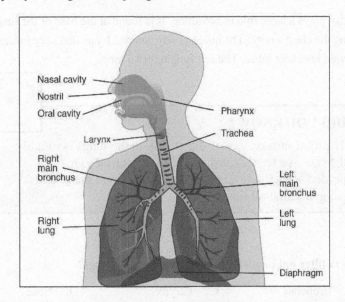

The respiratory organs can be divided into the upper and lower respiratory tract. The **upper respiratory tract** includes the nasal cavity, pharynx, and larynx. The trachea, bronchus, and lungs belong to the **lower respiratory tract**. The **nasal cavity** opens to the nose. The nose and nasal cavity warm and moisten air as a person breathes. As a defensive mechanism, tiny nose hairs and mucus produced by the epithelial mucosa cells in the nose help prevent particles in the air from entering the lungs.

Behind the nasal cavity is the **pharynx**. Both food and air pass through this long tube. Just below the pharynx is the **larynx**, or voice box. It channels air to the trachea and pushes food past the **epiglottis**, which covers the trachea during swallowing to prevent food from entering the lungs. Once food passes the epiglottis, it moves toward the esophagus. When air reaches the **trachea**, or windpipe, it travels down a long tube that branches into **bronchi**. The bronchi enter the lungs. As shown in the image, the bronchi branch into **bronchioles** before reaching tiny air sacs in the lung called **alveoli**. Gas exchange occurs in the alveolar region.

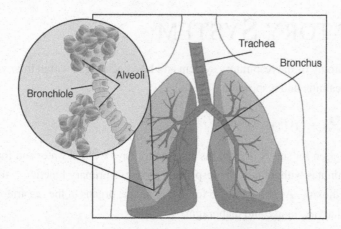

The **diaphragm** is a muscle that plays a large role in breathing. It is found at the base of the lungs and spreads across the bottom of the rib cage, forming the chest cavity. The human body has two lungs that vary in size and weight. The right lung, which is larger and heavier, has three lobes. The left lung has two lobes.

**DID YOU KNOW?**

The total surface area of the alveoli in the lungs is roughly the size of a tennis court. Such a large surface area is needed to facilitate gas exchange and ensure the body is oxygenated at all times.

## Example

**Which organ uses hairs to filter out particles that try to enter the lungs?**

A.  Alveoli          B.  Bronchus          C.  Larynx          D.  Nose

The correct answer is **D.** The nose is part of the upper respiratory tract. Because it is the site where air enters the body, nose hairs help prevent airborne particles from entering the lungs. **See Lesson: The Respiratory System.**

# Respiratory Functions and Breathing Mechanics

Recall that the primary function of the respiratory system is to provide oxygen to and remove carbon dioxide from the body. In addition to gas exchange, the respiratory system enables a person to breathe. Breathing, or inhalation, is essential to life. It is the mechanism that provides oxygen to the body. Without oxygen, cells are unable to perform their functions necessary to keep the body alive.

The primary muscle of **inspiration** is the diaphragm. Known as the chest cavity, this dome-shaped structure flattens when it contracts. The rib cage moves outward, allowing outside air to be drawn into the lungs. During relaxation, the diaphragm returns to its dome shape and the rib cage moves back to its natural position. This causes the chest cavity to push air out of the lungs.

The respiratory system can be functionally divided into two parts:

- **Air-conducting portion:** Air is delivered to the lungs. This region consists of the upper and lower respiratory tract—specifically, the larynx, trachea, bronchi, and bronchioles.

- **Gas exchange portion:** Gas exchange takes place between the air and the blood. This portion includes the lungs, alveoli, and capillaries.

Oxygen from the air enters the body through the respiratory system. But the cardiovascular system circulates oxygen throughout the body via the blood. As shown in the image, alveoli are surrounded by a capillary bed in the lung.

**Alveolus Gas Exchange**

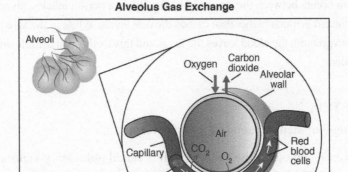

This anatomical structure allows blood to absorb oxygen and transport it through a network of blood vessels to cells in various tissues throughout the body. During the process of gas exchange, the blood system absorbs carbon dioxide from cells and carries it to the respiratory system, where it is exhaled from the body.

The respiratory system works closely with both the cardiovascular and nervous systems to maintain blood gas and pH **homeostasis**. The body must regulate blood pH levels. When there is too much carbon dioxide in the blood, it is acidic (that is, its pH value is too low). If there is not enough carbon dioxide in the blood, it will be too alkaline (its pH value will be too high).

**BE CAREFUL!**

When regulating blood gas and pH homeostasis levels, carbon dioxide, not oxygen, must be closely monitored.

## Example

**What structure is directly involved in gas exchange?**

A.  Alveolus           B.  Bronchiole           C.  Pharynx           D.  Trachea

The correct answer is **A.** The alveolus is a tiny air sac found in the lung. Its primary function is to help the respiratory system perform gas exchange. **See Lesson: The Respiratory System.**

# The Mechanics of Respiration

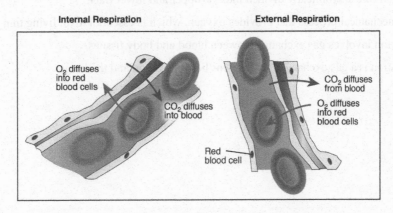

Internal Respiration

$O_2$ diffuses into red blood cells

$CO_2$ diffuses into blood

External Respiration

$CO_2$ diffuses from blood

$O_2$ diffuses into red blood cells

Red blood cell

As shown in the image, the process of gas exchange between the outside air and the body is called **respiration**. It occurs on two levels: internal and external.

- **External respiration** occurs between the lungs and blood. When a person inhales, alveoli fill with oxygen through **diffusion**. Oxygen content is much higher than carbon dioxide levels. While in the alveoli region, blood becomes oxygen-rich. Once oxygenated, the blood leaves the lungs and travels through the left side of the heart, where it is pumped into circulation.

---

**STEP-BY-STEP**

The following four steps summarize external respiration:

1. Air moves in and out of the lungs, which is called pulmonary ventilation.
2. Gases are exchanged between air and blood in the lungs by diffusion.
3. Gases are transported by circulation of the blood, with help from the heart.
4. Gases are exchanged by diffusion between blood and tissues throughout the body.

---

- **Internal respiration** occurs between the blood and tissues. Once blood enters circulation, it reaches the capillaries. Oxygen diffuses through the capillaries into the cells. Carbon dioxide diffuses from the cells into the capillaries. Because carbon dioxide content is higher than oxygen content in blood at this point, it is called oxygen-poor blood. This oxygen-poor blood travels to the right side of the heart. It moves through the pulmonary circuit, where external respiration begins.

## Example

**What happens during internal respiration?**

A. Air is inhaled into the body.

B. Oxygen-rich blood travels to the heart.

C. Air moves into and out of the pulmonary circuit.

D. Oxygen is exchanged for carbon dioxide in circulation.

The correct answer is **D**. During internal respiration, oxygen-poor blood is created as oxygen diffuses into the cells in exchange for carbon dioxide. **See Lesson: The Respiratory System.**

## Let's Review!

- The respiratory system supplies oxygen to the body and removes carbon dioxide.
- Blood pH levels are regulated by the respiratory, cardiovascular, and nervous systems.
- Respiratory organs are anatomically divided into the upper and lower tract.
- Breathing is a mechanical process that provides oxygen, which is essential to all living things.
- Internal respiration involves gas exchange between blood and body tissues.
- External respiration is a gas exchange that happens between blood and the lungs.

# THE GASTROINTESTINAL SYSTEM

This lesson introduces the structures and functions of the digestive system.

## Anatomy of the Digestive System

The following are the functions of the digestive system:

1. Take in food.
2. Break down food.
3. Absorb digested molecules.
4. Provide nutrients.
5. Eliminate wastes.

The digestive system consists of the **digestive tract**, which is a tube extending from the mouth to the anus, and the associated organs, which secrete fluids into the digestive tract. The term **gastrointestinal tract** technically refers to only the stomach and intestines.

## The Path of Food

Food takes the path outlined below as it moves through the body.

- The **oral cavity**, or the mouth, is the first part of the digestive system. It is bounded by the lips and cheeks and contains the teeth and tongue. Its primary function is to masticate, or chew, and moisten the food.
- The **pharynx**, or throat, connects the mouth to the esophagus.
- The **esophagus** is a muscular tube about 25 centimeters long. Food travels down it to the cardiac sphincter of the stomach.
- The **stomach** is an enlarged segment of the digestive tract.
  - The opening of the stomach is the **cardiac sphincter**.
  - The muscular layer of the stomach is different from other regions because it has folds called **rugae** that increase the surface area.
  - The exit of the stomach is the **pyloric sphincter**.
- The **small intestine** is about 6 meters long and consists of three parts: duodenum, jejunum, and ileum.
  - The duodenum has more **villi** (finger-like projections), has a larger diameter, and is thicker than the other two parts.
  - This increases the surface area in the duodenum, which allows for more absorption of nutrients.
  - The small intestine is the primary site for diffusion of nutrients into the blood.
- The **large intestine** consists of the cecum, colon, rectum, and anal canal. The cecum is located where the small and large intestine meet.
  - The colon is about 1.5 to 1.8 meters long and consists of four parts: the ascending, transverse, descending, and sigmoid colon.
  - The primary function of the large intestine is to compress the waste and collect any excess water that can be recycled.

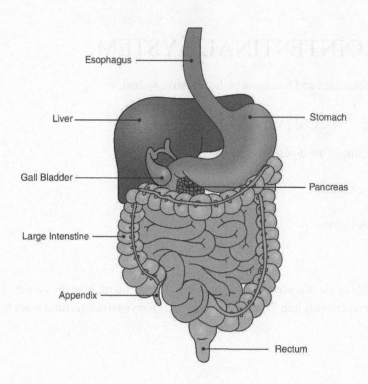

## Example

**Digestive organs include structures such as villi and rugae. Which of the following is a purpose they serve?**

A. Increase surface area

B. Increase blood supply

C. Increase mucus secretion

D. Increase bacterial content

The correct answer is **A.** Structures such as the rugae and villi increase surface area. This allows for greater absorption. **See Lesson: Gastrointestinal System.**

## Accessory Organs

**Accessory organs** contribute to the process of digestion. Food does not pass through these organs, but they play critical roles in the digestion of food. The accessory organs are listed below.

The **liver** weighs about 1.36 kilograms and is located in the upper-right quadrant of the abdomen. It is divided into two major lobes: the right lobe and left lobe. The liver has multiple functions:

- **Digestion:** Bile salts emulsify and help break down fats into fatty acids and glycerol.
- **Excretion:** Bile contains excretory products from the hemoglobin breakdown.
- **Nutrient storage:** The liver removes sugar from the blood and stores fats, vitamins, copper, and iron
- **Nutrient conversion:** The liver converts some nutrients into others. For example, it coverts amino acids to lipids or glucose
- **Detoxification of harmful chemicals:** The liver removes ammonia from the blood and converts it to urea.
- **Synthesis of new molecules:** The liver synthesizes new blood proteins such as albumins and fibrinogens.

The **pancreas** is a complex organ composed of both endocrine and exocrine tissues that perform several functions:

- It secretes bicarbonate ions, which neutralize acids.
- It secretes digestive enzymes that are important to all classes of foods.

- It produces insulin and glucagon, which regulate blood sugar levels.

The **gallbladder**, nestled under the liver, stores concentrated bile.

The **tongue** is a large, muscular organ that occupies most of the oral cavity. It moves food in the mouth and, in cooperation with the lips and cheeks, holds the food in place during mastication.

Saliva keeps the oral cavity moist and begins the process of chemical digestion with the enzyme amylase. There are three pairs of **salivary glands**:

- **Parotid** (largest, located in front of the ears)
- **Submandibular** (located below the mandible)
- **Sublingual** (smallest, located in the bottom of oral cavity)

These glands produce saliva, which is a mixture of serous (watery) and mucus fluids that contain digestive enzymes.

## Example

**Which of the following organs maintains a healthy pH level when a person eats an orange?**

A. Gallbladder

B. Liver

C. Pancreas

D. Tongue

The correct answer is **C.** One of the functions of the pancreas is to release bicarbonate ions, which neutralize acids.
**See Lesson: Gastrointestinal System.**

# Digestion

**Digestion** is the breakdown of food into molecules that are small enough to be absorbed into the bloodstream. There are two types of digestion: mechanical and chemical. **Mechanical digestion** breaks down large food particles into smaller ones and is evident as a person's teeth grind food into smaller pieces. During **chemical digestion**, digestive enzymes break covalent chemical bonds into organic molecules.

**Carbohydrates** are broken down into monosaccharides, **proteins** are broken down into amino acids, and **fats or lipids** are broken down into fatty acids and glycerol. Monosaccharides, amino acids, fatty acids, and glycerol molecules are small enough to diffuse across the membranes of the digestive system and enter the bloodstream, to be taken where they are needed.

**Absorption** begins in the stomach, where small, lipid-soluble molecules, such as alcohol and aspirin, can pass through the stomach epithelium into circulation. Most absorption occurs in the duodenum and jejunum, although some occurs in the ileum. Some molecules can diffuse through the intestinal wall. Others must be transported across the intestinal wall. Transport requires a carrier molecule. If the transport is active, energy is required to move the transported molecule across the intestinal wall.

**Enzymes**:

Most enzymes are recognizable by the *-ase* ending. Here are some of the most common enzymes:

- **Amylase** is produced in the mouth and breaks down carbohydrates.
- **Pepsin** is produced in the stomach and breaks down proteins.
- **Lipase** is produced in the pancreas and secreted into the small intestine to break down lipids.

- **Peptidase** is produced in the pancreas and secreted into the small intestine to brown down peptides into amino acids.

- **Sucrase** is produced in the small intestine and breaks down sucrose into glucose.

- **Lactase** is produced in the small intestine and breaks down lactose into glucose.

## Example

**What are the building blocks of carbohydrates?**

A. Glycerols

B. Fatty acids

C. Amino acids

D. Monosaccharides

The correct answer is **D.** Monosaccharides are the foundational units of carbohydrates.

**See Lesson: Gastrointestinal System.**

# Disorders of the Digestive System

The following are disorders of the digestive system.

**Stomach:**

- **Vomiting** results primarily from irritation of the stomach and small intestine. After the vomiting center has been stimulated, a sequence of events occurs that result in vomiting.

- **Ulcers** occur from a specific bacterium, *Helicobacter pylori*. Ulcers were previously thought to be caused by stress, but they can be treated successfully with antibiotics.

- **Peptic ulcer** is a condition in which the stomach acids digest the mucus lining of the duodenum. These ulcers are sometimes called **duodenal ulcers**. People who experience a great deal of stress tend to secrete as much as 15 percent more HCl than normal, which causes the **chyme**, semifluid food mass, to be highly acidic. There are not enough sodium bicarbonate ions to neutralize the acidic chime, and it eats away at the mucus lining, causing ulcers.

**Liver:**

- **Cirrhosis** is a disease characterized by damage or death of liver cells, which are replaced by connective tissue. This causes abnormal blood flow in the liver and interferes with normal liver functions.

- **Hepatitis** is an inflammation of the liver. Liver cells can die and be replaced with scar tissue.

**Intestine:**

- **Irritable bowel disease** is the general term for Crohn's disease or ulcerative colitis.

  o **Crohn's disease** includes a localized inflammatory degeneration that causes the wall of the small intestine to thicken. This disease causes diarrhea, abdominal pain, and weight loss.

  o **Ulcerative colitis** is limited to the mucosa of the large intestine. The involved mucosa exhibits inflammation, including edema, vascular congestion, and hemorrhaging.

- **Irritable bowel syndrome (IBS)** is a disorder of unknown cause in which intestinal mobility is abnormal. Patients exhibit pain in the left lower quadrant, especially after eating, and have alternating bouts of diarrhea and constipation.

- **Malabsorption syndrome** is a spectrum of disorders of the small intestine that result in abnormal nutrient absorption.

- **Appendicitis** is an inflammation of the appendix that usually occurs because of an obstruction.

## Example

**How is a duodenal ulcer different from an ulcer?**

A. Antibiotics are ineffective with ulcers.

B. A duodenal ulcer is only found in adults.

C. An ulcer can occur from a variety of bacteria.

D. An increase in stomach acids can produce a duodenal ulcer.

The correct answer is **D.** Duodenal ulcers can occur as a result of an increase in the acidic levels in the duodenum. Regular ulcers are caused by bacteria. **See Lesson: Gastrointestinal System.**

## Let's Review!

- The digestive system consists of the digestive tract, which is a tube extending from the mouth to the anus, and accessory organs.

- Accessory organs contribute to the process of digestion.

- Food does not pass through the accessory organs.

- Digestion is the breakdown of food into molecules that are small enough to be absorbed into the bloodstream.

- The two types of digestion are mechanical and chemical.

# THE REPRODUCTIVE SYSTEM

This lesson covers the human reproductive system. Through sexual intercourse, this system enables internal fertilization and delivery of an infant.

## The Male Reproductive System

Like all biological systems, the male reproductive system is comprised of several organs. These organs are located outside or within the pelvis.

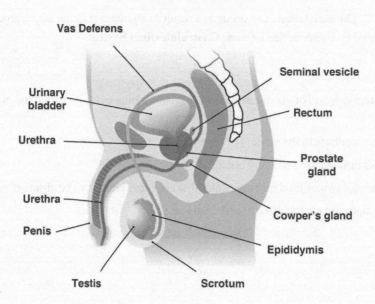

**Male Reproductive System**

The main male reproductive organs are the **penis** and the **testicles**, which are located external to the body. The penis is composed of a long shaft and a bulbous end called the glans penis. The glans penis is usually surrounded by an extension of skin called the foreskin (though this often is removed in a cosmetic procedure called **circumcision**). The penis has three internal compartments (the corpus cavernosum) that contain erectile tissue. When a male is sexually aroused, this tissue becomes suffused with blood, increasing pressure, and the penis becomes larger and erect.

The **testes** (analogous to the female ovaries), or testicles, are retained in a pouch of skin called the **scrotum**, with descends from the base of the penis. The scrotum contains nerves and blood vessels needed to support the testicles' functions. The scrotum also regulates the temperature of the testicles by contracting (drawing the testicles closer to the warmer body) or relaxing (allowing the testicles to move away from the warmer body).

Each testicle (or testis) produces **sperm** (analogous to the female ova), which are passed into a series of coiled tubules called the **epididymis**. The epididymis stores and nurtures sperm until they are passed into the **vas deferens**, a tubule that is about 30 centimeters long, extending from the testicle into the pelvis and ending at the ejaculatory duct. The epididymis and vas deferens are supported by several accessory glands (the seminal vesicles, the prostate gland, and the Cowper glands) that produce fluid components of **semen** and support the sperm cells. During male orgasm, semen passes through the ejaculatory duct into the urethra and is ejaculated from the penis through the urethral opening.

## Example

**Where is the male reproductive system located?**

A. The male reproductive system is located entirely within the pelvis.

B. The male reproductive system is located entirely outside the pelvis.

C. The male reproductive system is located primarily within the pelvis, though some components are outside the pelvis.

D. The male reproductive system is located primarily outside the pelvis, though some components are located within the pelvis.

The correct answer is **D.** Most of the components of the male reproductive system (penis, scrotum, testes, and epididymis) are external of the body, though some components (vas deferens and accessory glands) are located within the pelvis. The corpus cavernosum extends from within the pelvis into the penis. **See Lesson: Reproductive System.**

# The Female Reproductive System

Like all biological systems, the female reproductive system is comprised of several organs. These organs are located within the pelvis or external to the body.

The main female reproductive organs are the **uterus** (the "womb") and the **ovaries**, which are located in the pelvis. The ovaries (analogous to the male testes) produce several important hormones and the **ova** (analogous to the male sperm). After ovulation, the ovum is transported from the ovary to the uterus though the **Fallopian tube**. If sperm are present in the Fallopian tube, **fertilization** may occur. A fertilized **zygote** embeds in the endometrium of the uterus for gestation; an unfertilized ovum passes out of the body during subsequent menstruation.

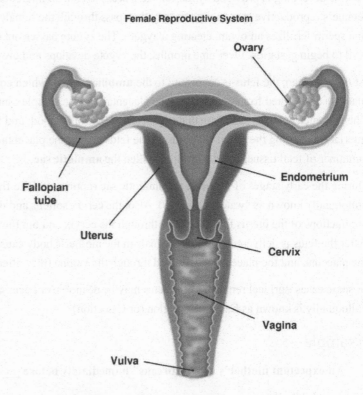

**Female Reproductive System**

- Ovary
- Endometrium
- Fallopian tube
- Uterus
- Cervix
- Vagina
- Vulva

The uterus has a lower opening called the **cervix**, which connects the uterus to the vagina. The female reproductive system has several organs that are external to the body, collectively known as genitals or, specifically, the vulva, including the labia (majora and minora), clitoris, and vaginal opening. When a female is sexually aroused, these external organs become suffused with blood, becoming larger and more erect, and the vagina becomes lubricated.

The uterus performs numerous critical functions during reproduction. It provides mechanical protection, nutritional support, and waste removal for the developing embryo (though a complex interfacing with the embryo's placenta). In addition, it is a powerful, muscular organ that is capable of contractions that push the fetus through the vagina at the time of birth.

HESI

## Example

**An embryo develops into a fetus in the _____.**

A. fallopian tube

B. ovary

C. uterus

D. vagina

The correct answer is **C.** The zygote implants into the endometrium (uterine wall) and develops into an embryo; the embryo then develops into a fetus within the uterus. **See Lesson: Reproductive System.**

# Reproduction

Human reproduce sexually, with a male partner (the "father") providing sperm and a female partner (the "mother") providing an ovum and all subsequent protection and nourishment until the fetus is delivered.

Post-natal feeding is provided by the female's breasts. Human intercourse consists of the male introducing sperm into the female's reproductive system. Sperm may then pass through the female's reproductive system to the Fallopian tubes where one sperm fertilizes an ovum, creating a zygote. The zygote passes out of the Fallopian tube and implants into the uterine wall to begin gestation. Over nine months, the zygote develops and grows into an **embryo** and then a **fetus**.

At the abdomen, the fetus is connected to the **umbilical cord**, which connects to the **placenta**. The umbilical cord and placenta are formed from fetal tissue. The placenta shares a complex interface with the endometrial lining of the uterus. The endometrium and uterus are maternal tissue. Hormones, food, and fetal waste all pass through the placental/uterine interface and along the umbilical cord. As the fetus grows, the placenta also grows. The fetus is encapsulated in a tough container of fetal tissue, filled with fluid, called the **amniotic sac**.

During the early stages of delivery, the amniotic sac ruptures and the fluid passes through the mother's vagina (this is colloquially known as "water breaking"). Also, the cervix softens and dilates to accommodate the fetus. Powerful muscular contractions of the uterus force the fetus through the cervix and out the vagina, normally with the head emerging first. After the fetus is delivered, hormonal signals in the mother's body cause the endometrial lining to quickly disconnect from the placenta, and the placenta is delivered through the vagina (the "afterbirth").

In some cases, surgical removal of the fetus may be desirable or necessary. This process delivers a live baby and colloquially is known as Caesarean section (or C-section).

## Example

**An expectant mother's water "breaks" immediately before _____.**

A. childbirth

B. fertilization

C. menstruation

D. puberty

The correct answer is **A.** The amniotic sac ruptures, releasing the amniotic fluid, in the early stages of childbirth. This rupturing releases a large amount of fluid and is colloquially known as "water breaking." **See Lesson: Reproductive System.**

# Development

Human newborn infants are unable to care for themselves and survive only with a large amount of parental care extending over at least the first several years of life. At birth, humans have all of the basic structures of the adult reproductive system, though some are undeveloped. At about 10–11 years old in females and about 11–12 years old in males, a child enters **puberty**, during which hormonal changes cause the reproductive system to develop fully. Puberty lasts for about 5–7 years.

**Menstruation** is a cyclical process occurring in the female body, especially the reproductive system, from about the end of puberty until menopause. During each period of menstruation, fluctuating hormone levels cause the uterus to change in anticipation of receiving a zygote. At the midpoint of the menstrual cycle, an ovum is released from an ovary and travels down the Fallopian tube. If the ovum is not fertilized, it passes out of the body along with the endometrium (lining of the uterus), causing menstrual bleeding. If the ovum is fertilized, the zygote implants in the endometrium and pregnancy follows.

There are significant differences between male and female bodies. The primary differences can be noted in the reproductive organs, but numerous other differences are the result of secondary sex characteristics. Male secondary sex characteristics include facial hair and a generally larger body. Female secondary sex characteristics include enlargement of the breasts and widening of the hips.

## Example

**Which statement best characterizes the changes that occur during puberty?**

A. Puberty is a recurring cycle involving fluctuating levels of hormones.

B. During puberty, the male's penis or the female's vulva develops basic structures.

C. During puberty, males and females reach sexual maturity and develop secondary sex characteristics.

D. Puberty occurs during the first trimester of pregnancy and results in the zygote developing into an embryo.

The correct answer is **C.** Puberty occurs during the early teenage years and results in sexual maturity. It is marked by the development of secondary sex characteristics. **See Lesson: Reproductive System.**

## Let's Review!

- The reproductive system enables sexual reproduction in humans.
- Components of the reproductive system are often known by multiple names, some of which are common or "slang" terms; the correct biological or medical terms are always preferred.
- The male reproductive system provides the sperm, the carrier of the genetic contribution from the father.
- The female reproductive system provides the ovum, or egg cell, which contains the genetic contribution from the mother. Additionally, the female reproductive system supports fertilization; provides the mechanical protection and nurturing environment needed for embryogenesis and gestation; and performs the actions necessary for the birth of the infant.
- The male testicles are analogous to the female ovaries. There are other similarities in the male and female reproductive systems.
- Sexual maturity occurs during puberty. Humans are capable of reproduction for several decades.

# THE URINARY SYSTEM

This lesson introduces the anatomy of the urinary system and how it functions. This lesson also explores the role of other body systems, particularly the circulatory and endocrine systems, in aiding with urinary excretion, absorption, and filtration.

## Anatomy of the Urinary System

Inside the body, the kidney, ureters, bladder, and urethra make up the **urinary system**, which is also called the renal system. The ureters, bladder, and urethra comprise the **urinary tract**. This system has many functions, some of which are outlined below:

- **Waste elimination:** Urea, creatinine, uric acid, and ammonium are the primary types of nitrogenous wastes excreted from the body. The urinary system also detects and excretes excess water from the blood and out of the body.
- **Osmoregulation of blood and water:** There must be a continual balance of water and salt in the blood. The urinary system, specifically the kidneys, help maintain this balance. It also balances levels of metabolites or electrolytes such as sodium, potassium, and calcium.
- **Hormone secretion:** The kidneys secrete several hormones to regulate processes that range from blood pressure and red blood cell production to calcium uptake via vitamin D.

Several of these functions are performed with help from other body systems, specifically the cardiovascular and respiratory systems.

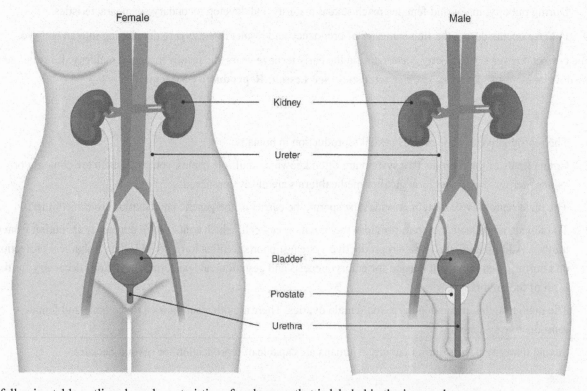

The following table outlines key characteristics of each organ that is labeled in the image above.

| Organ | Shape | Characteristics |
|-------|-------|-----------------|
| Kidney | Resembles beans, reddish-brown in color | The body has two kidneys, which excrete wastes in the urine out of the body. |
| Ureters | Tubular | Send urine from the kidney to the bladder. |
| Bladder | Pear (when emptied) | Stores urine until the body expels the fluid from the body. Has three openings: two for the ureters and one for the urethra. |
| Urethra | Tubular | Site where urine from the urinary bladder travels to an external opening. Removes urine from the body. |

The primary organ of the urinary system is the kidney. Blood from the heart flows through the kidneys via the **renal artery**. As blood drains from the kidney, it exits through a series of veins, the most prominent of which is the **renal vein**. When urine is produced, it does not drain through the tubes through which blood flows. Rather, urine flows through two ureters before emptying into the urinary bladder. The following steps outline how the urinary system works:

1. Kidney filters and excretes wastes from blood, producing urine.
2. Urine flows down the ureters.
3. Urine empties into the bladder and is temporarily stored.
4. Bladder, when filled, empties urine out of the body via the urethra.

**DID YOU KNOW?**

As a person ages, the kidneys and bladder change. This can affect functions such as bladder control and how well the kidneys filter blood. Kidney changes range from a decrease in kidney tissue to decreased filtration capacity. Bladder changes include decreased elasticity (which affects how much urine is stored) and weakened bladder muscles.

## Example

**Which organ of the urinary system filters blood?**

A.  Bladder        B.  Kidney              C.  Ureter              D.  Urethra

The correct answer is **B.** There are two kidneys in the body, which are located below the rib cage. The kidneys filter the blood that comes from the heart and remove wastes from the blood.

**See Lesson: The Urinary System.**

**BE CAREFUL!**

The kidneys do <u>not</u> make urine. They help regulate water balance, regulate levels of electrolytes such as sodium and potassium, and eliminate metabolic wastes. Urine is a byproduct of these functions.

# Nephrons and Urine Formation

The functional and structural unit of a kidney is a **nephron**. One kidney contains more than one million nephrons. An illustration of these functional units is shown below:

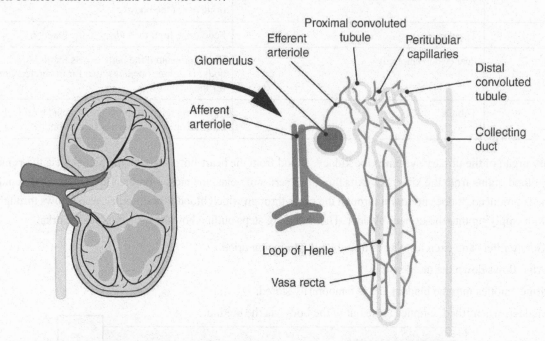

The nephron consists of two parts: the **renal corpuscle** and the **renal tubule**. The renal corpuscle can be divided into the **glomerulus** and **glomerular capsule** (or Bowman's capsule). The glomerulus is a type of capillary bed that functions as a filtration system, filtering solutes as blood enters the kidneys from the renal artery. Surrounding the glomerulus is Bowman's capsule. The renal tubule is a duct that connects to the glomerulus and terminates at the tip of the medullary pyramid. This tubule is divided into the following four regions: (1) **proximal convoluted tubule**, (2) **loop of Henle**, (3) **distal convoluted tubule**, and (4) **collecting duct**.

**KEEP IN MIND**

It is helpful to think of each nephron as a tiny filtering structure. Each nephron filters blood and forms urine. With more than one million nephrons in a single kidney, it is no wonder the kidneys are so efficient at filtering and excreting wastes from blood!

The components that make up the nephron filter blood and form urine. The following steps outline the pathway for urine formation. The steps are divided into three processes:

1. Glomerular filtration:

    A. Blood enters the kidney though the renal artery.

    B. This artery branches off into capillaries, allowing blood to flow into the glomerulus of the nephron.

    C. Blood pressure forces water and solutes (smaller than proteins) to diffuse from blood across the capillary walls and through pores of Bowman's capsule into the tubule.

2. Tubular reabsorption:

    A. The filtered fluid flows toward the proximal tubule. This is the major site of reabsorption of water and solutes such as glucose, amino acids, and certain ions.

    B. The fluid travels to the loop of Henle, which is another site of reabsorption.

    C. Next, the fluid reaches the distal convoluted tubule. Reabsorption and secretion take place in this segment.

3. Tubular secretion:

A. In the final segment, the collecting duct, fluid that remains in the duct is called urine. Reabsorption of some water and its return to the bloodstream may happen at this segment.

B. At this site, creatinine and other nitrogenous wastes are actively secreted into the urine so they can be excreted out of the body.

> **DID YOU KNOW?**
> About 180 liters of blood pass through the nephrons of the kidney each day. This explains why much of this fluid and its contents must be reabsorbed.

## Example

**Where does urine form?**

A. Loop of Henle

B. Collecting duct

C. Distal convoluted tubule

D. Proximal convoluted tubule

The correct answer is **B.** The nephron is the functional unit of the kidney. This structure consists of four major components: proximal and distal convoluted tubules, loop of Henle, and collecting duct. As blood travels through each of these segments, it is filtered to create urine in the collecting duct. **See Lesson: The Urinary System.**

# Urine Excretion and ADH

After blood is filtered through the nephron and the byproduct of urine is produced, urine accumulates in the collecting ducts of the nephron. Eventually, urine enters the ureters, which are muscular tubes. With help from muscle contractions, the ureters contract to move urine into the bladder. Urine is stored until the bladder is about half full.

Upon reaching this level, a neural impulse is transmitted telling a **sphincter** in the bladder to relax and allow urine to exit the bladder. Contraction of this sphincter, which is a muscular tube, is under involuntary control. Urine flows from the bladder into the urethra, which expels urine out of the body. A second sphincter enables urine to leave the body. This process is known as urination.

**BE CAREFUL!**

The urethra in males and females are different sizes due to the reproductive anatomy. The male urethra is about 20 centimeters long. It passes through the length of the penis and terminates at the end of the penis, where urine is removed from the body. The female urethra is about four centimeters long.

Recall that the urinary system works closely with the cardiovascular system to filter blood and return important substances back to the bloodstream during tubular reabsorption. To help maintain water and solute concentration either excreted from or reabsorbed by the body, the urinary system works with hormones that are part of the endocrine system to regulate this process. One of these hormones is the **antidiuretic hormone**, also known as ADH. This hormone is secreted from the posterior pituitary gland, which is found at the base of the brain.

One of the most important functions of ADH is to regulate urine concentration and volume by controlling how much water is reabsorbed in the tubules of the nephrons. The following image shows how ADH controls urine formation.

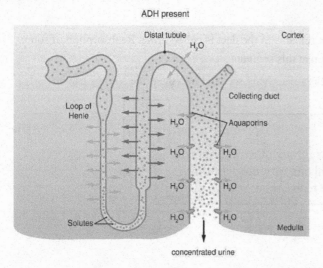
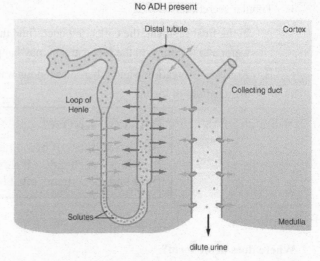

As shown in the image, when ADH is present, there is an increased permeability of water at the distal convoluted tubule and collecting duct. This causes more water to be reabsorbed and retained. It also decreases the volume of urine produced and concentrates the urine. The opposite occurs when ADH is not actively communicating with the kidneys and regulating urine formation.

**DID YOU KNOW?**

ADH control of urine formation is intimately connected to diabetes insipdus. When people have this disease, ADH does not communicate properly with the kidneys. As a result, symptoms include excessive thirst and frequent urination.

## Example

**The antidiuretic hormone primarily controls tubular reabsorption of which substance?**

A. Calcium          B. Creatinine          C. Urea          D. Water

The correct answer is **D.** Regulating how much water the body excretes or reabsorbs is a key function of the urinary system. To perform this function, kidneys must communicate with the hormone ADH, which is released from the posterior pituitary gland in the brain. **See Lesson: The Urinary System.**

# Urinalysis

Medical professionals can determine diseases that affect the urinary system by conducting a **urinalysis**. This type of test can reveal disease that does not necessarily present observable symptoms. Diseases confirmed through urinalysis include diabetes mellitus, different types of glomerulonephritis, and urinary tract infections. Both macroscopic and microscopic urinalysis can be performed.

- **Macroscopic urinalysis:** The first part of this testing involves visual observation of the urine. Normal fresh urine is pale to dark yellow in color. It is also clear and not cloudy. If the color is turbid or the urine is cloudy, there may be excess protein in the urine or the presence of a bacterial infection. Red or brown urine is considered abnormal. It could indicate that blood is present in the urine.

  An urine dipstick test is another type of macroscopic urinalysis. With this test, a plastic dipstick or paper strip is inserted into the urine sample. There are chemicals on the dipstick that cause it to change color when certain substances are present in the urine (at a specific concentration). Medical professionals can compare the color of the dipstick to a standard chart to analyze a urine sample.

- **Microscopic urinalysis:** This type of urinalysis requires the use of a light microscope. Typically, a urine sample is spun down, or centrifuged, in a test tube. This causes a sediment consisting of red blood cells, fat cells, and other large particles to aggregate and separate from the liquid portion of the urine.

When the liquid is removed, this sediment is mounted to a microscope slide and analyzed using a microscope. Typically, this test is performed to look at blood cells in the urinary tract, bacteria, parasites, or even tumor cells. This test also helps confirm the diagnosis of various urinary problems like kidney disease, cancer, microbial infections, and liver disease.

## Example

**What is most likely analyzed during microscopic urinalysis?**

A. Volume of water in urine

B. Amount of urea excreted

C. Sodium levels in the urine

D. Presence of white blood cells

The correct answer is **D.** During microscopic urinalysis, large substances like blood cells and bacteria are separated from the liquid portion of urine. These substances are placed on a microscopic slide and analyzed to make or confirm a diagnosis. **See Lesson: The Urinary System.**

## Let's Review!

- The urinary system eliminates wastes from the body, regulates blood and water levels, and secretes hormones that directly influence various physiological processes in the body.
- The circulatory and endocrine systems work with the urinary system to perform various functions.
- Nephrons are functional units and structures of the kidneys that play a large role in filtration, reabsorption, and secretion.
- After blood enters the kidneys through the renal artery, it is filtered in the glomerulus. Then, it travels through the proximal tubule, the loop of Henle, and the distal convoluted tubule before accumulating as urine in the collecting duct.
- The kidneys form urine as a byproduct, which travels through the ureter before being stored in the bladder and eventually excreted from the body via the urethra.
- Urinalysis is a method used to evaluate the quality of urine and help diagnose various urinary health problems.

# CHAPTER 11 HUMAN ANATOMY AND PHYSIOLOGY: ORGANIZATION OF SYSTEMS PRACTICE QUIZ

1. **What are the subdivisions of the dorsal cavity, located in the back of the human body?**

   A. Cranial and spinal

   B. Dorsal and ventral

   C. Lateral and proximal

   D. Inferior and superior

2. **Which of the following cavities contains the urinary bladder, part of the intestines, and the internal reproductive organs?**

   A. Abdominal

   B. Dorsal

   C. Pelvic

   D. Thoracic

3. **Which blood group is a universal acceptor?**

   A. A

   B. B

   C. AB

   D. O

4. **Which organ is responsible for producing oxygenated blood?**

   A. Heart

   B. Kidney

   C. Lung

   D. Stomach

5. **What structure channels food to the esophagus and air to the trachea?**

   A. Bronchiole

   B. Capillary

   C. Larynx

   D. Lung

6. **Which forms a network around the alveoli to facilitate gas exchange?**

   A. Rib cage

   B. Capillaries

   C. Bronchioles

   D. Epithelial cells

7. **What is the most common cause of appendicitis?**

   A. Spicy foods

   B. Poor nutrition

   C. An obstruction

   D. Inherited factor

8. **What organ of the digestive system has villi?**

   A. Pancreas

   B. Gallbladder

   C. Large intestine

   D. Small intestine

9. The ova are produced in the ___.

   A. vagina

   B. ovaries

   C. uterine wall

   D. Fallopian tube

10. Which statement about puberty is true?

    A. Puberty results from an unfertilized ovum.

    B. Males begin puberty at a younger age than females.

    C. Females begin puberty at a younger age than males.

    D. Puberty is a cyclical process occurring in the female body.

11. The antidiuretic hormone ADH is known to alter ____ concentration that is excreted from the urinary system.

    A. ammonia

    B. creatinine

    C. sodium

    D. urine

12. Where does fluid flow directly after leaving through the pores of Bowman's capsule?

    A. Bladder

    B. Glomerulus

    C. Loop of Henle

    D. Proximal convoluted tubule

# CHAPTER 11 HUMAN ANATOMY AND PHYSIOLOGY: ORGANIZATION OF SYSTEMS PRACTICE QUIZ – ANSWER KEY

**1. A.** The dorsal cavity has two subdivisions: the cranial cavity and the spinal cavity. **See Lesson: Organization of the Human Body.**

**2. C.** The pelvic cavity is a small space enclosed by the bones of the pelvis that contains the urinary bladder, part of the intestines, and the internal reproductive organs. **See Lesson: Organization of the Human Body.**

**3. C.** Type AB blood is a universal acceptor, while type O blood is a universal donor. **See Lesson: Cardiovascular System.**

**4. C.** The lungs contain oxygen that diffuses into the bloodstream, allowing deoxygenated blood to be converted to oxygenated blood. **See Lesson: Cardiovascular System.**

**5. C.** The larynx contains the voice box. It funnels air to the trachea and food past the epiglottis and down the esophagus. **See Lesson: The Respiratory System.**

**6. B.** Capillaries are blood vessels that form a network around the alveolar sacs to facilitate gas exchange between blood and the lungs. **See Lesson: The Respiratory System.**

**7. C.** The most common cause of appendicitis is an obstruction. **See Lesson: Gastrointestinal System.**

**8. D.** The small intestine has finger-like projections called villi covering the internal surface. **See Lesson: Gastrointestinal System.**

**9. B.** The ova are produced in the ovaries. **See Lesson: Reproductive System.**

**10.    C.** Females generally begin puberty at 10–11 years old; males generally begin puberty about a year later, at 11–12 years old. **See Lesson: Reproductive System.**

**11.    D.** The posterior pituitary gland at the base of the brain secretes the hormone ADH. This hormone alters how much water is excreted from urine by the kidneys. Thus, it controls the concentration and volume of urine in the body. **See Lesson: The Urinary System.**

**12.    D.** After filtered fluid leaves Bowman's capsule, which encloses the glomerulus, it travels to the proximal convoluted tubule before ending up in the loop of Henle. **See Lesson: The Urinary System.**

# Chapter 12 Human Anatomy and Physiology: Support and Movement

## The Skeletal System

This lesson introduces the anatomy and functions of the skeletal system. This lesson also explores how bone forms, remodels, and constantly changes as a person grows.

## Skeletal System Overview

A human is born with roughly 270 bones. As a person grows, this number decreases to approximately 206. This is because many of the bones fuse.

Anatomically, the skeletal system is divided into two major divisions: axial skeleton and appendicular skeleton. The **axial skeleton** consists of the bones of the skull, sternum, vertebral column, and ribcage. The **appendicular skeleton** comprises the bones of the upper and lower extremities and the associated girdles that connect the extremities to the vertebral column. The following table summarizes the number of bones found in each skeletal division.

> **FOR EXAMPLE**
>
> Half of the pelvic bone has three separate bones at birth: the ilium, ischium, and pubis. By adulthood, these bones fuse into one bone called the hipbone.

| Axial | 80 bones |
|---|---|
| Inner ear ossicles | 6 |
| Skull and hyoid | 23 |
| Sternum and ribs | 25 |
| Vertebral column | 26 |
| **Appendicular** | **126** |
| Pectoral girdle | 4 |
| Upper extremities | 60 |
| Pelvic girdle | 2 |
| Lower extremities | 60 |

Twenty-four of the bones in the vertebral column are called the pre-sacral vertebrae. These consist of 7 cervical, 12 thoracic, and 5 lumbar vertebrae. The last two bones of the vertebral column are the sacrum and coccyx.

The skeletal system consists of **bones**, **cartilage**, and **ligaments** that are tightly bound together to form a strong, yet flexible, framework. Bone is an active form of **connective tissue**. This tissue plays a role in many of the functions of the skeletal system:

- **Support:** Bones and cartilage support body posture because both structures are rigid. They also allow a person to remain upright and provide a framework to which soft tissues like muscles and organs can attach.

- **Movement:** Bones of the skeletal system interact with the muscular system to help he body move. Bones themselves cannot move. But when connected to each other by ligaments, along with the action of muscles, a human body can move.

- **Protection:** The skeletal system protects vital organs from external damage. The skull protects the brain, the vertebral column protects the spinal cord, and the sternum and ribcage protect the lungs.

- **Mineral storage:** Bone functions as a storage site for important minerals like calcium and phosphorus. These minerals are used for a variety of physiological functions in the body.

- **Hematopoiesis:** This is the process bones use to produce red blood cells and stem cells, which differentiate to a variety of different cell types in the body.

The following image illustrates the anatomy of the skeletal system.

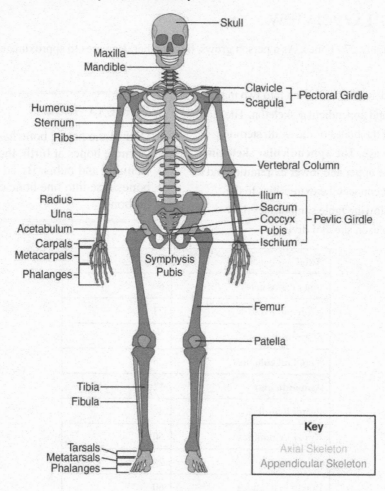

## Example

**Which of the following is part of the axial skeleton?**

A. Carpals      B. Femur      C. Patella      D. Skull

The correct answer is **D.** The axial skeleton consists of bones that do not belong to the upper and lower extremities: the skull, vertebral column, sternum, and ribcage. **See Lesson: Skeletal System.**

# Bone Shape and Structure

The overall structure of bone consists of an outer shell called **compact bone**. It encloses another type of bone tissue that is loosely organized called **spongy** or **cancellous bone**. Compact bone is made of units called **osteons**. These structures look like cylinders. They contain a mineral matrix and living bone cells. Each osteon also contains a **Haversian canal** that houses the bone's blood vessels and nerve fibers.

Surrounding the compact bone is a fibrous membrane called the **periosteum**. This consists of blood vessels, nerves, and lymphatic vessels that nourish the compact bone.

There are five types of bones in the human body: long, short, flat, irregular, and sesamoid. The following table details the characteristics of each and where they are found.

| Bone type | Appearance | Function | Example |
|---|---|---|---|
| Long | Elongated bones; longer than they are wide | Mechanical strength | Femur, tibia, clavicle, humerus, and metacarpals |
| Flat | Broad bones that are thin | Site of muscle attachment; provide protection | Scapula, hip bone (os coxa), sternum, nasal bone, and occipital/parietal/ frontal bones of the skull |
| Irregular | Have a non-uniform shape that cannot be classified as any other bone type | Mechanical support for the body | Vertebrae |
| Sesamoid | Small bones | Mechanical support; provide protection | Patella (kneecap) |
| Short | About same width as length | Provide support; little movement | Carpal and tarsal bones of the wrist and feet |

To visualize the anatomy of all bone types, it is helpful to view the anatomy of long bone. As shown in the following image, the long bone consists of three major sections: proximal epiphysis, diaphysis, and distal epiphysis.

- **Epiphysis:** This is found at each end of the long bone. It consists primarily of spongy bone with a thin layer of compact bone. Bone growth occurs at the epiphysis.
- **Articular cartilage:** This covers the epiphysis. It decreases frictions at the joints.
- **Diaphysis:** This is the longest part of the long bone. It consists primarily of compact bone.
- **Medullary cavity:** This is found inside the long bone. It is composed of red and yellow bone marrow. Red marrow is where hematopoiesis occurs. Yellow marrow consists primarily of fat cells.

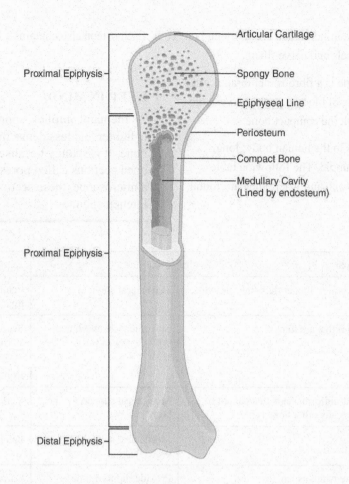

## Example

**A histologist cracks open a tibia. While viewing the inside, what does he see?**

A.  Diaphysis

B.  Soft tissue

C.  Spongy bone

D.  Proximal epiphysis

The correct answer is **C.** When looking inside a long bone, such as the tibia, the histologist sees the spongy bone. This is found at the proximal and distal ends of the epiphysis. **See Lesson: Skeletal System.**

# Ossification and Bone Remodeling

Although bone is a hard structure, it can grow. This is especially important in childhood. **Ossification** is the process of bone formation that occurs first during embryonic development. This process transforms soft, flexible cartilage to hard bone. It does so by replacing the cartilage with mineral deposits, specifically calcium and phosphorus. Ossification begins in the center of bones and spreads toward the end of the bones.

When a baby is born, a lot of cartilage is still found in the skeleton, particularly in the long bones. But there are **growth plates** at the end of long bones. This region is also made of cartilage. As the child grows, this area of cartilage at the growth plate experiences ossification to elongate the bone, enabling a person to grow taller.

Ossification also plays a role in **bone remodeling**. Mature bone tissue is constantly being broken down through a process called **bone resorption**. Through ossification, new bone tissue replaces this old bone. There are three types of bone cells:

- **Osteocytes:** These are bone cells. They produce collagen and other substances that create the extracellular matrix of bone.

266

- **Osteoblasts:** These are called bone-forming cells. They are found on the surface of bone and can be stimulated to differentiate into other type of bone cells called osteocytes.

- **Osteoclasts:** These are called bone-resorbing cells. They are found on the surface of bone. They dissolve the bone.

Recall that osteons are found in compact bone. As shown in the following image, the extracellular matrix of bone and osteocytes are found within the osteon. Osteoblasts and osteoclasts are found on the bone surface.

> **KEEP IN MIND**
>
> Bone resorption frees calcium and other minerals from bone for use in the body and clears out older pieces of bone. In doing so, this process promotes the deposition of new bone.

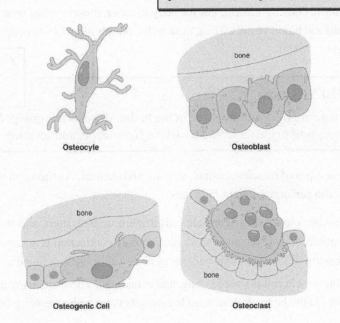

Osteocyte      Osteoblast

Osteogenic Cell      Osteoclast

## Example

**What bone cell is a bone-forming cell?**

A. Osteoblast      B. Osteoclast      C. Osteocyte      D. Osteon

The correct answer is **A.** Osteoblasts are bone-forming cells found on the bone's surface. They help form new bone as older bone is broken down through resorption. **See Lesson: Skeletal System.**

## Let's Review!

- The skeletal system provides structural support and protection, aids in movement, serves as a mineral reservoir, and helps produce cells.

- The appendicular skeleton consists of the upper and lower extremities.

- The axial skeleton consists of the skull, sternum, ribcage, and vertebral column.

- The five bone types in the human body are: long, short, flat, irregular, and sesamoid.

- Ossification is a bone-forming process typically performed in childhood.

- Bone remodeling is a process that involves replacing old, mature bone tissue with new bone.

- Osteons are bone cells found in compact bone that contain the Haversian canal, which is the site for blood vessels and nerve fibers.

- Osteoblasts are bone-forming cells, and osteoclasts are bone-dissolving or resorbing cells.

- Osteocytes are bone cells found deep within bone that produce substances like cartilage.

# THE MUSCULAR SYSTEM

This lesson introduces the anatomy of the muscular system, including the three different muscle tissues. This lesson also describes the role of the muscular system in movement and the physiology of muscle contraction.

## Anatomy of the Muscle

The **muscular system** is responsible for all types of body movement. Additional functions of this system include providing support, stabilizing joints, and generating heat for the body. All muscles consist of specialized cells known as **muscle fibers**, which contract to facilitate body movement. For the body to move, muscles must be attached to bones. Muscles are also attached to internal organs and blood vessels. Thus, most of the body's movements occur because of muscle contraction from muscle fibers.

> **DID YOU KNOW?**
> There are over 600 muscles in the body. Muscles are grouped according to characteristics such as size, shape, and location.

The body is comprised of three types of muscles: cardiac, smooth, and skeletal. As shown in the image below, these muscles look different. They also perform different functions.

- **Cardiac muscle:** This muscle consists of muscle cells that are striated, short, and branched. These cells contain one nucleus, are branched, and are rectangular. Cardiac muscle contraction is an involuntary process, which is why it is under the control of the autonomic nervous system. This muscle is found in the walls of the heart.

- **Skeletal muscle:** This muscle cell is striated, long, and cylindrical. There are many nuclei in a skeletal muscle cell. Attached to bones in the body, skeletal muscle contracts voluntarily, meaning that it is under conscious control.

- **Smooth muscle:** This muscle consists of non-striated muscle cells that are spindle-shaped. Like cardiac muscle cells, smooth muscle cells contain one nucleus. This muscle type is found in the walls of internal organs like the bladder and stomach. Smooth muscle contraction is involuntary and controlled by the autonomic nervous system.

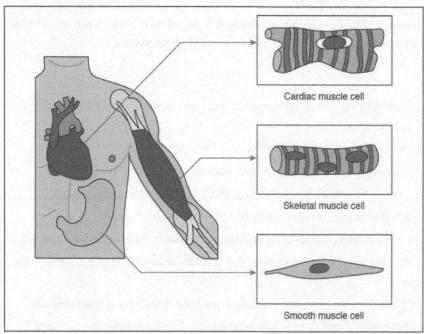

Cardiac muscle cell

Skeletal muscle cell

Smooth muscle cell

Despite the differences among cardiac, smooth, and skeletal muscles, they share four properties: excitability, contractility (muscle shortening), extensibility (muscle stretching), and elasticity.

## Example

**What is a purpose of the muscular system?**

A.  Connects one bone to another

B.  Helps the bones of the body move

C.  Protects the body from external injury

D.  Determines how blood circulates in the body

The correct answer is **B.** One of the primary functions of the muscular system is to aid in movement. Muscles help the bones of the skeletal system move. Muscles contract and relax to facilitate movement. **See Lesson: Muscular System.**

# Skeletal Muscle Anatomy

Bones move with the help of skeletal muscles, through contraction and extension. Skeletal muscles must be attached to the bones to pull on the bones and cause them to move. This movement is performed when the skeletal muscle shortens, or contracts.

As shown in the following image, connective tissue attaches skeletal muscle to bone or other tissues. Skeletal muscle consists of three types of connective tissue. The **endomysium** encases individual skeletal muscle fibers. These muscle fibers are bundled together by a connective tissue called the **perimysium**. Bundles of skeletal muscle fibers are called **fasciculi.** Each fascicle is bundled together by a strong connective tissue called the **epimysium.**

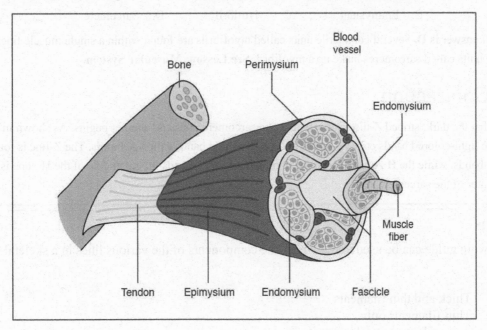

The cell membrane that surrounds a skeletal muscle fiber is called a **sarcolemma**. The cytoplasm of the skeletal muscle fiber is the **sarcoplasm**. One muscle fiber is filled with several long, cylindrical proteins called **myofibrils,** which are the contractile units of the fiber. The smallest contractile unit in a myofibril is a **sarcomere**. Several protein **myofilaments** make up a myofibril. There are two types of myofilaments: thick bands and thin bands. Thick bands, or myofilaments, are made of several protein molecules called **myosin**. Several protein molecules, called **actin,** link together to form the thin bands. These thin actin bands are attached to a **Z-disk** (or Z-line).

> **KEEP IN MIND**
>
> The connective tissue supports and protects muscle fibers. This tissue also provides a way for nerve and blood vessels to innervate the skeletal muscle.

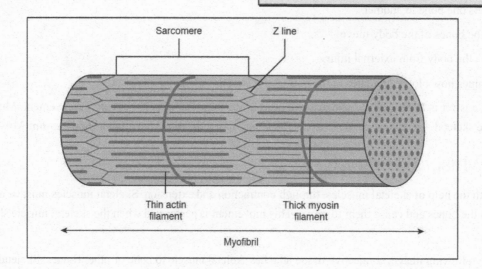

## Example

**What is the smallest contractile unit of skeletal muscle?**

A.  Actin          B.  Epimysium          C.  Myofibril          D.  Sarcomere

The correct answer is **D.** Several contractile units called myofibrils are found within a single muscle fiber. Smaller contractile units called sarcomeres make up a myofibril. **See Lesson: Muscular System.**

# Muscle Contraction

Keep in mind that the dark, striped Z-disc marks where one sarcomere ends and another begins. As shown in the image below, there are light-colored bands called **I-bands** and dark-colored bands called **A-bands**. The Z-line is found in the middle of the I-bands, while the **H zone** is found in the middle of the A-bands. In the middle of the H-zone is the **M line**, which is the center of the sarcomere.

> **TEST TIP**
>
> The following guide can be used to remember the components of the various lines in a skeletal muscle:
>
> A-band     Thick and thin filaments
> I-band     Thin filaments only
> Z-line     Actin filament attachment site
> H-band     Thick filaments only

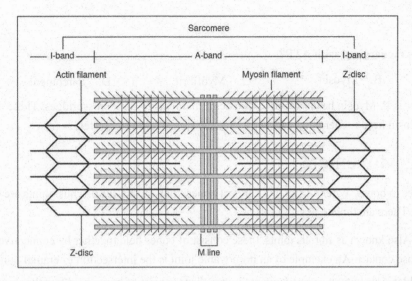

**Slide filament theory** explains muscle contraction. According to this theory, actin filaments slide past myosin filaments, pulling the actin filaments closer to the center of the sarcomere, or M line. As shown in the image below, this sliding action happens because of interactions between the heads of actin and myosin. The heads of myosin form attachments with the actin myofilaments. These attachments are known as **crossbridges**.

## KEEP IN MIND

The head of actin is a round protein shaped like a ball. Several of these round proteins link together to form a long chain, or thin myofilament. Myosin is a thick protein with a head that resembles a golf club. When several myosin proteins join together, they create a myosin filament, where the heads point outward.

With the help of energy in the form of ATP, the myosin heads are energized to attach to binding sites in actin and form a crossbridge. After energy in the myosin head is released, the myosin pulls actin myofilaments closer to the M line. This head can only form another crossbridge when another molecule of ATP attaches to the head, reenergizing it. Calcium also plays an important role in determining when contraction happens. This ion is found in the **sarcoplasmic reticulum**, which surrounds myofibrils.

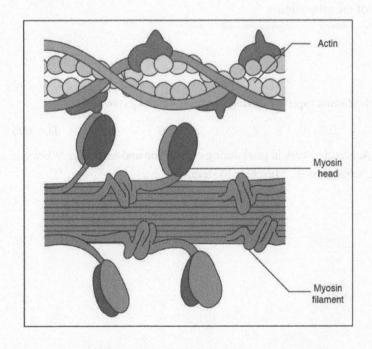

271

## Example

**What structure is reenergized with ATP?**

A.  Actin          B.  Myosin          C.  Myofibril          D.  Sarcomere

The correct answer is **B.** Myosin heads attach to thin actin filaments to form crossbridges. These attachments can only form when the myosin head is energized with ATP. **See Lesson: Muscular System.**

# Coordinating Movement

**Ligaments** attach bones to bones. Where ligaments connect bones, they form a **joint**. Thus, joints are the site where individual bones meet. There are three types of joints:

- **Immovable:** Also known as fibrous joints, these consist of bones held together by connective tissues. The bones are in very close contact. An example of an immovable joint is the intersection of cranial bones in the skull.

- **Partly movable:** Also known as cartilaginous joints, these consist of bones held together by cartilage. These joints allow some degree of movement. Partly movable joints include the vertebral discs in the spine.

- **Synovial:** These allow the largest freedom of movement because the bones are separated by a joint cavity. Examples of synovial joints are the hip and shoulder.

The muscular system works with the skeletal system to move the body. Thus, the muscles must be attached to bone. **Tendons** attach muscle to bone. Tendons consist of tough connective tissue that is found on either side of the joint where two bones are connected. Tendons work with skeletal muscles to move bones. When muscles contract, they shorten. This pulls on the bones, with the help of the tendon, to allow the body to move.

**FOR EXAMPLE**

Biceps and triceps muscles in the arm work together to bend and lengthen the elbow. As a biceps muscle contracts, the triceps muscle remains elongated, or relaxed. Thus, the biceps is the flexor and the triceps is the extensor of the elbow joint.

Muscles must work in pairs to move bones at the joint. The muscle that causes a joint to bend is called a **flexor muscle**. The muscle that contracts and causes a joint to straighten is called an **extension muscle**. If one muscle in the pair contracts, the other remains elongated.

## Example

**How many muscles must work together during contraction and extension?**

A.  2          B.  10          C.  206          D.  600

The correct answer is **A.** Muscles work in pairs during contraction and extension. When one muscle contracts, the other extends, or relaxes. **See Lesson: Muscular System.**

## Let's Review!

- A muscle is a fibrous tissue that aids in body movement, provides support, and generates heat energy for the body.

- Cardiac, smooth, and skeletal muscles are the three muscle types found in the body.

- Cardiac and smooth muscle are under involuntary control, while skeletal muscle is under voluntary control.

- Cardiac and skeletal muscles are striated, while smooth muscle is non-striated.

- Three types of muscle tissues comprise a skeletal muscle: epimysium, endomysium, and perimysium.

- A single skeletal muscle fiber consists of several contractile units called myofibrils, which consist of actin and myosin myofilaments.

- According to the slide filament theory, actin and myosin myofilaments form crossbridges to shorten a sarcomere, which shortens a skeletal muscle.

- Tendons attach muscle to bone and help bones move.

- Joints are the regions between bones that influence the degree of flexibility with body movement.

- Skeletal muscles move bones by working in muscle pairs to contract and elongate.

# THE INTEGUMENTARY SYSTEM

This lesson introduces the anatomy of the integumentary system, including the system's function. This lesson also describes the effects of aging and cancer on the integumentary system.

## The Skin's Many Layers

The **integumentary system** is a body system comprised of the skin and accessory structures, including the hair, sebaceous and sweat glands, and nails. This system protects the body, maintains homeostasis, and provides sensory information about the external environment.

The largest organ in the integumentary system is the skin. Often not thought of as an organ, the skin is made of four different tissues that work together to perform a variety of functions such as preventing toxic substances from entering the body and regulating body temperature.

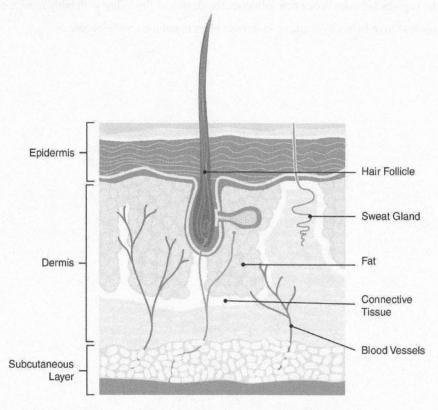

As shown in the image, the skin consists of several layers. These layers are divided into three regions: epidermis, dermis, and subcutaneous tissue. The **epidermis** is the outermost layer composed of **keratin** and stratified squamous epithelium tissue. Keratin is made of keratinocytes, which toughen and waterproof skin. Other cell types that make up the epidermis are melanocytes, which give skin its color, merkel cells, and Langerhans cells. The epidermis can have either four or five layers depending on where it is located on the body. As shown in the following image, these layers consist of the stratum basale (innermost layer), stratum spinosum, stratum granulosum, stratum lucidum, and stratum corneum.

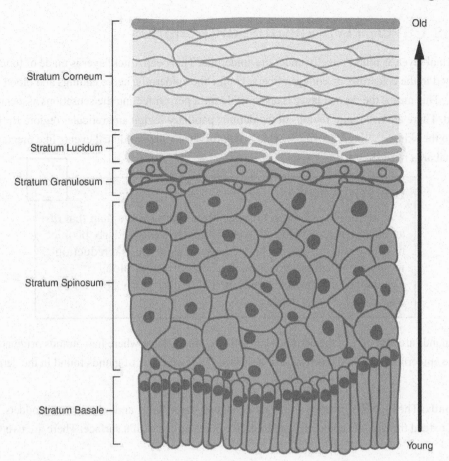

Nerve endings and blood vessels are not found in the epidermis. Epidermal cells are found deep in the stratum basale and constantly undergo mitosis to make new cells. As new cells are made, they travel to the outer skin surface, producing the protein keratin. Epidermal cells fill with keratin and die upon reaching the skin's surface. When this happens, the leftover keratin from the dead cells help form the stratum corneum, which is the waterproof layer. These dead epidermal cells are gradually shed from the skin and replaced with new cells.

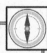

**FOR EXAMPLE**

The soles of the feet have five layers because they are exposed to a lot of friction as a person walks. The epidermis on the leg consists of only four layers.

## Example

**How many epidermal layers make up the face?**

A. 3          B. 4          C. 5          D. 6

The correct answer is **B.** The epidermis consists of either four or five layers. This depends on the part of the body where the epidermis is located. The soles of the feet and palms of the hand have five layers, and all other parts of the body, including the face, have four layers. **See Lesson: Integumentary System.**

# The Dermis Layer, Hypodermis, and Glands

The **dermis**, or dermal layer, is found directly under the epidermis. This deep, thick layer is made of tough connective tissue. It is connected to the epidermis by collagen fibers. Unlike the epidermis, nerve endings and blood vessels flow through the dermis. This means the dermal layer is responsible for a person feeling the sensations associated with touch, pain, heat, and cold. There are two major regions of the dermis: papillary region and reticular region. Both these regions provide elasticity to the skin, enabling it to stretch. This is helpful during physiological events like pregnancy, during which the abdominal area must stretch.

> **DID YOU KNOW?**
>
> The dermis layer of a young person is more elastic than that of an elderly person. This is because the dermis of elderly people has fewer elastic fibers. As the body ages, there is a reduction in physiological processes such as cell division, blood circulation, and muscle strength. These changes lead to a less elastic and thinner dermis.

Hair follicles and glands are also part of the dermis. Hair follicles are the sites where hair strands originate before protruding from the epidermal layer and onto the skin's surface. The two types of glands found in the dermis are detailed below:

- **Sweat glands:** These glands produce a fluid that contains water, salts, and other waste products. They are made of ducts that extend through the epidermis and look like pores on the skin's surface. There are two types of sweat glands:
  - **Apocrine:** These glands are found primarily in the armpits and groin area, where hair follicles are abundant. These glands are attached to hair follicles and create a watery fluid that contains proteins and fats. Apocrine glands are typically inactive until a person reaches puberty. They produce sweat when the body is anxious or experiencing stress.
  - **Eccrine:** These glands are found all over the body, primarily on the forehead, neck, palms, and soles of feet. They are not connected to hair follicles. They regulate body temperature with sweating if the body becomes too hot.
- **Sebaceous glands:** These oil-producing glands are typically attached to hair follicles. They release **sebum,** which is a fatty, oily substance. It waterproofs the hair and skin, preventing both structures from drying out. Sebum also has antimicrobial properties, which help the skin fight off infections.

> **DID YOU KNOW?**
>
> Sebaceous glands are found all over the body, but they are not found on the palms of the hands or soles of feet. The face and head contain the most sebum.

Right beneath the dermis is a third region of the integumentary system that contains subcutaneous tissue. This region is known as the **hypodermis**. It contains fat, or adipose tissue, that supplies energy for cells and provides insulation to regulate body temperature.

## Example

**Which structure produces sebum?**

A.  Hair follicles
B.  Eccrine glands
C.  Langerhans cells
D   Sebaceous glands

The correct answer is **D.** The dermis is made of sebaceous glands and sweat glands. Eccrine and apocrine glands are two types of sweat glands, neither of which produce sebum. Sebaceous glands produce sebum, which is a fluid that flows through a hair follicle. **See Lesson: Integumentary System.**

# Hair and Nails

Nails and hair are accessory organs of the integumentary system. Fingernails and toenails are made of keratin, which is also found in the hair and skin. In addition to mechanical functions such as grasping things and picking up objects, nails prevent injuries to the ends of fingers. As shown in the image below, the nail is made of several parts.

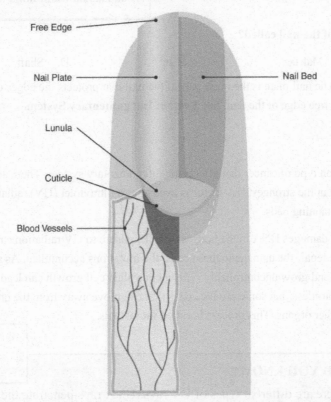

The nail plate is the hard outer part of the nail. Adjoining the nail plate is the free edge, which overhangs the fingertip. This is the part of the nail that is commonly groomed and cut down. The nail bed is a layer of skin found under the nail plate. This layer of skin is comprised of epidermal cells. The white space between the nail bed and **cuticle** is called the **lunula**. The cuticle is a layer of dead skin cells that accumulate and form a thick overhang layer at the base of the nail and around the nail edge. During nail care, cuticles are removed. Beneath the cuticle is the **matrix**, which is a layer of tissue that contains blood vessels and nerves.

# Hair

Hair consists of dead keratinized cells and grows from the dermis out of the epidermis and onto the surface of the body. This accessory organ provides insulation for the body, especially for the head.

Recall that within the dermis is the hair follicle. This is where hair strands in the epidermis originate. The **hair shaft** is not attached to the follicle. It consists of the hair that is exposed on the surface of the body. The **hair root** is attached to the follicles and found beneath the skin's surface. Extending beyond the root, deep beneath the skin is the **hair bulb**, which contains actively dividing basal cells.

**FOR EXAMPLE**

Consider eyelashes and eyebrows. These structures protect the eyes from irritants like dirt and water. In the nose, there are tiny hairs that trap dust particles and microorganisms to keep the air entering the lungs clean.

**KEEP IN MIND**

Aging affects the accessory organs. It causes hair and nails to thin over time.

## Example

**What is the outer layer of the nail called?**

A. Bed          B. Matrix          C. Plate          D. Shaft

The correct answer is **C.** The nail plate is the outer part of the nail that protects the edges of the finger. This structure is hard and connected to the free edge of the nail. **See Lesson: Integumentary System.**

# Skin Cancer

Skin cancer is the most common type of cancer that affects the integumentary system. There are many causes of skin cancer, including as genetics, but the strongest risk factor is exposure to ultraviolet (UV) radiation. Sources of UV radiation include sunlight and tanning beds.

Overexposure to UV radiation damages DNA in the body's cells. Exposure to UV radiation causes distinct mutations in skin cells. If the body does not repair the damage to these cells, the mutations accumulate. As a result, the cells can transform into cancerous cells and grow uncontrollably. The uncontrolled cell growth can lead to cancerous tumor formations. Most tumors are harmless, but some produce cells that can move away from the original site of DNA damage and establish new tumors in other organs. This process is called **metastasis**.

**DID YOU KNOW?**

There are different types of UV rays. UVA rays penetrate the dermis and can cause skin cancer. UVB rays penetrate the epidermis and cause damage to epidermal cells. UVB rays are responsible for sunburn and most skin cancers.

There are three types of skin cancer:

1. **Basal cell carcinoma:** This is the most common type of skin cancer that occurs in the basal cells of the epidermis. These cells are found in the stratum basale layer and divide to create keratinocytes. Basal cell carcinoma rarely spreads or undergoes metastasis.

2. **Squamous cell carcinoma:** This type of skin cancer occurs in the squamous cells of the epidermis. It affects the keratinocytes in the stratum spinosum. This is the second-most-common type of skin cancer. Because this type of skin cancer is more aggressive than basal cell carcinoma, if this carcinoma is not removed it can metastasize.

3. **Malignant melanoma:** This type of skin cancer occurs when there is an uncontrolled growth of melanocytes in the epidermis. Because melanocytes contribute to the pigmentation of the skin, melanoma is often associated with a dark patch on the body. It is the most dangerous and fatal type of skin cancer.

## Example

**What is a source of UV radiation?**

A.  Tanning bed

B.  Indoor lighting

C.  Topical products

D.  Outdoor irritants

The correct answer is **A.** Tanning beds and overexposure to the sun are common sources of UV radiation. UVA and UVB rays are known to cause skin cancer in people. **See Lesson: Integumentary System.**

## Let's Review!

- The integumentary system is a body system composed of the skin, hair and nails.

- Skin is the largest organ of the body that primarily functions to protect the body and maintain homeostasis.

- The epidermis, dermis, and subcutaneous layer are the three layers of skin.

- The epidermis has four or five layers: the stratum basale, stratum granulosum, stratum lucidum, stratum spinosum, and stratum corneum.

- Two types of glands, sebaceous glands and sweat glands, are found in the dermis.

- Eccrine glands are found all over the body. Apocrine glands are found mainly in the armpits.

- Hair, nails, and skin all contain keratin, which hardens and toughens each structure.

- Exposure to UV radiation can cause three types of skin cancer.

- Aging affects the integrity and structure of the skin, hair, and nails.

# CHAPTER 12 HUMAN ANATOMY AND PHYSIOLOGY: SUPPORT AND MOVEMENT
# PRACTICE QUIZ

1. **Which bone is classified as an irregular bone?**

   A. Coccyx

   B. Knee cap

   C. Humerus

   D. Nasal bone

2. **How many bones are in the adult human body?**

   A. 200

   B. 206

   C. 250

   D. 270

3. **Which muscle or region surrounded by a muscle is under voluntary control?**

   A. Bicep

   B. Heart

   C. Lung

   D. Stomach

4. **Which muscle causes a joint to bend?**

   A. Cardiac

   B. Extension

   C. Flexor

   D. Smooth

5. **The hypodermis primarily composed of ____ tissue.**

   A. adipose

   B. connective

   C. epithelial

   D. muscle

6. **Most common types of skin cancer directly affect the ____ of the skin.**

   A. dermis

   B. epidermis

   C. sebaceous glands

   D. subcutaneous layer

# CHAPTER 12 HUMAN ANATOMY AND PHYSIOLOGY: SUPPORT AND MOVEMENT PRACTICE QUIZ – ANSWER KEY

**1. A.** The coccyx is part of the vertebral column. This bone region is classified as an irregular bone. **See Lesson: Skeletal System.**

**2. B.** At birth, a human has roughly 270 bones. As some of these bones fuse, this number deceases to 206, the number of bones in the adult human body. **See Lesson: Skeletal System.**

**3. A.** A bicep is a muscle found in the upper arm. It is a skeletal muscle that helps move bones in the arm. A bicep is under voluntary control. **See Lesson: Muscular System.**

**4. C.** Flexor muscles are one part of a skeletal muscle pair that helps bones in the body move. They do so by causing a joint to bend. **See Lesson: Muscular System.**

**5. A.** The hypodermis is the subcutaneous layer beneath the dermis. It consists of fat, or adipose tissue, which serves as a layer of insulation deep inside the skin. This region also functions as an energy reservoir, supplying energy to cells. **See Lesson: Integumentary System.**

**6. B.** Basal cell carcinoma affects basal cells in the epidermis, while squamous cell carcinoma affects keratinocytes in the epidermis. Malignant melanoma affects melanocytes in the epidermis. **See Lesson: Integumentary System.**

# CHAPTER 13 HUMAN ANATOMY AND PHYSIOLOGY: INTEGRATION AND CONTROL

## THE NERVOUS SYSTEM

This lesson introduces the anatomy of the nervous system, including its functions and divisions. It also explores the parts of neuron, neural conduction, and synaptic transmission.

## What Is the Nervous System?

From perceptions to daily experiences, the **nervous system** controls many aspects of the human body. This system coordinates several activities in the body. It governs people's consciousness, their personalities, how they learn, and their ability to memorize. Working with the endocrine system, the nervous system regulates and maintains homeostasis.

The nervous system is anatomically divided into two parts:

1. **Central nervous system** (CNS): The central nervous system is comprised of the brain and spinal cord. It is where information processing and control occurs.

2. **Peripheral nervous system** (PNS): The peripheral nervous system is comprised of the nerves associated with the CNS. It connects all nerves of the body to the CNS. There are two types of fibers in the PNS: (a) **afferent fibers** that transmit impulses from organs and tissues of the body to the CNS; and (b) **efferent fibers** that transmit impulses from the CNS to the organs and tissues of the body.

The PNS is further divided into the somatic and autonomic nervous systems. The **somatic nervous system** primarily controls voluntary activities such as walking and riding a bicycle. Thus, this system sends information to the CNS and motor nerve fibers that are attached to skeletal muscle. The **autonomic nervous system** is responsible for activities that are non-voluntary and under unconscious control. Because this system controls glands and the smooth muscles of internal organs, it governs activities ranging from heart rate to breathing and digestion. The autonomic nervous system is further divided into the following:

- **Sympathetic nervous system:** The sympathetic nervous system focuses on emergency situations by preparing the body for fight or flight.

- **Parasympathetic nervous system:** The parasympathetic nervous system controls involuntarily processes unrelated to emergencies. This system deals with "rest or digest" activities.

**TEST TIP**

The first letter in the parasympathetic and sympathetic nervous system can be used to tell them apart:

**Sympathetic = stress**
**Parasympathetic = peace**

Based on the activities of the nervous system, this system can be functionally divided into three parts:

1. **Sensory:** Information is gathered (both internally and externally) and carried to the CNS. The senses gather the information that the sensory nervous system transmits.

2. **Integrative:** The integrative nervous system is where the CNS process and interprets information received from the sensory nerves.

3. **Motor:** Motor nerves convey information that is processed by the CNS to muscles and glands. The following flow chart summarizes the divisions of the nervous system:

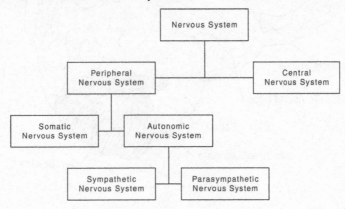

## Examples

1. **Which organ is part of the central nervous system?**

   A. Brain

   B. Heart

   C. Lung

   D. Stomach

   The correct answer is **A.** The nervous system is anatomically divided into two parts, the central and peripheral nervous systems. The central nervous system consists of the brain and spinal cord. **See Lesson: The Nervous System.**

2. **What part of the nervous system controls blood vessel contraction?**

   A. Autonomic

   B. Central

   C. Somatic

   D. Sympathetic

   The correct answer is **A.** The peripheral nervous system is divided into the somatic and autonomic nervous systems. The autonomic nervous system transmits neural signals to the smooth muscle found in the walls of internal organs and structures like blood vessels. **See Lesson: The Nervous System.**

# Anatomy of the Brain

The brain is a mass of tissue that is made of billions of nerve cells called neurons. This complex organ controls a wide range of processes and integrates information received from the five senses. Protected by the skull, the brain consists of four cavities called **ventricles**. These cavities are filled with **cerebrospinal fluid (CSF)**, which surrounds the CNS. This fluid serves many purposes such as protecting the brain from physical shocks and removing wastes from the neural tissue in the brain.

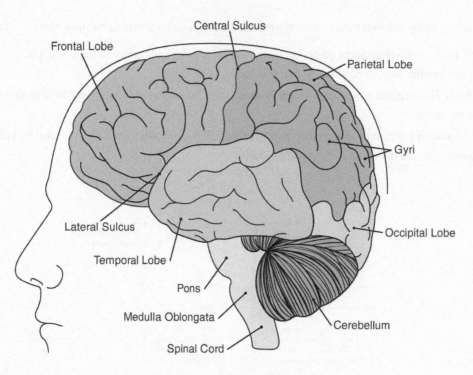

As shown in the above image, the brain is divided into the following three regions:

- **Cerebellum:** This is found beneath the cerebrum and behind the brainstem. It helps coordinate body movements, posture, and balance.

- **Brainstem:** This is found between the thalamus and the spinal cord. It is the lowest part of the brain that connects the brain with the spinal cord. Unconscious functions like breathing, heart rate, and blood pressure are controlled by the brainstem.

- **Cerebrum:** This part of the brain is the largest and part of the **forebrain**. The cerebrum controls higher-order functions such as interpreting touch, speech and language, reasoning, emotions, and fine motor control.

The **cerebral cortex** is **grey (or gray) matter** that surrounds the entire cerebrum. It is divided into a left and right hemisphere. The ridges of the cerebral cortex are called **gyri**, and the grooves are called **sulci**. The very large grooves are called **fissures**. The cerebral cortex is divided into four lobes: the frontal, parietal, temporal, and occipital lobe. The cerebral cortex is the most complex part of the brain, and each lobe has specific functions that are outlined in the following table.

**KEEP IN MIND**

The lobes are named after the bones of the skull that protect each lobe. For example, the frontal bone protects the frontal lobe.

| Lobe | Function |
| --- | --- |
| Frontal | Processes high-level cognitive skills, reasoning, concentration, motor skills, language, and functions as a control center for emotions. |
| Parietal | Integration site for visual perception and sensory information such as touch, pain, and pressure. |
| Temporal | Organizes sounds and processes language that is heard. Helps form memories, speech perception, and language skills. |
| Occipital | Interprets visual stimuli and information. |

## Example

**What lobe helps a person interpret information received from the retinas of eyes?**

A. Frontal        B. Occipital        C. Parietal        D. Temporal

The correct answer is **B**. The occipital lobe is part of the cerebrum. It interprets visual stimuli and information that comes from the eyes. **See Lesson: The Nervous System.**

# The Thalamus and Limbic System

Recall that the cerebral cortex is composed of grey matter. This mater is a type of neural tissue that contains three types of **neurons**, which are nerve cells that make up the nervous system:

- **Sensory neurons:** Afferent nerve cells that send information toward the CNS. This information is what is sensed, using the five senses, from the external environment.

- **Motor neurons:** Efferent nerve cells that carry impulses away from the CNS to the effectors, which are typically tissues and muscles of the body.

- **Interneurons:** Nerve cells that act as a bridge between motor and sensory neurons in the CNS. These neurons help form neural circuits, which helps neurons communicate with each other.

**BE CAREFUL!**

Grey matter is different from **white matter.** White matter is found in the spinal cord and surrounds the grey matter. It contains bundles of interneurons.

Another part of the forebrain incudes the **limbic system**, which controls emotions and memory. As shown in the image, this system is found right beneath the cerebral cortex and sits above the brainstem.

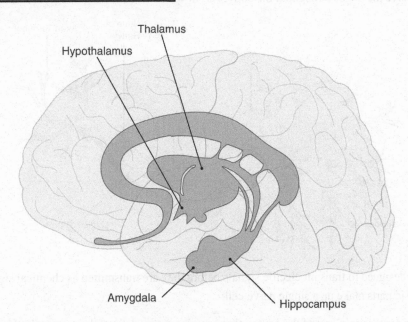

Four major structures of the brain comprise the limbic system:

- **Hypothalamus:** Found below the thalamus, this structure plays a role in regulating the autonomic nervous system. It is primarily concerned with homeostasis and regulates various activities such as hunger, anger, and the response to pain. The hypothalamus works with the pituitary gland from the endocrine system. This gland uses hormones, or chemical messengers, to generate responses in the body.

285

- **Amygdala:** Recognized as the aggression center, areas of this region produces feelings such as anger, violence, fear, and anxiety.

- **Thalamus:** Different sensory inputs come through the nerves and end at the thalamus, which directs this information to various parts of the cerebral cortex. The sense of smell is the only sense that bypasses the thalamus. Information related to movement is also processed by the thalamus.

- **Hippocampus:** Helps convert short-term memory to long-term memory. If the hippocampus is destroyed, new memories cannot be formed but old memories are retained.

---

**DID YOU KNOW?**

Kluver-Bucy syndrome is a condition that includes destruction of the amygdala. This means a person will present with erratic emotional behavior symptoms like hypersexuality, compulsive eating, and putting objects in the mouth.

---

## Example

**Which structure controls memory?**

A. Amygdala          B. Hippocampus          C. Hypothalamus          D. Thalamus

The correct answer is **B.** All these structures are part of the limbic system and perform specific functions in the body. The hippocampus converts short-term memory into long-term memory. **See Lesson: The Nervous System.**

# Anatomy of a Neuron

Recall that the nervous system is comprised of specialized cells called neurons. A large network of neurons work together to quickly send and receive messages throughout the body. As shown in the following image, a neuron has several parts.

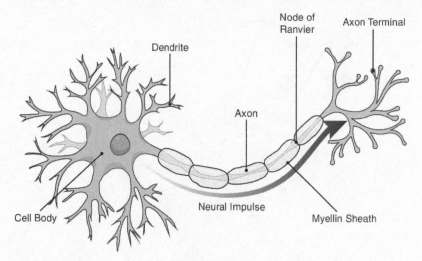

A neuron's structure is designed to transmit electric signals before they are transmitted as chemical signals to a target cell. The following three basic parts make up a single nerve cell:

- **Cell body:** This is the main part of the neuron that contains the nucleus of the nerve cell. Also called the soma, other organelles are also found in the cell body.

- **Dendrites:** These are appendages attached to the cell body that receive signals from other neurons.

- **Axon:** This is the long structure attached to the cell body. It conducts and transmits information to other cells. Branches at the end of the axon form **axon terminals**. These branches facilitate communication between neurons and target cells.

Also shown in the image is a **myelin sheath** and **node of Ranvier**. The myelin sheath is a protein and lipid structure produced by a type of glial cell called a **Schwann cell**. This sheath functions like a blanket that provides a layer of insulation around the axon of a neuron, increasing the speed of electrical signal transmission. Regularly spaced gaps called nodes of Ranvier are found between the myelinated sheaths. Electric signals jump from one node to the next, thereby increasing the speed of signal transmission.

**DID YOU KNOW?**

Several diseases cause degeneration of the myelin sheath, or **demyelination**. One example is multiple sclerosis. When demyelination occurs, it can lead to severe neurological problems like motor and cognitive function. Demyelination reduces the speed at which neural impulses are transmitted along the axon.

## Examples

1. **What structure receives information from another neuron?**

   A. Axon      B. Dendrite      C. Myelin      D. Soma

   The correct answer is **B**. Dendrites are appendages attached to the cell body, or soma, of a neuron. They receive information from other neurons and transmit this information to the cell body.
   **See Lesson: The Nervous System.**

2. **How many types of neuroglia are found in the CNS?**

   A. 2      B. 4      C. 11      D. 17

   The correct answer is **B**. Neuroglia are cells that support neurons in the body. More neuroglia are present in the body than neurons. Four types are found in the CNS, and two types are found in the PNS. **See Lesson: The Nervous System.**

## Synaptic Transmission and Nerve Impulses

The electric signals neurons transmit are called **neural impulses**. Neurons must be excited to create a nerve impulse. A stimulus triggers excitation. At the resting state, the inside of the neuron is more negatively charged, while the outside of the neuron is more positively charged. This difference in electrical charge because of potassium and sodium ions establishes the **resting potential**.

**DID YOU KNOW?**

As a person ages, the rate of **neuroplasticity**, or ability for the brain to form neural connections through synapses, decreases. Neuroplasticity is important because it helps the brain adapt to new stimulation, damage, or changes in the environment.

During an **action potential**, a reverse in electrical charge occurs across the membrane of a neuron in its resting state. As shown in the following image, this happens when a neuron receives a neural impulse by way of a stimulus or a chemical signal from another neuron. The inside of the neuron becomes more positively charged, while the outside of the neuron becomes more negatively charged. This reverse in charge travels down the axon as an electric current.

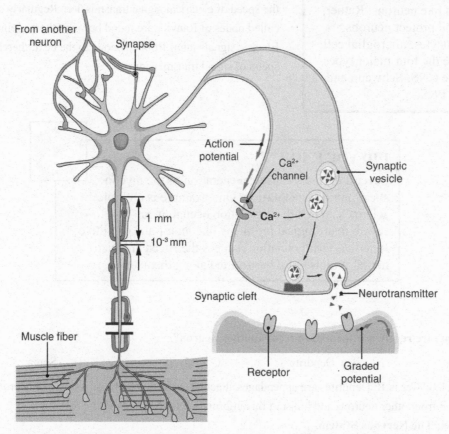

Once the action potential reaches the terminal bulbs of the axon terminal, the synaptic transmission process begins. The sequential numbers in the image outline the steps of synaptic transmission. The details of each numbered step are outlined below:

1.  An action potential travels down the axon and reaches the terminal branches of the axon. Voltage gated sodium gates open, causing sodium to enter the axon terminal bulb.

2.  Voltage gated $Ca^{2+}$ channels open at the same time.

3.  Calcium ions move into the axon terminal bulb of the presynaptic neuron.

4.  Calcium ions bind with proteins on synaptic vesicles that carry chemical messages called **neurotransmitters**.

5.  This binding causes the vesicles to contract and move to the presynaptic membrane.

6.  Neurotransmitters are released from the vesicles via exocytosis and diffuse across the **synaptic cleft**.

7.  Neurotransmitters bind with receptors on the postsynaptic membrane of a neuron, gland, or muscle.

8.  Depending on what the postsynaptic target cell is, the following responses will happen:

    *   Axon to dendrite: Action potential travels to next neuron.

    *   Axon and muscle cell: Muscle contraction.

    *   Axon and gland: Hormones released from gland.

## Example

**Which ion helps establish an action potential along an axon?**

A. Barium       B. Calcium       C. Magnesium       D. Potassium

The correct answer is **D.** Electrical impulses travel along the axon of a neuron when the inside of a cell is positively charged and the outside of a cell is negatively charged. This difference in charge is due an exchange in the flow of sodium and potassium ions in and out the cell. **See Lesson: The Nervous System.**

## Let's Review!

- The nervous system is divided into the central nervous system (CNS) and peripheral nervous system (PNS).
- The somatic nervous system controls voluntary activities, while the autonomic nervous system is responsible for involuntary activities under unconscious control.
- The nervous system performs sensory, integrative, and motor functions.
- The three major regions of the brain are the cerebrum, brainstem, and cerebellum.
- Four lobes comprise the cerebral cortex, which is grey matter that surrounds the cerebrum.
- The limbic system consists of the hypothalamus, thalamus, hippocampus, and amygdala, each of which has different purposes.
- Neurons are made of dendrites, a cell body, an axon, and an axon terminal.
- Myelin sheaths insulate the axon of neuron, increasing the spread of electric signal transmission.
- A neuron must be excited from a stimulus to create a nerve impulse.
- Resting potentials are established when the outside of a nerve cell is more positively charged than the inside of a nerve cell.
- Action potentials are established when the reverse of a resting potential occurs.
- Synaptic transmission occurs in several steps and only occurs following an action potential.
- Neurotransmitters are chemical messengers released during an electrically stimulated synaptic transmission process.

# THE ENDOCRINE SYSTEM

This lesson introduces the endocrine system and the role it plays in the maintenance of homeostasis.

## Functions of the Endocrine System

The endocrine system works with the nervous system to regulate the activities critical to the maintenance of homeostasis. The following are the main functions of the endocrine system:

- Water balance
- Uterine contractions and milk release
- Growth, metabolism, and tissue maturation
- Ion regulation
- Heart rate and blood pressure regulation
- Blood glucose control
- Immune system regulation
- Reproductive functions control

## Chemical Signals

Chemical signals, or **ligands**, are molecules released from one location that move to another location to produce a response. **Intracellular chemical signals** are produced in one part of a cell, such as the cell membrane, and travel to another part *of the same cell* and bind to receptors, either in the cytoplasm or in the nucleus. **Intercellular chemical signals** are released from one cell, are carried in the intercellular fluid, and bind to receptors that are found in *other* cells, but usually not in all cells of the body.

Intercellular chemical signals can be placed into functional categories on the basis of the tissues from which they are secreted and the tissues they regulate.

**Autocrine chemical signals:** These chemical signals are released by cells and have a local effect on the same cell type. Example: prostaglandin-like chemicals that are secreted in response to inflammation.

**Paracrine chemical signals:** These chemical signals are released by cells and have effects on other cell types. Example: somatostatin, secreted by the pancreas, inhibits the release of insulin by other cells in the pancreas.

**Neuromodulators and neurotransmitters:** These chemical signals are secreted by nerve cells and aid the nervous system. Example: acetylcholine produced during stressful encounters.

**Pheromones:** These chemical signals are secreted into the environment and modify the behavior and physiology of other individuals. Example: those produced by women can influence the length of the menstrual cycle of other women.

## Example

**Which chemical signal would respond to the redness caused by an infected wound?**

A. Autocrines

B. Neuromodulators

C. Paracrines

D. Pheromones

The correct answer is **A**. Autocrine chemical signals include prostaglandin-like chemicals that are secreted in response to inflammation, which can indicate an infection. **See Lesson: Endocrine System.**

# Receptors

Chemical signals bind to proteins or glycoproteins called **receptor molecules** to produce a response. The shape and chemical characteristics of each receptor site allow only certain chemical signals to bind to it. This tendency is called **specificity**.

There are two major types of receptor molecules that respond to an intercellular chemical signal:

**Intracellular receptors:** These receptors are located in either the cytoplasm or the nucleus of the cell. Signals diffuse across the cell membrane and bind to the receptor sites on intracellular receptors.

**Membrane-bound receptors:** These receptors extend across the cell membrane, with their receptor sites on the outer surface of the cell membrane. They respond to intercellular chemical signals that are large, water-soluble molecules that do not diffuse across the cell membrane.

When an intercellular signal binds to a membrane-bound receptor, three general types of responses are possible:

**Receptors that directly alter membrane permeability:** For example, acetylcholine (adrenaline) from nerve fiber endings binds to receptors that are part of the membrane channels for sodium ions.

**Receptors and G proteins:** A G proteins (guanine nucleotide-binding proteins) are found on the inner surface of the plasma membrane and function as receptors of hormones. For example, chemical signals include cyclic adenosine monophosphate glycerol and inositol triphosphate that bind to receptor molecules in the cell and alter their activity to produce a response.

**Receptors that alter the activity of enzymes:** For example, increasing the activity of an enzyme responsible for the breakdown of glycogen into glucose makes glucose available as an energy source for muscle contractions.

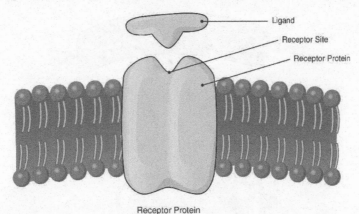

Some intercellular chemical signals diffuse across cell membranes and bind to intracellular receptors. Because these intracellular chemical signals are relatively small and soluble in lipids, they can diffuse through the cell membrane. The chemical signal and the receptor bind to DNA in the nucleus and increase specific messenger RNA synthesis in the nucleus of the cell. The messenger RNA then moves to the ribosomes, then to the cytoplasm, where new proteins are produced.

In contrast, intercellular chemical signals that bind to membrane-bound receptors produce rapid responses. For example, a few intercellular chemical signals can bind to their membrane-bound receptors, and each activated receptor can produce many intracellular chemical signal molecules that rapidly activate many specific enzymes inside the cell. This pattern of response is called the **cascade effect**.

## Example

**A friend is changing the tire on her car, and the jack breaks. Her hand is caught under the car. A passerby notices, runs over, and lifts the car off her hand. Which type of intercellular signal has responded?**

A. Receptors and G proteins

B. Receptors that alter the activity of enzymes

C. Receptors that directly alter membrane permeability

D. Receptors that indirectly alter membrane permeability

The correct answer is **C.** Nerve fiber endings bind to receptors that are part of the membrane channels for sodium ions to enable adrenaline to respond. **See Lesson: Endocrine System.**

# Hormones

The term **endocrine** implies that intercellular chemical signals are produced within and secreted from endocrine glands, but the chemical signals have effects at locations that are away from, or separate from, the endocrine glands that secrete them. The intercellular chemical signals, or hormones, are transported in the blood to tissues some distance from the glands. **Hormones** are produced in minute amounts by a collection of cells to influence the activity of those tissues in a specific way. For example, **neurohormones** are hormones secreted from cells of the nervous system.

Hormones are distributed in the blood to all parts of the body, but only certain tissues, called **target tissues**, respond to each type of hormone. Target tissue is made up of cells that have receptor molecules for a specific hormone. Each hormone can only bind to its receptor molecules and cannot influence the function of cells that do not have receptor molecules for the hormone.

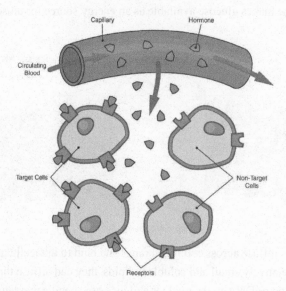

## Regulation of Hormone Secretion

The secretion of hormones is controlled by negative-feedback mechanisms. Negative-feedback mechanisms keep the body functioning within a narrow range of values consistent with life. Hormone secretion is regulated in three ways:

1. **Blood levels of chemicals:** The secretion of some hormones is directly controlled by the blood levels of certain chemicals. For example, blood glucose levels control insulin secretion.

2. **Hormones:** The secretion of some hormones is controlled by other hormones. For example, hormones from the pituitary gland act on the ovaries and the testes, causing those organs to secrete sex hormones.

3. **Nervous system:** These hormones are controlled by the nervous system. For example, epinephrine is released from the adrenal medulla as a result of nervous system stimulation.

## Example

**The negative-feedback mechanism that regulates the level of glucose in a person's blood is an example of what type of hormone secretion regulation?**

    A.  Hormone regulation

    B.  Nervous system regulation

    C.  Blood levels of chemical regulation

    D.  Intercellular ion concentration regulation

The correct answer is **C.** The blood levels of certain chemicals, such as insulin, directly control the secretion of some hormones. **See Lesson: Endocrine System.**

# Endocrine Glands and Their Secretions

The endocrine system consists of ductless glands that secrete hormones directly into the blood. An extensive network of blood vessels supplies the endocrine glands. The following is a table of hormones secreted by the anterior pituitary gland.

| Anterior Pituitary Gland | | |
|---|---|---|
| **Hormone** | **Target** | **Response** |
| Growth hormone | Most tissues | Increases protein synthesis |
| Thyroid-stimulating hormone | Thyroid gland | Increases thyroid hormone secretion |
| Adrenocorticotropic | Adrenal cortex | Increases secretion of cortisol |
| Melanocyte-stimulating hormone | Melanocytes in skin | Increases melanin production to make skin darker |
| Luteinizing hormone | Females: ovaries<br>Males: testes | Females: promotes ovulation<br>Males: promotes sperm cell production |
| Follicle-stimulating hormone | Females: ovarian follicles<br>Males: seminiferous tubules | Females: promotes follicle maturation<br>Males: promotes sperm cell production |
| Prolactin | Ovary and mammary glands | Prolongs progesterone secretion |

Additional common hormones are listed in the chart below.

| Gland | Hormone | Target Tissue | Response | Under- or Overproduction of Hormone |
|-------|---------|---------------|----------|-------------------------------------|
| Thyroid gland | Thyroid hormone | Most cells of the body | Increases metabolic rate | Hypothyroidism Hyperthyroidism |
| Adrenal medulla | Epinephrine | Heart, blood vessels, liver, adipose cells | Increases cardiac output and blood flow | Addison's disease |
| Pancreas | Insulin and glucagon | Liver, skeletal muscles, and adipose tissue | Insulin: increases uptake and use of glucose Glucagon: increases breakdown of glycogen | Diabetes |

## The Effects of Aging

The aging process affects hormone activity in one of three ways: their secretion can decrease, remain unchanged, or increase.

Hormones that decrease secretion include the following:

- Estrogen (in women)
- Testosterone (in men)
- Growth hormone
- Melatonin

In women, the decline in estrogen levels leads to menopause. In men, testosterone levels usually decrease gradually. Decreased levels of growth hormone may lead to decreased muscle mass and strength. Decreased melatonin levels may play an important role in the loss of normal sleep-wake cycles (circadian rhythms) with aging.

Hormones that usually remain unchanged or slightly decrease include the following:

- Cortisol
- Insulin
- Thyroid hormones

Hormones that may increase secretions levels include the following:

- Follicle-stimulating hormone
- Luteinizing hormone
- Norepinephrine
- Epinephrine, in the very old
- Parathyroid hormone

## Example

**Which of the following is an effect of aging on hormone secretion?**

A.  Weak teeth

B.  Loss of appetite

C.  Trouble sleeping

D.  Loss of body hair

The correct answer is **C.** The reduction of melatonin can result in the inability to sleep. **See Lesson: Endocrine System.**

## Let's Review!

- The endocrine system functions with the nervous system to regulate the many activities critical to the maintenance of homeostasis.

- Chemical signals, or ligands, are molecules released from one location that move to another location to produce a response.

- Chemical signals bind to proteins or glycoproteins called receptor molecules to produce a response.

- A hormone is an intercellular chemical signal that is produced in minute amounts by collections of cells to influence the activity of those tissues in a specific way.

- Hormones are distributed in the blood to all parts of the body, but only certain tissues, called target tissues, respond to each type of hormone.

- Negative-feedback mechanisms control the secretion of hormones.

- The endocrine system consists of ductless glands that secrete hormones directly into the blood.

- The aging process affects hormone activity.

# The Lymphatic System

This lesson introduces the structure and function of the lymphatic system, which is commonly referred to as the immune system. It also examines the common diseases and disorders of this system.

## The Key Players in the Lymphatic System

Components of the lymphatic system are the spleen, tonsils, adenoids, appendix, thymus gland, and lymph nodes. The **spleen** helps fight certain types of bacteria. The **tonsils**, **adenoids**, and **appendix** were once believed to be vestigial organs, meaning they are remnants left over from human evolution. Now, scientists have found they have active functions. The **thymus gland** is located directly above the heart. It secretes hormones that stimulate the maturation of killer T cells. This gland is only active from birth through puberty. After puberty, it decreases in size and functionality.

The body initiates a battle as soon as a **pathogen**, or a foreign body, enters. Two types of **lymphocytes**, B cells and T cells, are white blood cells that target the pathogen. Macrophages, another type of white blood cell, join in the invasion.

**Killer T cells** attack and kill infected cells. **B cells** label invaders for later destruction by macrophages. **Helper T cells** activate killer T cells and B cells. **Macrophages** consume pathogens and infected cells. These four kinds of white blood cells exchange information and correlate their activities as an integrated system.

When someone comes down with the flu, influenza viruses enter the body in small water droplets inhaled into the respiratory system. If the mucous membranes do not ensnare them, they slip past patrolling macrophages and begin to infect and kill mucous membrane cells, which makes the person feel sick. Macrophages initiate an "alarm" signal that activates the helper T cells, which serve as the "generals" of the lymphatic system. Helper T cells activate killer T cells and B cells and produce defensive proteins.

The body now initiates a robust attack against the flu virus. Using a second chemical signal, the helper T cells call into action killer T cells, which recognize and destroy body cells that the virus has infected. The T cells have receptors that recognize tiny bits of the virus's proteins and release enzymes into the infected cells that encourage the cells to destroy themselves.

The protein the helper T cells releases also activates the B cells. Like killer T cells, B cells have receptor proteins called **antibodies** on their surfaces. The B cells can release copies of these antibodies into the bloodstream or attach them directly to pathogens, marking pathogens for destruction. These B cells also secrete antibodies that attach to any invading pathogen into the bloodstream.

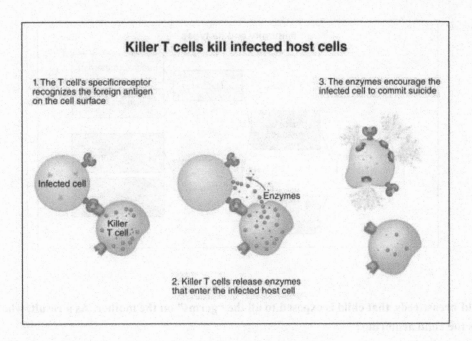

## Examples

1. **Which of the following is the correct series of the lymphatic system's defense mechanisms?**

   A.  B cell and T cell → Macrophage → Helper T cell

   B.  Helper T cell → T cell → B cell → Macrophage

   C.  Macrophage → Helper T cell → B cell → T cell

   D.  Macrophage → Helper T cell → B cell and T cell

   The correct answer is **D.** Once the macrophages sound the alarm, the helper T cells simultaneously activate the B cells and T cells. **See Lesson: The Lymphatic System.**

2. **The B cells do not directly attack pathogens or infected cells. Instead, they**

   A.  mark the pathogens for destruction by macrophages and B cells.

   B.  mark the antibodies for destruction by B cells and natural killer cells.

   C.  mark the antibodies for destruction by macrophages and killer T cells.

   D.  mark the pathogens for destruction by macrophages and natural killer cells.

   The correct answer is **D.** The B cells do not directly attack pathogens or infected cells. Instead, they mark the pathogens for destruction by macrophages and natural killer cells. When a B cell encounters a foreign microbe with a surface protein that matches the shape of its antibodies, it attaches an antibody to the microbe. **See Lesson: The Lymphatic System.**

# Types of Immunity

The four types of immunity are natural/passive, natural/active, artificial/passive, and artificial/active. The following are examples of these types of immunities:

- Natural/passive – Babies receive immunities from breastmilk.

- Natural/active – The body produces antibodies to combat an illness when a person becomes sick.

- Artificial/passive – This immunity is temporary and requires doses of serum to maintain the immunity.

- Artificial/active – A vaccination provides artificial/active immunity.

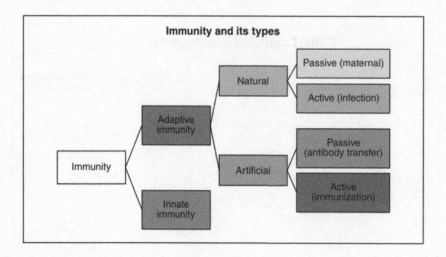

Immunity and its types

## Example

**When a child breastfeeds, that child is exposed to all the "germs" on the mother. As a result, what type of immunity is the child acquiring?**

A. Artificial/active

B. Artificial/passive

C. Natural/active

D. Natural/passive

The correct answer is **D.** The child acquires this immunity without the baby's body experiencing an illness. The baby is not born with this immunity and does nothing to acquire it. Therefore, it is passive. **See Lesson: The Lymphatic System.**

# Vaccination Prepares the Lymphatic System

**Vaccination** is the introduction into the body of a dead or disabled pathogen or of a harmless microbe with the protein of a pathogen on its surface. Vaccination triggers the lymphatic system response against the pathogen without an infection occurring. Afterward, the bloodstream of the vaccinated person contains memory cells that are directed against the pathogen. The vaccinated person is immunized against the disease. Vaccinations have dramatically reduced the incidence of many bacterial and viral diseases, including polio, tetanus, and diphtheria. An intensive vaccination program led to the elimination of the deadly disease smallpox in the 1970s.

## Example

**Sometimes, people complain they have become sick because of a vaccination. Why is this impossible?**

A. The pathogen is dead.

B. The pathogen was originally harmless.

C. The pathogen is only viable for a short time.

D. The pathogen has been disabled by sterilization.

The correct answer is **A.** Vaccination is the introduction into the body of a dead or disabled pathogen or of a harmless microbe with the protein of a pathogen on its surface. **See Lesson: The Lymphatic System.**

# Diseases and Disorders of the Lymphatic System

The ability of killer T cells and B cells to distinguish cells of the body from foreign cells is crucial to the fight against pathogens. In **autoimmune diseases**, this ability breaks down, causing the body to attack its own cells. The following chart gives examples of autoimmune conditions.

| Diseases | Areas affected | Symptoms |
| --- | --- | --- |
| Systemic Lupus Erythematosus | Connective tissue, joints, kidneys | Facial, skin rash; painful joints; fever; fatigue; kidney problems; weight loss |
| Type I Diabetes | Insulin-producing cells in the pancreas | Excessive urine production; blurred vision; weight loss; fatigue; irritability |
| Graves' Disease | Thyroid | Weakness; irritability; heat intolerance; increased sweating; weight loss; insomnia |
| Rheumatoid Arthritis | Joints | Crippling inflammation of the joints |

## Age

As people age, their bodies produce fewer B and T cells. As a result, their bodies' ability to defend themselves against viruses and bacteria lessens.

## Allergies

Sometimes, the body's immune system works too well and attacks itself. This is known as an **allergy**. Hay fever is an example.

**Mast cells**, attached to white blood cells, line entrances to the body. When they encounter matching antibodies, they initiate an **inflammatory response,** which releases histamines. **Histamines** cause capillaries to swell and increase mucous membrane production.

## HIV/AIDS: Lymphatic System Collapse

HIV/AIDS is a result of a mutation that occurred in a virus that affects chimpanzees. It destroys macrophages and helper T cells.

## How Is HIV Transmitted?

Because there is no cure for AIDS, prevention is key. HIV/AIDS can only survive in blood or body fluids because macrophages are located there. The primary means of transmission is through sexual intercourse.

HIV is not transmitted through the air, on toilet seats, or by any other medium where a macrophage cannot survive. It cannot be transmitted through shaking hands, sharing food, or drinking from a water fountain because macrophages cannot be transmitted through casual contact.

## Example

**Why is AIDS a devastating disease?**

A. It targets red blood cells.

B. It targets respiratory lining cells.

C. It targets many different types of cells.

D. It targets the cells in the lymphatic system that target pathogens.

The correct answer is **D.** A mutation arose in the chimpanzee virus that allowed it to recognize a human cell surface receptor on certain immune system cells, primarily the macrophages and helper T cells. **See Lesson: The Lymphatic System.**

## Let's Review!

- This lesson explored the lymphatic system's keys components and the major disease and disorders of the system.
- The lymphatic system provides immunity against pathogens.
- Several organs work together to make the lymphatic system efficient.
- Killer T cells recognize and destroy body cells that have been infected with a virus.
- B cells do not directly attack pathogens or infected cells.
- B cells have receptor proteins on their surface called antibodies.
- Vaccination is the introduction into the body of a dead or disabled pathogen or of a harmless microbe with the protein of a pathogen on its surface.
- In autoimmune diseases, the ability to distinguish cells of the body from foreign cells breaks down, causing the body to attack its own cells.
- Age has a negative effect on the lymphatic system.

# CHAPTER 13 HUMAN ANATOMY AND PHYSIOLOGY: INTEGRATION AND CONTROL PRACTICE QUIZ

1. **Which of the following is a characteristic of an interneuron?**

   A. Forms neural circuits

   B. Interacts with effectors

   C. Sends impulses to the CNS

   D. Functions as an efferent nerve cell

2. **Nodes of Ranvier are**

   A. spaces between myelin sheaths.

   B. cavities in the brain filled with fluid.

   C. dendrites that receive sensory inputs.

   D. chemical messages carried in vesicles.

3. **Neurohormones are hormones secreted from cells of the ____system.**

   A. circulatory

   B. digestive

   C. integumentary

   D. nervous

4. **The shape and chemical characteristics of each receptor site allow only certain chemical signals to bind to it. This is called ____.**

   A. conductivity

   B. memory

   C. permeability

   D. specificity

5. **Which of the following can transmit HIV?**

   A. Air

   B. Toilet seats

   C. Water fountains

   D. Infected intravenous syringes

6. **Why is sexual intercourse the most common method of spreading HIV?**

   A. Because T cell are located in semen and vaginal secretions

   B. Because B cells are located in semen and vaginal secretions

   C. Because proteins are located in semen and vaginal secretions

   D. Because macrophages are located in semen and vaginal secretions

# CHAPTER 13 HUMAN ANATOMY AND PHYSIOLOGY: INTEGRATION AND CONTROL
# PRACTICE QUIZ – ANSWER KEY

**1. A.** The interneuron is a type of nerve cell that bridges a connection between motor and sensory neurons to create neural circuits. This bridge facilitates communication between the neurons. **See Lesson: The Nervous System.**

**2. A.** Nodes of Ranvier are the gaps in myelin sheaths that increase the speed of an electrical neural signal down the axon of a neuron. **See Lesson: The Nervous System.**

**3. D.** Neurohormones are secreted by the nervous system. **See Lesson: Endocrine System.**

**4. D.** Specificity is the characteristic that causes chemical signals to connect only to the correct receptors. **See Lesson: Endocrine System.**

**5. D.** HIV can be transmitted through infected intravenous syringes, semen, vaginal secretions, and blood. **See Lesson: The Lymphatic System.**

**6. D.** Because semen and vaginal secretions are rich in macrophages, a person can become infected with HIV through sexual intercourse with an infected person. **See Lesson: The Lymphatic System.**

# SECTION VIII
# PHYSICS

# Physics: 25 questions, 50 minutes

**Areas assessed:** Motion, Friction, Kinetic Energy, Electricity and Magnetism, and Waves and Sound

## *PHYSICS TIPS*

- Review general physics concepts: acceleration, average speed, energy, friction, gravitation, light, motion, optics, projectile, and rotation.

- Know Newton's Laws of Motion.

# CHAPTER 14 PHYSICS

# NATURE OF MOTION

This lesson introduces the basics of motion and the application of simple physical principles and basic vector math to problems involving moving bodies. It culminates with an introduction to projectile motion and a presentation of Newton's laws of motion, which summarize the classical view of physics.

## Section 1: Nature of Motion

The space that people perceive is filled with objects of various sizes and shapes, but these objects are not always in the same places. They change their distances and orientations relative to observers and to one another, although these changes do not take place all at once. Such changes are called **motion,** and they are measured as differences in position or orientation over time.

Systematically measuring motion requires standards of **distance** and **time**—two concepts that people use and understand in everyday situations but may have difficulty defining independently. Instead of tackling the philosophical problem of what time and distance are, most people take the pragmatic approach to using these concepts by employing a generally agreed-upon standard. For example, in the metric (SI) system, the **meter** (m) is the fundamental unit of length. Comparing the relative locations of objects to that standard enables an observer to measure the distance between them and report it in a way that others can understand.

Time is more esoteric. A standard for time requires reference to some periodic event (a concept that is itself based on some understanding of time). For example, the revolution of Earth around the sun (a year), the full rotation of Earth on its axis (a day), or even something as mundane as the drip of a faucet (a duration that depends on numerous factors) are periodic events that can be used as standards for time. In the metric (SI) system, the fundamental unit of time is the **second** (s). The critical point is that the event be periodic. Because it occurs at unchanging intervals, it provides a common standard of time to which everyone can refer.

**Simple Motion Measurement**

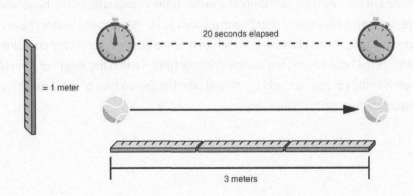

305

## Example

**Which approach would best serve as a common standard for measuring motion?**

A.  Comparing changes in distance using a peach and a sundial

B.  Comparing changes in distance using a yardstick and a heartbeat

C.  Comparing changes in distance using a quarter and a dripping faucet

D.  Comparing changes in distance using an index card and a metronome

The correct answer is **D.** To measure motion in a way that is meaningful to others and consistent in different locations and on different days, the standards of time and distance must be consistent and reproducible. Although a quarter, a yardstick, and an index card all have consistent dimensions, peaches vary. A sundial and a metronome can provide consistent indications of time's passage, but heartbeats and dripping faucets vary. Thus, the best answer is an index card and a metronome. **See Lesson: Nature of Motion.**

# Section 2: Vectors and Scalars

Determining the change in the distance or orientation of an object with respect to some standard of time yields a measurement of the object's motion. Motion has two general characteristics: its direction and its quickness. Therefore, **vectors** are helpful in quantifying motion. A vector is a quantity that has a direction and a length (or magnitude) but no defined location. It is often depicted as an arrow that begins at one point (called the **tail**) and ends at another point (called the **head**). Because a vector has no location, it can move anywhere and remain the same vector. Variables representing vectors often appear in boldface (e.g., $v$) or with a small arrow above them (e.g., $\vec{v}$).

In a rectangular coordinate system, one representation of a vector is the coordinates of the head when the tail is at the origin. For example, a vector in two dimensions might be expressed as $(3, -5)$. Because vectors have no location, however, the same vector can have its tail elsewhere. To return it to the origin, subtract the coordinates of the tail from the respective coordinates of the head to yield the standard vector form. To find the length of a vector expressed in standard form, square each of the coordinates, add them, and take the square root of the sum. This process is an application of the Pythagorean theorem for right triangles.

306

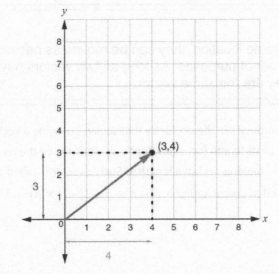

Length of (3,4) is

$$\sqrt{3^2 + 4^2} = \sqrt{9 + 16}$$
$$= \sqrt{25} = 5$$

In contrast with a vector is a **scalar,** which has a magnitude but no direction. A simple number such as 5 or 10.2 is a scalar. The length of a vector, for example, is a scalar.

## Example

**What is the length of a vector that has its head at (1, 3) and its tail at (−2, 7)?**

A.  1                    B.  5                    C.  9                    D.  25

The correct answer is **B.** First, convert the vector to standard form by subtracting the tail coordinates from the corresponding head coordinates: (1 − [−2], 3 − 7) = (3, −4). Then, calculate the length by squaring each coordinate, adding them, and taking the square root of the sum:

$$\sqrt{(3)^2 + (-4)^2} = \sqrt{9 + 16} = \sqrt{25} = 5$$

**See Lesson: Nature of Motion.**

# Section 3: Basic Vector Operations

Adding two or more vectors yields a **resultant.** Graphically, adding two vectors involves placing the tail of one on the head of the other (and continuing this process when adding more vectors). The resultant is a new vector starting at the tail of the first and ending at the head of the second. Because the resultant vector is the same regardless of which way the vectors are added, vector addition is **commutative** (meaning $\vec{a} + \vec{b} = \vec{b} + \vec{a}$). Adding vectors in coordinate form just requires adding the respective coordinates of each. For example, (7, 1) + (2, −3) = (7 + 2, 1 + [−3]) = (9, −2).

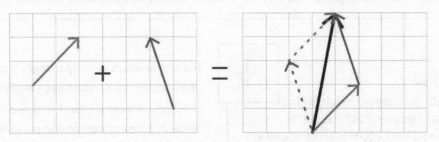

Subtracting vectors follows similar rules: for example, (7, 1) − (2, −3) = (7 − 2, 1 − [−3]) = (5, 4).

**KEY POINT!**

Remember that because vectors have no location, they can be moved as necessary to aid in visualization, addition, or any number of purposes. As long as two vectors have the same direction and length (magnitude), they are the same vector.

To multiply a vector by a scalar, multiply each coordinate in the vector by that scalar. To divide a vector by a scalar, divide each coordinate by that scalar. Dividing a vector by its length (or, equivalently, multiplying by the reciprocal of its length) yields a new vector that has the same direction as the original but a length 1. Such a vector is called a **unit vector.** These rules also allow vector subtraction to be expressed as vector addition: $\vec{a} - \vec{b} = \vec{a} + ([-1] \times \vec{b}) = \vec{a} + (-\vec{b})$. They also enable easier graphical addition of vectors.

## Example

**If $\vec{u} = (2, 5)$ and $\vec{v} = (3, -1)$, what is $2\vec{u} - 3\vec{v}$?**

A.  (−5, 13)    B.  (−1, 6)    C.  (1, −6)    D.  (13, 7)

The correct answer is **A.** First, perform the multiplication of each vector by its respective scalar:
$$2\vec{u} - 3\vec{v} = 2(2, 5) - 3(3, -1) = (4, 10) - (9, -3)$$
Next, either convert to addition or simply subtract the respective coordinates:
$$(4, 10) - (9, -3) = (4 - 9, 10 - [-3]) = (-5, 13)$$

**See Lesson: Nature of Motion.**

# Section 4: Velocity and Acceleration

Because motion has a direction and a magnitude of some type, vectors are a way to quantify it. One measurement of how quickly an object is moving is **speed:** the distance from one point to another divided by the travel time. For instance, if a plane moves 252 meters in 2.00 seconds, its speed is 252 meters ÷ 2.00 seconds = 126 meters per second (m/s). But for passengers on that plane, the direction of flight is just as important as the speed. Thus, multiplying the speed by a unit vector in the direction of travel yields a vector called **velocity.**

**KEY POINT!**

The *velocity* of an object is a vector: it quantifies both the magnitude and the direction of the object's motion. The *speed* of an object is a scalar: it is just the magnitude of its motion. Therefore, two objects can have the same speed but different velocities.

**KEEP IN MIND**

These simple mathematical definitions of *velocity* and *acceleration* assume constant speed and acceleration scalars, respectively, over the time period in the calculation. If the speed or acceleration is changing, they yield *average* values for that time period.

The rate at which velocity changes is called **acceleration.** Like velocity, acceleration has a magnitude and a direction, so it can be expressed as a vector. (Note that the term *acceleration* can also mean the magnitude of the acceleration vector, which is a scalar. The context of the problem will generally clarify whether the term refers to a vector or a scalar.) For instance, if a truck moving in a straight line is speeding up, its acceleration is in the same direction as its velocity; if the truck is slowing down, its acceleration is in the direction opposite to its velocity. Quantitatively, the magnitude of the acceleration is the difference in speed divided by the elapsed time.

## Example

**A runner finishes a 1,600-meter race in 5 minutes and 20 seconds. What was his average speed?**

A. 1 m/s        B. 5 m/s        C. 64 m/s        D. 320 m/s

The correct answer is **B.** The average speed of the runner is the distance divided by the running time. Before calculating the speed, convert the time to seconds: because 5 minutes is equal to 300 seconds, the total time is 320 seconds.

$$\frac{1{,}600 \text{ m}}{320 \text{ s}} = 5 \text{ m/s}$$

**See Lesson: Nature of Motion.**

# Section 5: Projectile Motion

One special case of motion involves an object moving under the influence of gravity—for example, when a player hits a baseball or a cannon fires a cannonball. Ignoring any other forces (including air resistance), such an object moves in two dimensions, generally combining a horizontal component of motion and a vertical component. It experiences downward acceleration of 9.8 meters per square second ($m/s^2$) but no horizontal acceleration.

Given a horizontal speed $v_x$ and an initial horizontal position (coordinate) $x_i$, the object's horizontal position (assuming a starting time of $t = 0$) is $x(t) = x_i + v_x t$. However, the object's vertical distance from its starting point is complicated by the acceleration due to gravity. Some basic calculus shows that given an initial vertical speed $v_y$ and an initial vertical position (coordinate) $y_i$, the object's vertical position (assuming a starting time of $t = 0$) is $y(t) = -\frac{1}{2}gt^2 + v_y t + y_i$. Note that $g$ is the acceleration due to gravity (9.8 $m/s^2$) and that the quadratic term is negative because gravity accelerates an object downward. Plotting the coordinates of the object at various times shows that it traces a parabola.

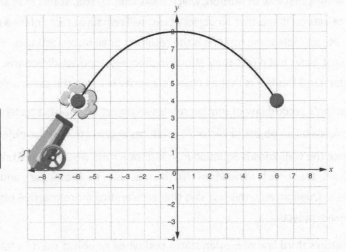

**BE CAREFUL!**
Make sure you know the height of the ground when analyzing projectile motion. Generally, an object won't be able to go any lower than ground level!

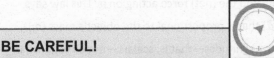

## Example

**A child throws a ball directly upward from the ground with an initial speed of 45 meters per second. How long will the ball take to return to the ground?**

A. 1.4 seconds     B. 2.0 seconds     C. 3.0 seconds     D. 9.2 seconds

The correct answer is **D**. Because the ball has no horizontal velocity, just use the equation for height with respect to time. The initial vertical velocity is 45 meters per second, and the initial height of the ball is 0. Also recall that the acceleration due to gravity is 9.8 m/s².

$$y(t) = -\frac{1}{2}gt^2 + v_y t + y_i = -\frac{1}{2}(9.8)t^2 + (45)t + 0 = -4.9t^2 + 45t$$

Next, set the height y equal to 0 and solve for t by factoring.

$$y(t) = 0 = -4.9t^2 + 45t$$
$$0 = t(-4.9t + 45)$$

Note that the ball is at ground level at t = 0 (the factor t), but the solution to this problem is for t greater than 0 (the factor –4.9t + 45). Set the latter equal to 0 and solve for t.

$$-4.9t + 45 = 0$$
$$4.9t = 45$$
$$t = 9.2$$

The solution is 9.2 seconds. **See Lesson: Nature of Motion.**

# Section 6: Newton's Laws of Motion

**Newton's laws of motion** summarize the qualitative characteristics of moving objects. These laws refer to two important concepts in physics: **force** and **mass.** A force is a "push" or "pull" that an object experiences or exerts on another object; it is also a vector with a direction and magnitude. Mass is in some sense resistance to movement (or "displacement") by a force; it is a scalar. Thus, given a certain force, an object with less mass will move more than an object with more mass.

**Newton's first law of motion,** which deals with **inertia,** states that an object in motion will remain in motion unless a **net force** acts on it and that an object at rest will remain at rest unless a net force acts on it. Note that *net force* just means the object feels some force: it is the resultant of all forces acting on the object. If two people push with the same force against a cart but direct their efforts in precisely opposite directions, the cart will feel no net force. Another way to understand this law is that an object's velocity will stay the same unless a force acts on the object.

**Newton's second law of motion** relates an object's mass, its acceleration, and the (net) force acting on it. This law says the force on an object (a vector $\vec{F}$) produces acceleration of the object ($\vec{a}$) that is proportional to the object's mass (m). Hence the well-known equation $\vec{F} = m\vec{a}$ (or F = ma when dealing only in magnitudes—that is, scalars—not directions.) In SI units, the force is in newtons (N), the mass is in kilograms (kg), and the acceleration is in meters per square second (m/s²). Qualitatively, this law says that accelerating more-massive objects requires a greater force than accelerating less-massive objects.

**Newton's third law of motion** states that when an object exerts a force on another object, it experiences a force of equal magnitude but opposite direction from that other object. This law is sometimes expressed by saying that for every action, there is an equal and opposite reaction.

## Example

**A 2.0-kilogram object experiences a net force of 144 newtons. What is its acceleration?**

A. 36 m/s²            B. 72 m/s²            C. 140 m/s²            D. 290 m/s²

The correct answer is **B.** Use Newton's second law of motion: $F = ma$. (Vectors are unnecessary because the problem only deals with scalars.) Plug in the numbers and solve for $a$, noting that it will be in meters per square second.

$$F = ma$$
$$144\ \text{N} = (2.0\ \text{kg})a$$
$$a = \frac{144\ \text{N}}{2.0\ \text{kg}} = 72\ \text{m/s}^2$$

**See Lesson: Nature of Motion.**

## Let's Review!

- Motion is the change in an object's position or orientation over time.

- Measurement of motion requires a consistent, accessible standard of distance and time.

- A vector is a quantity with magnitude and direction but no location; a scalar has a magnitude but no direction.

- The standard notation form of a vector is the coordinates of its head when its tail is at the origin of the coordinate system. If the vector is shown elsewhere, subtract the coordinates of the tail from the respective coordinates of the head to get the standard form.

- To multiply a scalar and a vector, multiply each coordinate of the vector by the scalar: $a \times (x, y) = (ax, ay)$.

- To calculate the resultant, or sum, of two vectors, add the respective coordinates of those vectors: $(a, b) + (c, d) = (a + c, b + d)$.

- To find the length of a vector, square its coordinates, add them, and take the square root.

- Vector addition is commutative: $\vec{a} + \vec{b} = \vec{b} + \vec{a}$.

- Velocity is a vector that represents how quickly an object is moving. Speed is the magnitude of that vector (it is a scalar).

- Acceleration is a vector that represents how quickly the velocity is changing.

- Projectile motion is the motion of an object under the influence of gravity. Such an object follows a parabolic path. Its horizontal position at time $t$, given initial horizontal velocity $v_x$ and initial horizontal position $x_i$, is $x(t) = x_i + v_x \times t$. Its vertical position at time $t$, given initial vertical velocity $v_y$ and initial vertical position $y_i$, is $y(t) = -\frac{1}{2}gt^2 + v_yt + y_i$.

- Newton's laws of motion summarize motion in classical physics.

- Newton's first law is that an object at rest stays at rest and an object in motion stays in motion, unless a net force acts on the object.

- Newton's second law is that the net force, object mass, and acceleration are related by $\vec{F} = m \times \vec{a}$ (or $F = m \times a$ when dealing only in magnitudes).

- Newton's third law is that an object exerting a force on another object feels the same force, but in the opposite direction.

# FRICTION

This lesson discusses different types of motion. Then, it examines uniform circular (rotational) motion and centripetal acceleration. It also introduces the concept of friction and its effect on motion in real-world situations.

## Types of Motion

According to Newton's first law of motion, an object moving with a given velocity (even if it is zero) will maintain that velocity indefinitely unless some net force acts on it. Absent any net force, the object will move in one direction along a line (assuming a nonzero speed). In this case, the object exhibits **linear motion** because its movement is in only one spatial dimension. If a force acts on the object and that force is parallel with the dimension in which the object is moving, the acceleration will be parallel or antiparallel (exactly opposite in direction) to the velocity. Thus, even though the object will speed up or slow down, its motion will remain linear.

If a force acts on an object in a direction that is not parallel to the object's velocity, the object no longer moves along a line; it exhibits **nonlinear motion.** Passengers riding in a car, for example, can tell the difference between linear and nonlinear motion by the direction of the force they feel as they ride. If the car speeds up or slows down linearly, they will feel only a backward force (positive acceleration) or a forward force (negative acceleration, or deceleration). If it turns (nonlinear motion), the passengers will feel a force toward either side as the car turns in some direction.

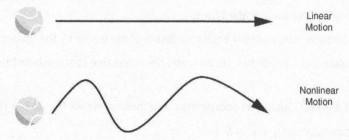

In general, mathematically analyzing nonlinear motion requires vector calculus. However, in certain cases, nonlinear motion can be described using only algebra. One case is **rotational motion**, which involves objects spinning on an axis or moving in a circle around some central point. Because rotational motion involves circular geometry, it is also commonly called **circular motion**.

### Example

**An object has a constant nonzero speed but a randomly varying velocity. Which term best describes its motion?**

A. Linear                    B. Nonlinear

C. Rotational                D. Stationary

The correct answer is **B.** If the object has a fixed speed greater than zero but its velocity changes randomly, then its direction of motion changes randomly. Therefore, the object is exhibiting nonlinear motion. Because the changes are random, however, it cannot be rotational motion, which is nonlinear but also determinate with regard to changes in velocity. **See Lesson: Friction.**

## Uniform Circular Motion

An object that rotates about an axis or revolves circularly around some point exhibits **rotational motion** (or **circular motion**). A simple case that provides a foundation for more-complex analysis is an object moving in a circle around some point outside its surface. For example, consider a ball tied to the end of a stick by a string. If someone holds the stick and causes the ball to move a circle, the ball will always be a fixed distance from the end of the stick—that distance is the length of the string. If such an object moves with a constant speed, its movement is called **uniform circular motion.**

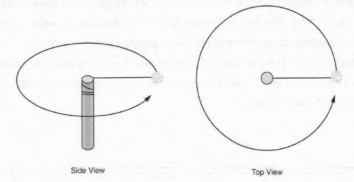

Side View                    Top View

The speed of an object in uniform circular motion is, like in linear motion, a distance divided by the time required to traverse that distance. A simple expression is the circumference of the circle divided by the time the object takes to go around one full time. Given a radius $r$ and a time $T$ to go around the circle, the speed $v$ is

$$v = \frac{2\pi r}{T}$$

This time $T$ is also called the object's **period,** and its inverse $(\frac{1}{T})$ is the **frequency,** often expressed as $f$. The frequency measures how often the object completes a revolution around the circle, and its unit (when $T$ is in seconds) is hertz (Hz). Another useful quantity is the **angular frequency,** $2\pi f$, which is often expressed as $\omega$ and may also use hertz. Employing this definition, the velocity is $\omega r$. Therefore, the velocity $v$ is also equal to $2\pi f r$.

**DID YOU KNOW?**

In the case of a ball on a string, if at any point the string is removing the force acting on the ball, the ball will immediately begin moving linearly at the same speed with which it was moving circularly. Its direction will be tangential to the circle— that is, the direction of its velocity at the moment the string is cut.

## Example

An electron in a magnetic field moves in a circle of radius 0.030 meters. If the angular frequency of its rotational motion is 2,400 hertz, what is its velocity?

A.   $1.3 \times 10^{-5}$ m/s          B.   72 m/s

C.   452 m/s                              D.   80,000 m/s

The correct answer is **B.** The velocity of the electron is the following:

$$v = \frac{2\pi r}{T}$$

Because $\frac{2\pi}{T}$ is equal to $2\pi f$, it is the angular frequency ($\omega$). Thus, the velocity in meters per second is

$$v = \omega r = (2{,}400 \text{ hertz})(0.030 \text{ m}) = 72 \text{ m/s}$$

**See Lesson: Friction.**

# Centripetal Acceleration

Although the *speed* of an object in uniform circular motion is constant, its *velocity* is always changing: it is at all points tangent to the circular path. By Newton's first law of motion, therefore, the object is experiencing acceleration and thus a force. This acceleration—called **centripetal acceleration**—always points toward the center of the circle. A simple example is a planet, such as Earth, orbiting a star. The star exerts a gravitational force that pulls the planet toward the star, and the planet moves (ideally) in a circle around the star. The derivation of centripetal acceleration ($a_c$) is complicated, but the formula is simple given a speed $v$ and a radius $r$:

$$a_c = \frac{v^2}{r}$$

---

**TEST TIP**

If you are unsure whether you correctly remember a formula, such as centripetal acceleration, you can increase your confidence by checking the units. For instance, using metric units, acceleration is in units of $m/s^2$. Velocity squared yields units of $m^2/s^2$, and the radius is in units of m. Dividing the squared velocity units by the radius units yields $m/s^2$, which is the same as for acceleration. This check is not sufficient to prove the formula is correct, but it can identify an erroneous formula.

---

By Newton's second law of motion, the **centripetal force** $F_c$ on an object of mass $m$ is therefore

$$F_c = ma_c = \frac{mv^2}{r}$$

**Centrifugal force** is a "ghost" force. For example, a passenger in a car that turns right feels a leftward force. But by Newton's first law of motion, the passenger's body tries to keep moving straight when the car turns right, causing the car to push the passenger to the right. The feeling, however, is of another force pushing the passenger leftward into the car rather than the car pushing the passenger rightward toward the center of rotational motion. The centrifugal force is therefore equal in magnitude but opposite in direction to the centripetal force.

## Example

A 75-kilogram passenger on a rotating theme-park ride experiences a centripetal force of 230 newtons. If she is 12 meters from the center of rotation, what is her velocity?

A.  6.1 m/s          B.  6.2 m/s          C.  37 m/s          D.  38 m/s

The correct answer is **A.** Use the formula for centripetal force with respect to mass, velocity, and radius of rotation:

$$F_c = \frac{mv^2}{r}$$
$$v^2 = \frac{F_c r}{m}$$
$$v = \sqrt{\frac{F_c r}{m}}$$

Use the given quantities to get the velocity in meters per second:

$$v = \sqrt{\frac{(230)(12)}{75}} = \sqrt{37} = 6.1 \text{ m/s}$$

**See Lesson: Friction.**

# Friction

Newton's first law of motion seems to break down in everyday life: rolling cars come to a stop, falling objects stop accelerating at a certain speed despite the force of gravity, and so on. The cause of the apparent breakdown is another force that resists the motion of objects: **friction**. For example, a plane that turns off its engines loses horizontal speed because of **air resistance**, which is a type of friction. A heavy piece of furniture is often difficult to slide across a floor because it experiences friction wherever it touches the floor. Friction can also act on nonmoving objects. For instance, it can prevent an object from sliding down an incline despite the force of gravity.

Because friction is a force, it causes acceleration. For moving objects, the friction force generally has a direction opposite that of the velocity. When an object decelerates because of friction, byproducts of this deceleration can be motion of something else (such as waves or eddies when the object is moving in water) or **heat**. Heat is another type of motion that involves movement of the atoms and molecules that constitute matter. For example, people with cold hands may rub them together briskly to warm them. For stationary objects, the force of friction is opposite to what would otherwise be a net force, such as gravity.

A common example of friction is an object sliding on a surface. The force due to friction is proportional to the object's mass because the mass determines the object's **weight** (which is the force it experiences from gravity). The weight of an object causes it to "push" against the surface, and when the object slides, that vertical push creates the resistance to horizontal motion (that is, friction) because of surface imperfections and irregularities.

> **KEEP IN MIND**
>
> Calculating the friction force can be difficult because it involves many factors, such as the roughness of surfaces (in the case of sliding objects) and the fluid characteristics of air (in the case of air resistance). For this reason, problems often assume friction is negligible—an assumption that often still allows a good approximation of the solution.

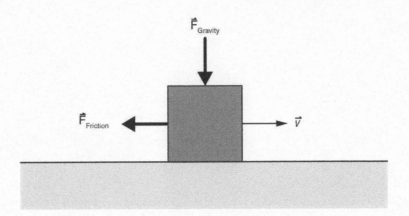

## Example

**A car is moving east at 20 meters per second. In what direction is the force of friction?**

A. East          B. North          C. South          D. West

The correct answer is **D.** Friction is generally in the direction opposite to the direction of motion—hence, a car that coasts in neutral, for example, will slow down without changing direction. For a car moving east, the friction force is directed west. The car's speed is unimportant to determining the direction of the force of friction. **See Lesson: Friction.**

# Let's Review!

- Linear motion is movement along a line; the velocity and acceleration may vary, but they are always parallel to the line.

- Nonlinear motion is movement that is not confined to a line; the velocity and acceleration can be any quantity.

- Rotational (circular) motion is movement around an axis or along a circular path.

- The period ($T$) of an object in uniform circular motion is the time it takes to travel once around the circle. The inverse of the period is the frequency ($f$), and the angular frequency ($\omega$) is $2\pi f$.

- Centripetal acceleration ($a_c$) is the acceleration an object experiences when in uniform circular motion. It is equal to $\frac{v^2}{r}$, where $v$ is the object's velocity and $r$ is the radius of the circle of motion.

- The centripetal force on an object in uniform circular motion is the object's mass times its centripetal acceleration.

- Centrifugal force is a "ghost force" in which an object undergoing centripetal acceleration "feels" like it is being pushed away from the center of rotation.

- Friction is resistance to motion. It is a force that is generally directed opposite to a moving object's velocity.

- Friction causes heat and/or motion of surrounding materials as a byproduct of its force on a moving object.

- Friction can prevent motion by acting opposite to other forces, such as gravity.

# WAVES AND SOUND

This lesson reviews a simple model of the atom and its role in the materials of everyday life. It then discusses waves in general and mechanical and electromagnetic waves in particular and applies these principles to optics.

## Matter and Atomic Structure

The materials that are common to human experience (through sight, touch, and the other senses) have an invisible, microscopic structure that experimenters can probe using scientific instruments. The fundamental unit of this structure is the **atom,** which comprises a central, heavy **nucleus** (plural **nuclei**) surrounded ("orbited") by lighter **electrons.** The nucleus is composed of **protons,** which carry a positive electric charge, and **neutrons,** which carry no electric charge (they are electrically neutral). Together, the protons and neutrons are sometimes called **nucleons.** Electrons carry a negative electric charge. Below is a simple representation of the structure of an atom.

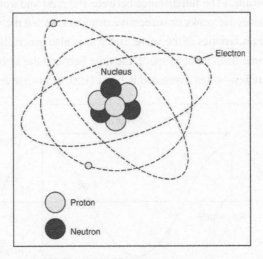

Electric charge (or just "charge") is a property of matter that relates to attraction or repulsion through the **electric force.** Charge comes in two known varieties; although scientists use *positive* and *negative* to describe charge, these terms are just conventions that have some mathematical utility. They do not describe a fundamental "signed" property of charge. The main qualitative rule is that like charges repel and unlike charges attract.

The electric force holds the atom together through the attraction of the negatively charged electrons to the positively charged nucleus. When an atom has the same number of electrons as protons, it is electrically neutral because the amount of charge on an electron is the same as that on a proton, but they are unlike, causing electrical attraction. The result is the simplistic model of an atom that shows electrons orbiting the nucleus like planets orbit the sun.

The number of protons in a nucleus determines the **element** that the atom represents: hydrogen (1 proton), helium (2), carbon (6), oxygen (8), iron (26), and so on. The number of neutrons in a nucleus can vary. Instances of an element with different neutron counts are called **isotopes** of that element. As a rule, isotopes of common elements have about as many neutrons as protons.

If the number of electrons in an atom differs from the number of protons, that atom has a net electric charge: positive if it has more protons than electrons, and negative if it has more electrons than protons. An atom with a net electric charge is called an **ion.**

Although not all matter is composed of atoms—physicists claim to have discovered a variety of particles that can exist apart from atoms—an understanding of atomic structure informs numerous fields, including chemistry and semiconductor physics. Moreover, the nucleons of an atom appear to have a deeper internal structure, a topic that researchers are exploring.

## Example

**A certain isotope of magnesium has 13 neutrons and 12 protons. If an atom of this isotope is electrically neutral, how many electrons does it have?**

A.  12                    B.  13                    C.  25                    D.  50

The correct answer is **A.** An electrically neutral atom must have the same number of protons as electrons. Because they carry no charge, neutrons have no electrical effect on the atom. **See Lesson: Waves and Sounds.**

# Properties of Waves

A universally recognizable example of waves is in water—whether in the ocean, a pool, or a small container. It is possible to visualize many aspects of invisible and conceptual, or mathematical, waves by observing how waves act in water. For example, the highest part of an ocean wave is the **crest** (or **peak**), the lowest part is the **trough,** and half the distance between these two points is the **amplitude.** (The full distance between the crest and trough is called the **peak-to-peak amplitude.**) The distance between successive peaks or successive troughs is called the **wavelength.** These parameters describe the spatial (space-related) characteristics of the wave. But waves also generally have temporal (time-related) characteristics. For example, given some fixed point in space, the time between the arrival of successive waves is the **period,** and its reciprocal is the **frequency**—often expressed in hertz (Hz), or inverse seconds ($s^{-1}$).

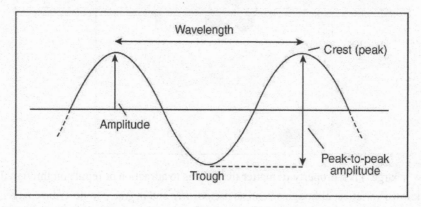

The wavelength ($\lambda$), frequency ($f$), and **wave speed** ($v$) are related by the equation $v = \lambda f$.

Although these spatial and temporal properties are the most intuitive, waves can have other, less intuitive properties. For instance, if a light source increases and decreases in intensity over time, its intensity can be described as a wave whose frequency is temporal and whose amplitude is intensity (rather than height). Mechanical (e.g., sound and water) and electromagnetic (e.g., visible light and radio) waves are additional examples.

Water waves also demonstrate some of the general behaviors of waves. When they strike a wall or other fairly stationary object, for example, the result is **reflection**: some or all of the wave "bounces" off the object. Waves that pass through a medium with changing material properties may bend, a phenomenon called **refraction.** The changing depth of the ocean floor, for instance, causes ocean waves to bend and usually arrive perpendicular to shore, regardless of their original direction. Another behavior of waves is **diffraction**: waves traveling in a certain direction can "turn" around sharp edges.

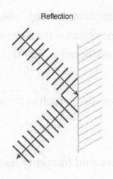

Reflection

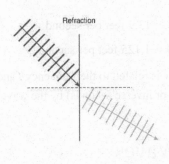

Refraction

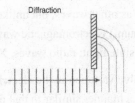

Diffraction

## Example

**An oceanographer has set a post in the water near shore to study waves before a hurricane. If she finds that the waves are 75 feet apart and a trough arrives every 25 seconds, what is the frequency?**

A.  0.013 Hz          B.  0.040 Hz          C.  25 Hz          D.  75 Hz

The correct answer is **B.** The frequency of a wave is the reciprocal of its period: the time between arrival of successive troughs or peaks. In this case, the frequency is $\frac{1}{25\text{ s}} = 0.040\text{ s}^{-1} = 0.040$ Hz. **See Lesson: Waves and Sounds.**

# Mechanical Waves

Waves that propagate in matter—for example, water waves—are called **mechanical waves.** They can involve variation in height, as in water waves, or variation in pressure, as in acoustic/sound waves. Earthquakes involve mechanical waves similar to sound waves: these seismic waves cause the ground to shake as they travel from the source of the quake.

In the case of sound, what the ear detects as **pitch** is essentially the frequency of the wave, and the **volume** is essentially the amplitude. Characteristics of the wave, including its speed, depend on the properties of the **medium** (or substance/material) that carries it. In the case of sound, for example, the wave speed depends on the **density** of the medium—how many atoms are packed into a unit volume—and the **compressibility** of the medium—how much the medium can be compacted given a certain force or pressure. The denser and less compressible a material, the faster sound waves will travel through it. Because water is denser and less compressible than air, for instance, sound travels faster in the former than in the latter. Similarly, waves in a rope will travel faster if the rope is taut than if it is loose.

Depending on the type of mechanical wave and the medium through which it travels, the wave speed may be apparent to the human senses. For example, at a sufficiently large distance from the observer, an event such as a hammer strike or gunfire is visible before it is audible. This delay occurs because light travels much faster than sound. Therefore, distant events are often seen before they are heard.

Mechanical waves exhibit the same phenomena as other waves, such as reflection, refraction, and diffraction.

## Example

**If a sound wave in air at a certain temperature and humidity has a frequency of 125 Hz and a wavelength of 9.00 feet, what is its wave speed?**

A.  0.0720 feet per second

B.  13.9 feet per second

C.  134 feet per second

D.  1,125 feet per second

The correct answer is **D.** The wave speed $v$ is related to the frequency $f$ and wavelength $\lambda$ by the formula $v = \lambda f$. Multiply the frequency (which is in hertz, or inverse seconds) by the wavelength to get the wave speed in feet per second. **See Lesson: Waves and Sounds.**

# Electromagnetic (Light) Waves

**Electromagnetic waves** exhibit the same behavior as other waves, but unlike mechanical waves, they require no medium to propagate. (That is, they can propagate in a vacuum.) Electromagnetic waves result from the movement—specifically, the acceleration—of a charge. Examples include visible light, radio waves, X-rays, microwaves, and infrared radiation.

As their name implies, electromagnetic waves involve variation in the **electric field** and the **magnetic field** around the source charge(s). These fields mutually oscillate in a manner similar to that of mechanical waves, although the oscillation is in field intensity and direction rather than, for example, wave height or material pressure.

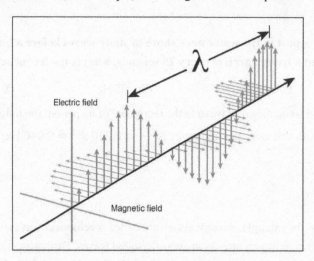

In a vacuum, the speed of an electromagnetic wave (or the **speed of light,** sometimes labeled $c$) is a constant: approximately 186,000 miles per second, which is much faster than the speed of sound in air—roughly 0.2 miles per second, or about 770 miles per hour. When traveling in a material, the speed of an electromagnetic wave decreases by a factor of $1/n$, where $n$ is the material's **refractive index** (or **index of refraction**). Therefore, the speed of light $v$ in a material of refractive index $n$ is $v = c/n$. The refractive index depends on the electrical and magnetic properties of the material.

## Example

**A radio wave is passing through a material with a refractive index of 2.00. What is its speed?**

A.  2,000 miles per second

B.  93,000 miles per second

C.  186,000 miles per second

D.  372,000 miles per second

The correct answer is **B.** The speed of light in a medium (material) is the speed of light in a vacuum ($c = 186,000$ miles per second) divided by the refractive index (2.00, in this case). The result is 93,000 miles per second. **See Lesson: Waves and Sounds.**

# Optics

In situations where the dimensions of a problem are much larger than the wavelength of the electromagnetic waves, those waves can often be accurately approximated as **rays**: directed line segments that represent the waves. Some simple rules enable analysis of electromagnetic-wave behavior in media that involve mirrors and in materials with different refractive indices. This model is a straightforward, often effective way to study **optics,** which is the subset of physics that examines the behavior of light.

**DID YOU KNOW?**

A laser acts as like nearly ideal ray because it maintains a very narrow beam over long distances. When used with caution (specifically, eye protection), low-power lasers are excellent for clearly seeing the principles of optics in action.

Many problems in optics can be analyzed using two simple rules. First, for a reflective surface (mirror), the **angle of incidence** of a ray is equal to the **angle of reflection**. Both angles are measured from a line perpendicular—or **normal**—to the surface and passing through the point at which the ray meets that surface. In the case of reflection, the angles can also be measured relative to a line parallel to the surface at that point. Second, for a ray passing from a material with one refractive index to a material with a different refractive index, the formula below relates the angle of incidence ($\theta_i$) to the **angle of refraction** ($\theta_r$), where $n_i$ is the refractive index of the material from which the ray originates and $n_r$ is the refractive index of the material into which the ray transmits. This relationship is called **Snell's law** and is responsible for the magnification of objects using lenses.

$$\frac{\sin \theta_i}{\sin \theta_r} = \frac{n_r}{n_i}$$

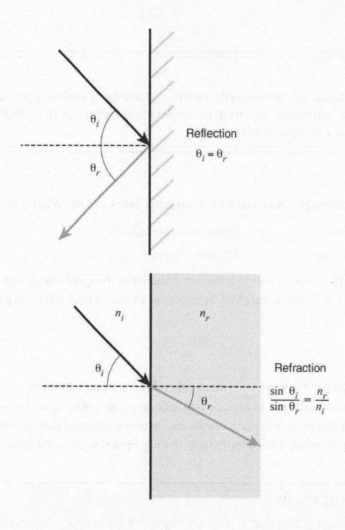

Reflection

$\theta_i = \theta_r$

Refraction

$$\frac{\sin \theta_i}{\sin \theta_r} = \frac{n_r}{n_i}$$

## Example

**If a light ray hits a mirror with a 30° angle of incidence relative to the normal, what is its angle of reflection relative to the normal?**

A. 30°          B. 40°          C. 60°          D. 90°

The correct answer is **A**. The angle of incidence is equal to the angle of reflection, as long as both angles are measured from the same line (normal or parallel). **See Lesson: Waves and Sounds.**

## Let's Review!

- The matter that appears in everyday life is largely composed of atoms; each atom has a central nucleus made of positively charged protons and uncharged neutrons that is surrounded by "orbiting" negatively charged electrons.

- The elements are each a type of atom with a different number of protons in its nucleus. A given element with a given number of neutrons is an isotope.

- The electric force binds the electrons to the nucleus of an atom.

- Waves occur throughout nature in different forms, but they have common properties and behaviors.

- A wave is defined by its amplitude, frequency, and wavelength. The wave speed is equal to the product of the frequency and the wavelength ($v = \lambda f$).

- Common wave behaviors include reflection (when the wave "bounces" off an object), refraction (when it bends in a medium), and diffraction (when it turns around an edge).

- Mechanical waves are waves in a material—solid, liquid, or gas. Examples include sound waves, seismic waves, and ocean waves.

- The speed of a mechanical wave depends on the compressibility and density of a material. As these values increase, so does the wave speed.

- Electromagnetic waves are a back-and-forth oscillation of the electric and magnetic fields owing to acceleration of a charge. They can propagate without a medium (that is, in a vacuum).

- The speed of an electromagnetic wave in a material is equal to the speed of light in a vacuum ($c$) divided by the refractive index of that material.

- In optics, the angle of incidence of a light ray is equal to the angle of reflection.

- Refraction of a ray is described by Snell's law: $\frac{\sin \theta_i}{\sin \theta_r} = \frac{n_r}{n_i}$, where $\theta_i$ is the angle of incidence, $\theta_r$ is the angle of refraction, $n_i$ is the refractive index in the material from which the ray is traveling, and $n_r$ is the refractive index in the material to which the ray is traveling.

# KINETIC ENERGY

This lesson introduces the concept of mechanical energy as the sum of kinetic energy and potential energy. The lesson also examines objects in motion and the effects of changing velocities and forces on moving objects. Finally, the lesson discusses how the force of gravitation affects objects in the universe.

## Mechanical Energy

Energy is the ability to do work. Mechanical energy can be divided into two types: kinetic energy and potential energy.

**Kinetic energy** of an object is represented by the equation $KE = \frac{1}{2}mv^2$, where $m$ is the mass of the object and $v$ is the velocity. The kinetic energy is proportional to the object's mass. A 7.26 kg shot thrown through the air has much more kinetic energy than a 145 g baseball with the same velocity. The kinetic energy of an object is also proportional to the square of the velocity of the object. A car traveling at 40 m/s has four times the kinetic energy of the same car moving at 20 m/s. This is the result of the squared velocity term in the formula. Kinetic energy, like work, is measured in **joules**.

Consider a group of boulders perched high on a cliff. These boulders have energy in a stored condition because gravity could cause them to fall. This is called gravitational potential energy (there are other types of stored energy, such as chemical and electrical). Potential energy of an object is stored energy due to the object's configuration or position relative to a force acting on it. The formula for calculating gravitational potential energy is $PE = mgh$, where $m$ is the mass of the object, $g$ is the acceleration of gravity on Earth (9.8 m/s$^2$), and $h$ is the object's height above Earth's surface. The unit for potential energy is also **joules**. Potential energy is an energy of position because much of the way this quantity can be changed is due to height.

Falling objects provide an interesting case for mechanical energy calculations. If we assume that there is no wind resistance, then all potential energy an object has before falling turns into kinetic energy as the object falls. Once the object impacts Earth's surface, there are different calculations to be done. We will simplify things by considering the object at the moment before impact.

### Example

**If a boulder falls off a 65 m high cliff, at what height, in meters, does the boulder have zero potential energy?**

A.  0                 B.  0.010              C.  32                 D.  65

The correct answer is **A**. Potential energy is defined as $PE = mgh$. Only at $h = 0$ will the equation equal 0. **See Lesson: Kinetic Energy.**

## Linear Momentum and Impulse

The **momentum** of an object depends upon its mass and velocity. **Momentum** is defined as $p = mv$, where $m$ is the mass and $v$ is the velocity. The unit for momentum is kg·m/s and does not have a special name. This concept can be illustrated by a simple example: Most people would rather try stopping a child's tricycle rolling at 0.5 miles per hour than a loaded dump truck at the same speed. The difference is the dump truck's greater momentum as a result of its much larger mass.

Newton's second law of motion explains how the momentum of an object is changed by a net force acting upon it. Newton's second law of motion, $F = ma$, can be rewritten by using the definition of acceleration as the change in velocity divided by the time interval.

$$F = ma = m\left(\frac{\Delta v}{\Delta t}\right)$$

Multiplying both sides of the equation by the time interval results in the following equation:

$$F\Delta t = m\Delta v$$

The left side, $F\Delta t$, is the product of the average force and the time interval over which it acts. This product is called the **impulse**, and an impulse is found by determining the area under the curve of a force-time graph, as shown below.

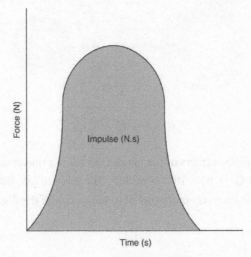

**Impulse-Momentum Theorem:** $F\Delta t = p_2 - p_1$

This equation is called the **impulse-momentum theorem**. The impulse on an object is equal to the change in momentum that it causes. If the force is constant, the impulse is just the product of the force and the time interval over which it acts.

What happens to a driver when a crash suddenly stops a car? An impulse is needed to bring the driver's momentum to zero. The steering wheel can exert a large force during a short period of time. An airbag reduces the force exerted on the driver by greatly increasing the length of the time over which the force is exerted.

Refer to the equation: $F = (m\Delta v)/\Delta t$. In the equation, $\Delta v$ is the same with or without the airbag. However, the airbag reduces $F$ by increasing $\Delta t$. Less force on a person during a crash is a good thing.

## Example

**What is the mass of a student's phone, in grams, if a pillow on the floor provides 7.71 N in 0.100 s while reducing the falling phone's speed from 4.43 m/s to rest?**

A.   0.174             B.   1.74                        C.   17.4                           D.   174

The correct answer is **D.** Use the impulse-momentum theorem to solve for mass.

$$\frac{F \cdot \Delta t}{v} = m; \quad \frac{7.71\,N \cdot 0.100\,s}{4.43\,\frac{m}{s}} = 0.174\,\text{kg} = 174\,\text{g}$$

**See Lesson: Kinetic Energy.**

# Universal Gravitation

Newton used mathematical arguments to show that if the path of a planet is an ellipse, then the magnitude of the force, $F$, on the planet resulting from the sun must vary inversely with the square of the distance between the center of the planet and center of the sun.

Newton later stated that the sight of a falling apple made him think about the motion of planets. He recognized that the apple fell straight down because Earth attracted it. He wondered whether this force might extend beyond the trees to the clouds, to the moon, and beyond. Could gravity also be the force that attracts the planets to the sun? Newton hypothesized that the force on the apple must be proportional to its mass. In addition, according to Newton's third law of motion, the apple would also attract Earth. Thus, the force of attraction must be proportional to the mass of Earth. The attractive force that exists between all objects is known as **gravitational force**.

Newton assumed that the same force of attraction would act between any two masses, $m_1$ and $m_2$. He proposed his **law of universal gravitation**, which is represented by the following equation:

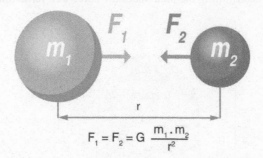

$$F_1 = F_2 = G \; \frac{m_1 \cdot m_2}{r^2}$$

In the equation, **r** is the distance between the centers of the masses, and **G** is a universal constant—that is, it is the same everywhere. The gravitational constant $G = 6.67 \times 10^{-11}$ N·m²/kg². The force of gravitation is directly proportional to the masses of the objects. However, force is inversely proportional to the square of the distance between the objects.

## Example

**What is the force of gravitational attraction, in newtons, between Mars ($6.39 \times 1023$ kg) and its inner moon Phobos ($10.6 \times 10^{15}$ kg) $6.00 \times 10^6$ m away?**

A. $1.25 \times 10^{16}$        B. $4.37 \times 10^{16}$        C. $2.42 \times 10^{17}$        D. $8.93 \times 10^{18}$

The correct answer is **A**. Use the formula to calculate the force:

$$F = G \left( \frac{m_1 m_2}{r^2} \right)$$

$$F = \left( 6.67 \times 10^{-11} \frac{N \cdot m^2}{kg^2} \right) \left( \frac{(6.39 \times 10^{23} kg)(10.6 \times 10^{15} kg)}{(6.00 \times 10^6 m)^2} \right) = 1.25 \times 10^{16} N.$$

**See Lesson: Kinetic Energy.**

## Let's Review!

- Kinetic energy, or the energy of motion, of an object is represented by the equation $KE = \frac{1}{2}mv^2$.

- The potential energy of an object is stored energy due to the object's configuration or position relative to a force acting on it. Gravitational potential energy is defined as $PE = mgh$. Near Earth's surface, gravitational acceleration is measured to be $g = 9.8$ m/s².

- Newton's second law of motion explains how the momentum of an object is changed by a net force action on it.

- The impulse on an object is equal to the change in momentum that it causes.

- The attractive force that exists between all objects is known as gravitational force. That force is directly related to the product of the two masses and inversely related to the square of the distance between the masses.

- $F = G \left( \frac{m_1 m_2}{r^2} \right)$ where $G = 6.67 \times 10^{-11} \frac{N \cdot m^2}{kg^2}$

# ELECTRICITY AND MAGNETISM

This lesson reviews the nature and relationship of electricity and magnetism and how these forces enable many modern technologies.

## Electric Forces and Fields

Objects that have an **electric charge** attract or repel other electrically charged objects depending on whether the charges are like (repel) or unlike (attract). **Coulomb's law** describes the **electric force** $F_E$ that an object carrying charge $Q_1$ exerts on an object carrying charge $Q_2$:

$$F_E = k\frac{Q_1 Q_2}{r^2}$$

where $r$ is the distance between the objects and $k$ is the electric constant. When using SI units—that is, the force is measured in newtons (N), distance in meters (m), and charge in coulombs (C)—$k$ is approximately $9 \times 10^9$. To aid the math, electric charge is described as either positive (like the charge on a proton) or negative (like the charge on an electron).

When studying and describing light (and other electromagnetic waves), defining the **electric field** is helpful. The electric field is the force that an object with a charge of 1 coulomb experiences at a given distance $r$ from an object with charge $Q$. The formula for this field ($E$) is similar to Coulomb's law:

$$E = k\frac{Q}{r^2}$$

The field is measured in newtons per coulomb.

Generally, the electric force and field are vectors, meaning they have both a magnitude and direction. Correctly adding forces therefore requires adding the vectors, not just the magnitudes. As a result, for example, if two forces acting on a charged object have equal magnitudes but opposite directions, their sum is zero—the object experiences no net force.

> **BE CAREFUL!**
> Charged objects only exert a force on other charged objects. Uncharged objects—for example, neutrons and many everyday objects—neither experience nor exert an electric force (at least under typical conditions).

> **KEEP IN MIND**
> Generally, if Coulomb's law yields a negative value for the electric force, that force is attractive; if it yields a positive value, that force is repulsive.

## Example

**What is the magnitude of the attractive electric force, in newtons, that an object with a charge 5.0 C exerts on another object with a charge –8.0 C that is $1.2 \times 10^2$ meters away?**

A. $-2.7 \times 10^{-3}$    B. $-3.3 \times 10^{-1}$    C. $-2.6 \times 10^7$    D. $-3.0 \times 10^9$

The correct answer is **C.** Using Coulomb's law:

$$F_E = k\frac{Q_1 Q_2}{r^2}$$

$$F_E = (9 \times 10^9)\frac{(5.0) \times (-8.0)}{(1.2 \times 10^2)^2}$$

$$F_E = (9 \times 10^9)\frac{-40}{1.4 \times 10^4} = -2.6 \times 10^7 \text{ newtons}$$

**See Lesson: Electricity and Magnetism.**

# Magnetism

**Magnetism** manifests through forces and fields in a manner similar to electricity, but the mathematics are more complicated. Qualitatively, a simple model of magnetism is relatively easy to understand. **Magnetic fields** and **magnetic forces** arise from moving charges—that is, any charged object with a nonzero velocity produces a magnetic field (and thus can exert a magnetic force on another moving charge). For instance, a wire that carries an **electric current**—which is the movement of negatively charged electrons through the wire—creates a magnetic field around that wire. The movement of electrons around the nucleus of an atom also creates a magnetic field, and in some elements (such as iron), the result can be powerful magnetic properties. Earth has a magnetic field that allows navigation using a compass, which uses a small magnetic needle to detect the direction of the field.

**DID YOU KNOW?**

Because electric currents create magnetic fields, they can deflect a compass needle. For instance, if you connect a wire across the terminals of a battery, causing an electric current to flow, you can see the effect of magnetism if you bring a compass near it. An accidental observation of this phenomenon led to the discovery of the link between electric current and magnetism.

Like electric charge, magnetism has two "polarities" (or **poles**) called **north** and **south**. Unlike electric charge, however, a magnetic object (or **magnet**) always has a magnetic north and a magnetic south—north and south never exist by themselves. (Positive and negative electric charges can exist by themselves.) In addition, like polarities repel, and unlike polarities attract.

**BE CAREFUL!**

Remember that any motion of charge creates a magnetic field, but only charge *acceleration* creates electromagnetic waves.

## Example

**Which of the following events produces a magnetic field?**

A. An accelerating electron

B. A wire in an electric field

C. A neutron moving through space

D. A positively charged object in a stationary position

The correct answer is **A.** Magnetic fields result from moving charges. Of the possible choices, only A involves a charged object (neutrons have no net charge) that is also in motion. **See Lesson: Electricity and Magnetism.**

# Electric and Magnetic Flux

**Electric flux** is the "flow" of the electric field through a given surface. To envision this concept, drawing **electric field lines** is helpful. Field lines show the direction of the electric force in space—specifically, the path a positive "test charge" would follow if it were initially stationary at some arbitrary point in space. By convention, field lines are generally shown flowing out from positive charges and in to negative charges. The illustration below shows a positive charge in empty space, a negative charge in empty space, and a positive and negative charge in close proximity.

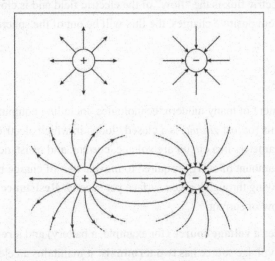

The more field lines that flow through an area, the greater the flux. Higher field-line density indicates a stronger field or force in that region. Although field lines are conceptual rather than physical, they are a helpful way to represent how electricity and magnetism permeate the space around charged objects.

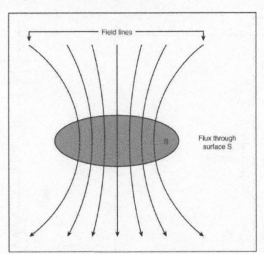

**Magnetic flux** and **magnetic field lines** are analogous to electric flux and field lines, but they represent magnetism rather than electricity. The same general principles apply.

One aspect of electricity and magnetism underlying much of today's technology is **electromagnetic induction.** This phenomenon occurs when an electrical conductor such as a wire experiences a changing magnetic field: the result is an electric force in that conductor. The strength of the electric force around a conducting loop is proportional to the rate at which the magnetic flux through that loop is changing. For example, spinning a coil of wire positioned between powerful magnets (or vice versa) is essentially how power companies produce electricity. Electrically driven motors apply the same principles, but in reverse.

## Example

**A positively charged object is inside a sphere that has no effect on electric fields. In what direction will the electric flux be?**

A. Into the sphere                                 B. Out of the sphere

C. Along the surface of the sphere                 D. Both into and out of the sphere

The correct answer is **B.** The electric flux is the "flow" of the electric field and is closely related to the field lines. Because the field lines go out from positive charges, the flux will be out of the sphere in this case. **See Lesson: Electricity and Magnetism.**

# Electric Circuits

Electric circuits are a critical component of many modern technologies, including computing technology and electrical power distribution. An **electric circuit** (or just *circuit*) is a closed "loop" in which electric charge experiences an electric force around the loop. Important parameters in a circuit are voltage, current, and resistance. **Voltage,** also called the **electric potential difference,** is the amount of energy required to move a unit of charge between two points in a circuit. **Current** is the amount of charge flowing through a given surface per second. **Resistance** is a measure of how much an electrical component impedes the flow of current.

A simple example of a circuit includes a **voltage source** (for example, a battery) and a **resistor** (for example, a light bulb) connected by metal wires. A simple voltage source has two **terminals:** it maintains an electric potential difference across those terminals so that charge will try to flow from the higher-voltage ("positive") terminal to the lower-voltage ("negative") terminal.

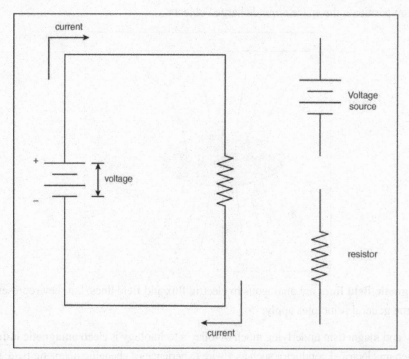

Voltage is usually measured in **volts** (V); current is usually measured in **amperes** (A) or **amps,** which are coulombs per second; and resistance is usually measured in **ohms** ($\Omega$). Materials, such as metal, that allow the free flow of electric charge are called **conductors.** Materials, such as many plastics, that do *not* allow the free flow of electric charge are called **insulators.**

**DID YOU KNOW?**

By convention, current is defined as the flow of positive charge. But because *negative* charge (electrons) is what actually flows in basic circuits, the mathematical assignment of a negative sign to the electron's charge created a historical dilemma. Mathematically, the flow of positive charge in one direction is equal to the flow of negative charge in the opposite direction, so the common practice is to discuss the flow of positive charge even though electrons often constitute the current.

## Example

**Which of the following best describes an electric current?**

A.  The storage of electric charge

B.  The movement of electric charge

C.  The energy required to move electric charge

D.  The impedance of electric charge's movement

The correct answer is **B.** Electric current is the flow of electric charge. **See Lesson: Electricity and Magnetism.**

# Ohm's Law

Circuit analysis can become extremely complex when the circuit involves many components, but a ew basic principles can aid the process, especially for simple circuits. One example is **Ohm's law,** which relates the current *I* through and voltage *V* across a component with a given resistance *R: V = IR.*

**FOR EXAMPLE**

If a circuit involves a 10-volt battery connected to a 100-ohm resistor, you can find the current through the resistor using Ohm's law:

$$V = IR$$

$$I = \frac{V}{R} = \frac{10 \text{ volts}}{100 \text{ ohms}} = 0.1 \text{ amps}$$

Two important rules also help in analyzing circuits. The first rule is that at any point (or **node**) in the circuit, the current flowing into that point must equal the current flowing out of that point. Thus, if three wires join at a node, the sum of the currents flowing in must equal the sum of the currents flowing out. The second rule is that for any closed loop in the circuit, the sum of the voltages around the loop must equal zero. For this rule, going around the entire loop in the same direction is critical. One convention is that going from a higher voltage to a lower voltage represents a positive voltage change (or voltage "drop"), whereas going from a lower voltage to a higher voltage represents a negative voltage change. Thus, in a circuit containing just a battery and a resistor, the voltage change across the resistor must be equal in magnitude but opposite in sign to the voltage change across the battery (when going either clockwise or counterclockwise around the circuit).

## Example

**If 0.2 amps are flowing through a 1,000-ohm resistor, what is the voltage across that resistor?**

A.  0.0002 volts

B.  200 volts

C.  1,000 volts

D.  5,000 volts

The correct answer is **B.** Use Ohm's law:

$$V = IR$$
$$V = (0.2 \text{ amps}) \times (1{,}000 \text{ ohms}) = 200 \text{ volts}$$

**See Lesson: Electricity and Magnetism.**

## Let's Review!

- Electric charges, which can be either positive or negative, create electric fields and exert an electric force on other charges.

- The electric force between two charges ($Q_1$ and $Q_2$) obeys Coulomb's law: $F_E = k \frac{Q_1 Q_2}{r^2}$, where $k$ is the electric constant (about $9 \times 10^9$ when working in SI units) and $r$ is the distance between the charges.

- The electric field from a charge $Q$ is $E = k \frac{Q}{r^2}$.

- Magnetic fields and forces result from moving charges (an electric current). Magnets have north and south polarities, but unlike electricity where negative and positive charges can appear separately, these magnetic polarities always appear together.

- Electric flux is the "flow" of the electric field, which can be visualized using electric field lines.

- Magnetic flux is the "flow" of the magnetic field, which can be visualized using magnetic field lines.

- Changing magnetic flux through a surface creates an electric field through that surface—a phenomenon that enables electricity generation.

- Electric circuits involve current flowing through resistors and other electrical components, driven by an electric potential difference (voltage).

- The voltage across a resistor is equal to the product of the resistance and the current (Ohm's law). Common units for these parameters are volts, amperes, and ohms.

# CHAPTER 14 PHYSICS PRACTICE QUIZ

1. **Which description best summarizes inertia?**

   A. The force on an object due to gravity

   B. The speed of an object with a changing velocity

   C. The acceleration of an object due to a net force

   D. The constant velocity of an object in the absence of a net force

2. **A vector has its tail at (9, 4) and its head at (0, 3). Which representation of the vector is correct?**

   A. $(-9, -1)$

   B. $(-9, 1)$

   C. $(-9, 7)$

   D. $(-9, 12)$

3. **Surface imperfections cause a horizontally sliding block to come to a halt. Which of the following remains as a result?**

   A. Heat

   B. Velocity

   C. Air resistance

   D. Horizontal force

4. **Which of the following best describes the behavior of an object in uniform circular motion?**

   A. Constant speed, constant velocity, constant acceleration vector

   B. Changing speed, changing velocity, constant acceleration vector

   C. Constant speed, constant velocity, changing acceleration vector

   D. Constant speed, changing velocity, changing acceleration vector

5. **Which of the following affects the speed of a mechanical wave in a material?**

   A. The wave's source

   B. The material's density

   C. The material's refractive index

   D. The wave's peak-to-peak amplitude

6. **Which term best describes two atoms that have the same number of protons but different numbers of neutrons?**

   A. Elements

   B. Ions

   C. Isotopes

   D. Nuclei

7. **The gasoline in automobiles can be considered what type of energy?**

   A. Electrical

   B. Kinetic

   C. Potential

   D. Thermal

8. **The chemical bonds found in sugar are an example of what type of energy?**

   A. Kinetic

   B. Magnetic

   C. Potential

   D. Thermal

9. **Which situation represents an attractive magnetic force?**

   A. Two north poles in close proximity

   B. Two south poles in close proximity

   C. Any two magnetic poles in close proximity

   D. A north pole and a south pole in close proximity

10. **A scientist is using a compass to detect magnetic fields. Which experiment will deflect the compass needle?**

    A. Holding a charged object stationary near the compass

    B. Moving a charged object quickly away from the compass

    C. Holding an uncharged object stationary near the compass

    D. Moving an uncharged object quickly away from the compass

# CHAPTER 14 PHYSICS
# PRACTICE QUIZ – ANSWER KEY

**1. D.** Inertia is the tendency of an object to maintain the same velocity as long as no net force acts on it. Thus, a moving object will move in the same direction and at the same speed, and an object at rest will stay at rest, unless a net force acts on the object. **See Lesson: Nature of Motion.**

**2. A.** The standard form of a vector is the head coordinates minus the tail coordinates: $(0 - 9, 3 - 4) =$ (–9, –1). **See Lesson: Nature of Motion.**

**3. A.** Once the block has come to a stop, it no longer has any velocity or acceleration. It is therefore experiencing no net force. Likewise, without any velocity, air resistance no longer applies. But as the block slowed, it created heat because of friction, and that heat remains—just like when people who feel cold rub their hands together briskly to warm them up. **See Lesson: Friction.**

**4. D.** An object in uniform circular motion has a constant speed, but as it moves, its velocity and its acceleration vector change direction. **See Lesson: Friction.**

**5. B.** The speed of a mechanical wave in a material depends on the material's density and compressibility. **See Lesson: Waves and Sounds.**

**6. C.** If two atoms have the same number of protons, they are the same element. If two atoms of the same element have different numbers of neutrons, they are isotopes. **See Lesson: Waves and Sounds.**

**7. C.** The gasoline, which is a form of stored, potential energy, is converted into kinetic energy when it is burned. **See Lesson: Kinetic Energy.**

**8. C.** When the bonds are broken, the potential energy stored in them is converted to kinetic energy. **See Lesson: Kinetic Energy.**

**9. D.** As with electric charge, magnetic polarities (or poles) attract if they are different and repel if they are like. Therefore, a north pole attracts a south pole (and vice versa), but north poles repel each another, as do south poles. **See Lesson: Electricity and Magnetism.**

**10.    B.** A magnetic field will deflect the compass needle. Magnetic fields result from moving charges, eliminating answers C and D (which involve uncharged objects). Answer B involves a moving charged object, which will deflect the compass needle. **See Lesson: Electricity and Magnetism.**

# SECTION IX
# FULL-LENGTH
# PRACTICE EXAMS

# HESI Practice Exam 1

## Section I. Mathematics

*You have 50 minutes to complete 50 questions*

1. Evaluate the expression 275 − 198.

   A. −77　　　　　　　　B. 77

   C. 198　　　　　　　　D. 473

2. Which percent is closest to the ratio 7:3?

   A. 23%　　　　　　　　B. 43%

   C. 73%　　　　　　　　D. 233%

3. Simplify $(x^2y^3z^{-1})^3$.

   A. $\dfrac{z^3}{x^6y^9}$　　　　　　B. $\dfrac{x^6z^3}{y^9}$

   C. $\dfrac{x^6y^9}{z^3}$　　　　　　D. $x^6y^9z^3$

4. Which decimal is the greatest?

   A. 1.3741　　　　　　　B. 1.7413

   C. 1.4371　　　　　　　D. 1.1743

5. Multiply $2\frac{1}{4} \times 1\frac{1}{3}$.

   A. 1　　　　　　　　　B. 2

   C. 3　　　　　　　　　D. 4

6. Multiply $1\frac{1}{4} \times 1\frac{1}{2}$.

   A. $1\frac{1}{8}$　　　　　　　B. $1\frac{1}{3}$

   C. $1\frac{2}{3}$　　　　　　　D. $1\frac{7}{8}$

7. Multiply $1\frac{1}{2} \times 2\frac{1}{3}$.

   A. $3\frac{1}{6}$　　　　　　　B. $3\frac{1}{5}$

   C. $3\frac{1}{4}$　　　　　　　D. $3\frac{1}{2}$

8. Which ratio is equal to 31%?

   A. 3:10　　　　　　　　B. 31:100

   C. 3:1　　　　　　　　D. 31:1

9. Solve $x^3 = 343$.

   A. 6　　　　　　　　　B. 7

   C. 8　　　　　　　　　D. 9

10. The landmass of the United States is about $4 \times 10^6$ square miles, and the landmass of Alaska is about $7 \times 10^5$ square miles. How many times larger is the landmass of the United States than the landmass of Alaska?

    A. 1　　　　　　　　　B. 3

    C. 4　　　　　　　　　D. 6

11. A biologist has captured only two kinds of snakes, ringnecks and garters. If she has 6 ringneck snakes and 13 snakes total, how many garter snakes does she have?

    A. 6　　　　　　　　　B. 7

    C. 13　　　　　　　　D. 19

12. Write $\frac{1}{5}$ as a percent.

    A. 15%　　　　　　　　B. 20%

    C. 25%　　　　　　　　D. 30%

**13. Which statement is true?**

A. The sum of a positive number and a negative number is always negative.

B. The sum of a positive number and a negative number is always positive.

C. The sum of a positive number and a negative number is always zero.

D. None of the above.

**14. Which math statement is true?**

A. $3 \div 1 = 0$

B. $0 \div 3 = 1$

C. $3 \div 0 = 3$

D. None of the above

**15. Divide $2\frac{9}{10} \div 3\frac{1}{2}$.**

A. $\frac{2}{7}$

B. $\frac{9}{20}$

C. $\frac{2}{3}$

D. $\frac{29}{35}$

**16. What is the product of 8:15 and 25%?**

A. $\frac{8}{375}$

B. $\frac{2}{15}$

C. $\frac{15}{2}$

D. $\frac{375}{8}$

**17. Solve the system of equations, $\begin{aligned} y &= x \\ x^2 + y^2 &= 10 \end{aligned}$.**

A. (3, 3) and (−3, −3)

B. (3, −3) and (−3, 3)

C. (2.2, 2.2) and (−2.2, −2.2)

D. (2.2, −2.2) and (−2.2, 2.2)

**18. How many whole numbers are less than 3 but greater than −3?**

A. 2

B. 3

C. 4

D. 5

**19. When dealing with a series of multiplication and division operations, which is the correct approach to evaluating them?**

A. Evaluate all division operations first.

B. Evaluate the expression from left to right.

C. Evaluate all multiplication operations first.

D. None of the above.

**20. Which number is less than all the others?**

A. −223

B. −18

C. 0

D. 223

**21. Evaluate the expression 462 ÷ 53.**

A. 1R3

B. 8R0

C. 8R38

D. 8R53

**22. Evaluate the expression 26 ÷ 9.**

A. 2

B. 2R8

C. 3R1

D. 35

**23. Evaluate the expression −3 × 5.**

A. −15

B. −2

C. 2

D. 15

**24. Write 0.21 as a percent.**

A. 2.1%

B. 20%

C. 20.1%

D. 21%

**25. Write $0.\overline{1}$ as a percent.**

A. $0.\overline{1}\%$

B. $1.\overline{1}\%$

C. $11.\overline{1}\%$

D. $111.\overline{1}\%$

**26. Change $7\frac{13}{20}$ to a decimal. Simplify completely.**

A. 7.55

B. 7.6

C. 7.65

D. 7.7

27. The number 36 is what percent of 16?

   A. 31%    B. 44%

   C. 69%    D. 225%

28. If 1 out of every 250 people will contract a certain disease, what percent of people will contract it?

   A. 0.004%    B. 0.4%

   C. 2.5%    D. 25%

29. Convert 8 liters to quarts.

   A. 6.94 quarts    B. 7.55 quarts

   C. 8.48 quarts    D. 9.06 quarts

30. Convert 16,000 ounces to tons.

   A. 0.5 ton    B. 1 ton

   C. 1.5 tons    D. 2 tons

31. Convert 14 centimeters to inches.

   A. 5.51 inches    B. 11.46 inches

   C. 16.54 inches    D. 35.56 inches

32. Convert 4 tons to pounds.

   A. 2,000 pounds

   B. 4,000 pounds

   C. 8,000 pounds

   D. 10,000 pounds

33. Solve the inequality for the unknown, $\frac{2}{3}x - 4 \le \frac{4}{5}x + 2$.

   A. $x < -45$    B. $x > -45$

   C. $x < 90$    D. $x > 90$

34. Solve the equation for the unknown, $\frac{1}{2}x + 3 = \frac{1}{4}x - 2$.

   A. $-20$    B. $-10$

   C. $10$    D. $20$

35. Solve the equation for the unknown, $3x - 8 + 5 + 2x = 4x - x + 6$.

   A. $-\frac{9}{2}$    B. $-\frac{2}{9}$

   C. $\frac{2}{9}$    D. $\frac{9}{2}$

36. Solve the equation for $h$, $SA = 2\pi rh + 2\pi r^2$.

   A. $2\pi rSA - 2\pi r^2 = h$    B. $2\pi rSA + 2\pi r^2 = h$

   C. $\frac{SA - 2\pi r^2}{2\pi r} = h$    D. $\frac{SA + 2\pi r^2}{2\pi r} = h$

37. Solve the equation for $c$, $2a(b + c) = c$.

   A. $\frac{2ab}{1 - 2a} = c$    B. $\frac{2ab}{1 + 2a} = c$

   C. $\frac{2ab}{2a} = c$    D. $\frac{2ab}{a} = c$

339

**38.** Solve the system of equations by graphing, $\begin{array}{l} 3x + 4y = -5 \\ -2x + 2y = 8 \end{array}$.

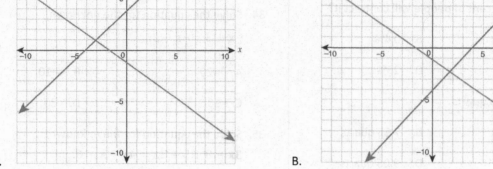

A.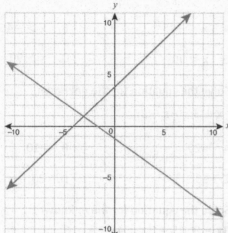

B.

C.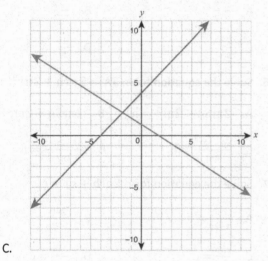

D.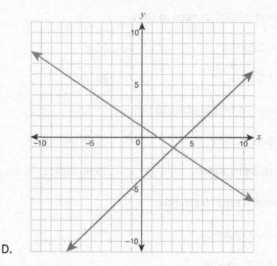

**39.** Solve the system of equations, $\begin{array}{l} 3x + 5y = 19 \\ 5x - 2y = 42 \end{array}$.

A. (8, −1)

B. (−8, 1)

C. (2, 3)

D. (3, 2)

**40.** Solve the system of equations, $\begin{array}{l} -4x + 5y = 32 \\ 4x - y = 0 \end{array}$.

A. (2, 2)

B. (8, 8)

C. (2, 8)

D. (8, 2)

**41.** Simplify $(9x^{-2}y^3)^2$.

A. $\dfrac{1}{81x^4y^6}$

B. $\dfrac{81y^6}{x^4}$

C. $\dfrac{81x^4}{y^6}$

D. $81x^4y^6$

**42.** One recipe calls for $\frac{3}{4}$ cup of sugar, and another calls for $2\frac{1}{2}$ cups of sugar. The first recipe is tripled, and the second recipe is halved. How many cups of sugar are needed?

A. 1

B. $1\frac{3}{4}$

C. 3

D. $3\frac{1}{2}$

**43.** Karida has a part-time job. She works 4.25 hours on Thursday and Friday and 6.5 hours on Saturday and Sunday. What is her hourly rate if her check is $268.75?

A. $8.50

B. $12.50

C. $14.50

D. $21.50

44. John spends $21.25 at the movies. His ticket is $7.75, and he buys popcorn, a pretzel, and a drink. If each snack costs the same, what is the price of the pretzel?

A. $3.58      B. $4.50

C. $6.00      D. $7.08

45. Jayden rides his bike for $2\frac{3}{4}$ miles. He takes a break and rides another $3\frac{1}{3}$ miles. How many miles does he ride?

A. $5\frac{1}{12}$      B. $5\frac{4}{7}$

C. $6\frac{1}{12}$      D. $6\frac{4}{7}$

46. In a backyard, $\frac{1}{6}$ of the yard is a garden, $\frac{2}{5}$ is landscaped, and $\frac{1}{3}$ is for play. How much of the yard is available for other use?

A. $\frac{1}{10}$      B. $\frac{2}{15}$

C. $\frac{13}{15}$      D. $\frac{9}{10}$

47. Multiply, $(3x^2 - 2)(x - 3)$.

A. $3x^3 + 9x^2 - 2x + 6$

B. $3x^3 - 9x^2 - 2x + 6$

C. $3x^3 + 9x^2 - 2x - 6$

D. $3x^3 - 9x^2 - 2x - 6$

48. Multiply, $(2x + 3)(x^2 - 3x - 4)$.

A. $2x^3 + 3x^2 - x - 12$

B. $2x^3 - 3x^2 - x - 12$

C. $2x^3 + 3x^2 - 17x - 12$

D. $2x^3 - 3x^2 - 17x - 12$

49. Multiply, $-4x^2y^2(5xy^3)$.

A. $-20x^2y^5$      B. $-20x^3y^5$

C. $-20x^2y^6$      D. $-20x^3y^6$

50. Apply the polynomial identity to rewrite $9x^2 - 30x + 25$.

A. $(3x + 5)(3x - 5)$      B. $(3x - 5)^2$

C. $(3x - 5)(3x - 1)$      D. $(3x - 5)(3x + 1)$

# SECTION II. READING COMPREHENSION

*You have 50 minutes to complete 47 questions*

**Read the following text and answer questions 1-6.**

WiseWear gear provides you with cutting-edge technology to enhance your performance and optimize your training. WiseWear products include sensors to track your heart rate, activity level, and calorie burn during workouts. Information is automatically uploaded to your phone and organized so you can track your improvement over time with just a tap of the screen.

Concerned about comfort? We've got you covered. WiseWear clothing is made with high-tech synthetic compression fabrics to promote circulation and wick away sweat while you work out.

Top-level pro athletes, like ultra-marathoner Uri Schmidt, rely on WiseWear for training and competition. Shouldn't you do the same?

1. **What is the most likely purpose of a popular science book describing recent advances in genetics?**

   A.  To decide

   B.  To inform

   C.  To persuade

   D.  To entertain

2. **The purpose of this passage is to:**

   A.  decide.

   B.  inform.

   C.  persuade.

   D.  entertain.

3. **With which statement would the author of this passage most likely agree?**

   A.  Americans who work out put too much emphasis on performance and not enough on enjoyment.

   B.  People who do not buy high-end exercise gear do not deserve to get a good workout and stay healthy.

   C.  The best way to achieve a healthy body is to follow a simple exercise plan and avoid hyped-up gadgets.

   D.  Consumers want help pushing their bodies to the limit and gathering information about their exercise performance.

4. **The author most likely includes the detail about a famous ultra-marathoner in order to make readers:**

   A.  understand that WiseWear gear is factually the best on the market.

   B.  take a weak position when they attempt to argue against the point.

   C.  trust that scientists have really studied WiseWear gear and proven it worthy.

   D.  feel an association between WiseWear products and a person they admire.

5. **Which detail from the passage, if true, is factual?**

   A.  WiseWear transforms the user into a better and more informed athlete.

   B.  WiseWear gear is the most comfortable exercise clothing on the market.

   C.  WiseWear products contain sensors that track the user's body signals.

   D.  WiseWear users are bound to improve at the sport of their choice over time.

6. The author of the passage includes details about WiseWear's comfort and ease of use in order to appeal to the reader's:

   A. reason.     B. trust.

   C. feelings.     D. knowledge.

**Please read the text below and answer questions 7-11.**

A global temperature change of a few degrees is more significant than it may seem at first glance. This is not merely a change in weather in any one location. Rather, it is an average change in temperatures around the entire surface of the planet. It takes a vast amount of heat energy to warm every part of our world—including oceans, air, and land—by even a tiny measurable amount. Moreover, relatively small changes in the earth's surface temperatures have historically caused enormous changes in climate. In the last ice age 20,000 years ago, when much of the northern hemisphere was buried under huge sheets of ice, mean global temperatures were only about five degrees Celsius lower than they are now. Scientists predict a temperature rise of two to six degrees Celsius by 2100. What if this causes similarly drastic changes to the world we call home?

7. Which sentence is the topic sentence?

   A. What if this causes similarly drastic changes to the world we call home?

   B. A global temperature change of a few degrees is more significant than it may seem at first glance.

   C. It takes a vast amount of heat energy to warm every part of our world—including oceans, air, and land—by even a tiny measurable amount.

   D. In the last ice age 20,000 years ago, when much of the northern hemisphere was buried under huge sheets of ice, mean global temperatures were only about five degrees Celsius lower than they are now.

8. In the paragraph above, global temperature change is:

   A. the topic.

   B. the main idea.

   C. a supporting detail.

   D. the topic sentence.

9. Which sentence summarizes the main idea of the paragraph?

   A. A small change in weather at any one location is a serious problem.

   B. The author is manipulating facts to make global warming sound scary.

   C. People should be concerned by even minor global temperature change.

   D. It takes an enormous amount of energy to warm the earth even a little.

10. What function does the information about temperature differences in the last ice age play in the paragraph?

   A. Topic

   B. Opinion

   C. Main idea

   D. Supporting detail

11. Which sentence would *best* function as a supporting detail in this paragraph?

   A. Electricity and heat production create one quarter of all carbon emissions globally.

   B. The world was only about one degree cooler during the Little Ice Age from 1700 to 1850.

   C. China has surpassed the United States as the single largest producer of carbon emissions.

   D. Methane emissions are, in some ways, more concerning than carbon dioxide emissions.

**Read the following sentence and answer questions 12-14.**

Numerous robotic missions to Mars have revealed tantalizing evidence of a planet that may once have been capable of supporting life.

12. **Imagine this sentence is a *supporting detail* in a well-developed paragraph. Which of the following sentences would best function as a *topic sentence*?**

    A. Venus is an intensely hot planet surrounded by clouds full of drops of sulfuric acid.

    B. Of all the destinations within human reach, Mars is the planet most similar to Earth.

    C. Liquid water—a necessary ingredient of life—may once have flowed on the planet's surface.

    D. Space research is a costly, frivolous exercise that brings no clear benefit to people on Earth.

13. **Imagine this sentence is the *topic sentence* of a well-developed paragraph. Which of the following sentences would best function as a *supporting detail*?**

    A. Of all the destinations within human reach, Mars is the planet most similar to Earth.

    B. Venus is an intensely hot planet surrounded by clouds full of drops of sulfuric acid.

    C. Space research is a costly, frivolous exercise that brings no clear benefit to people on Earth.

    D. Liquid water—a necessary ingredient of life—may once have flowed on the planet's surface.

14. **How could this sentence function as a *supporting detail* in a persuasive text arguing that space research is worth the expense and effort because it teaches us more about Earth and ourselves?**

    A. By using statistics to back up an argument that needs support to be believed

    B. By showing how a space discovery could earn money for investors here on Earth

    C. By providing an example of a space discovery that enhances our understanding of life

    D. By developing the main idea that no space discovery can reveal information about Earth

**Read the following paragraphs and answer questions 15-21.**

The idea of raising children in prison is controversial, but well-run prison nursery programs can actually be beneficial. A study of preschool age children showed that anxiety and depression are common among young children who are separated from their mothers at birth and reunited later. In contrast, babies who spent brief sentences of two years or less behind bars with their mothers showed greater resilience and stronger attachments.

According to a nationwide analysis of women who participated in prison nursery programs, the benefits for mothers are even clearer than the benefits to children. Women who were allowed to remain with their infants during prison sentences were less likely to be convicted of another crime and less likely to use drugs in the five years after release. They were more likely to continue their education in prison and more likely to find employment on the outside. Mothers involved in prison nursery programs also reported better mental health and greater confidence in their own parenting skills.

15. **Which statement expresses an opinion?**

    A. A study of preschool age children showed that anxiety and depression are common among young children who are separated from their mothers at birth and reunited later.

    B. The idea of raising children in prison is controversial, but well-run prison nursery programs can actually be beneficial.

    C. Mothers involved in prison nursery programs also reported better mental health and greater confidence in their own parenting skills.

    D. Women who were allowed to remain with their infants during prison sentences were less likely to be convicted of another crime and less likely to use drugs after release.

16. **Consider this sentence from the passage. Is the following statement a fact or an opinion? Why?**

    Mothers involved in prison nursery programs also reported better mental health and greater confidence in their own parenting skills.

    A. An opinion because it shares information about confidence, which is an emotion.

    B. A fact because it states verifiable information about how women reported they felt.

    C. A fact because it focuses on information from medical records rather than faulty memories.

    D. An opinion because it relies on human input rather than objective sources like computer records.

17. **What is the primary argument of the passage?**

    A. Young children should not be forced to live in prisons.

    B. Society must promote the health and safety of children.

    C. Letting imprisoned mothers keep their babies can be helpful.

    D. It is bad for children but good for mothers if children live in prison.

18. **What is one assumption behind the passage?**

    A. Imprisoned mothers should take parenting classes to learn how to raise children.

    B. Some people disagree with the idea of allowing mothers to raise children in prison.

    C. The needs of incarcerated mothers are more important than the needs of their babies.

    D. Society should protect the health and wellbeing of children born to incarcerated mothers.

19. **Which sentence responding to the passage displays faulty reasoning?**

    A. Although prison nursery programs have benefits, they do not justify the costs.

    B. Putting babies in jail is wrong because people that young do not belong in prison.

    C. Further research is necessary before it becomes a common practice to incarcerate babies.

    D. Society needs to find a better solution than prison for babies with incarcerated mothers.

20. The paragraph in the passage about benefits to mothers contains faulty reasoning because it:

   A.  suggests a cause-and-effect relationship without proving it.

   B.  causes readers to question the mothers' mental health outcomes.

   C.  does not prove factually that women in the program are better mothers.

   D.  fails to show that it is beneficial to participate in prison education programs.

21. Read the following sentences:

   We must provide funding to expand prison nursery programs to serve all women who give birth in prison. To do otherwise would cause babies to suffer needlessly.

   This would be an *ineffective* conclusion to the passage above because:

   A.  it uses circular reasoning.

   B.  it uses either/or reasoning.

   C.  its language includes insults.

   D.  its language displays gender bias.

22. Which of the following is *not* clearly a form of faulty reasoning?

   A.  Either/or fallacy

   B.  Circular reasoning

   C.  An overgeneralization

   D.  A statement of opinion

23. What is the best definition of the word *argument* in the context of reading and writing?

   A.  An eloquent summary

   B.  An angry conversation

   C.  A persuasive point in a text

   D.  An object or direct object phrase

24. Which of the following could *not* be a primary source?

   A.  An oil painting

   B.  A personal email

   C.  An autobiography

   D.  An encyclopedia entry

25. Which source would provide the most credible information to a researcher interested in studying changes in farming technology since the beginning of the millennium?

   A.  A current advertising pamphlet produced by a tractor company

   B.  A recent post about a tractor accident on the blog *Farmer Joe's Farmin' Life*

   C.  A book published in 1950 about improvements in farm equipment over time

   D.  A recent article comparing features of farm equipment in a journal for farm owners

26. Which of the following is *not* a primary source on Charles Darwin?

   A.  Charles Darwin's field notes from his travels

   B.  *On the Origin of Species* by Charles Darwin

   C.  An online database of Charles Darwin's writings

   D.  A blog post about Charles Darwin's contributions

27. A source is considered credible if readers can _____it.

   A.  trust                    B.  publish

   C.  analyze                  D.  decipher

28. Which type of evidence would not be considered credible to back up arguments in a persuasive text?

   A. Logic
   B. Statistics
   C. Scare tactics
   D. Firsthand accounts

29. What type of source is an online video of a conference presentation by a scientist reporting on the results of her research?

   A. Primary
   B. Secondary
   C. Tertiary
   D. None of the above

30. _____provide insight and commentary on the topic but may also introduce biases or errors.

   A. Primary sources
   B. Secondary sources
   C. Tertiary sources
   D. Quaternary sources

31. Which sources are usually considered most trustworthy?

   A. Primary sources
   B. Secondary sources
   C. Tertiary sources
   D. Quaternary sources

**Study the graphic elements below and answer questions 32-34.**

A high school student is presenting research on how gender affects participation in her political science class.

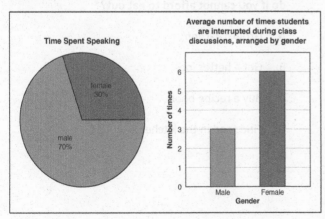

32. Male students spend _____of class time speaking.

   A. 3%
   B. 6%
   C. 30%
   D. 70%

33. Which statement accurately describes the average number of interruptions during each class discussion?

   A. Male students are interrupted an average of six times.
   B. Female students are interrupted an average of six times.
   C. Male students interrupt others an average of three times.
   D. Female students interrupt others an average of three times.

34. Which argument does the information in the graphs best support?

   A. Female students do not have as many ideas about political science as male students.
   B. The class should make a greater effort to give students of both genders a fair chance to speak.
   C. Contrary to popular belief, male students face greater gender discrimination in school settings.
   D. There is no substantial difference between male and female students' class participation in discussions.

35. A _____restates the main idea of a text in different words, attributing the ideas to the author.

   A. summary
   B. sequence
   C. topic sentence
   D. graphic element

347

**Read the text below and answer question 36.**

Before I came to America, I couldn't have known how difficult it would be. I knew I would miss my mother and my friends and my language, but I didn't know I would have to scrabble so desperately for so long to earn my place. Even when I had managed to make a living, I overworked myself with an animal terror. When I left home, I thought I was leaving poverty behind, but eventually I came to understand that I had escaped physical poverty by stepping into a poverty of the soul.

**36. Which sequence accurately describes what happened first, second, and third in the passage?**

A. Arriving in America, overworking, escaping physical poverty.

B. Coming to America, escaping physical poverty, stepping into a poverty of the soul.

C. Knowing how difficult America would be, leaving home, stepping into a poverty of the soul.

D. Expecting to miss friends, knowing how difficult America would be, arriving in America.

**37. A _____ would be most helpful for showing how many units of various products a business has sold.**

A. diagram     B. pie chart

C. bar graph     D. flowchart

**Study the flowchart below and answer questions 38-39.**

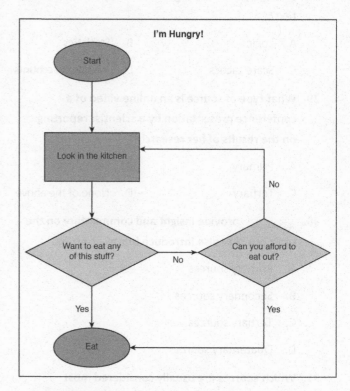

**38. What is the first thing the chart asks you to do if you are hungry?**

A. Eat.

B. Look in the kitchen.

C. Consider whether you can afford to eat out.

D. Consider whether you want to eat what you have.

**39. According to the flowchart, what do you need to do if you cannot afford to eat out?**

A. Grow a garden.

B. Get a better job.

C. Buy a recipe book.

D. Find food in the kitchen.

348

**40. Read the sentences below. What is the function of the <u>underlined</u> transition word in sentence two?**

My tame wolf is not a danger to humans. <u>Despite</u> her size and alarming appearance, she is basically a big, warm hearted puppy.

A. To express a contrast

B. To provide an example

C. To add emphasis to a point

D. To indicate time or sequence

**41. Read the sentences below. Which words or phrases should be inserted into the blanks to provide clear transitions between these ideas?**

Shaniqua shows clearly that she is driven to succeed as a student. _____I have often noticed her waiting outside the library before it opens at 6:00 a.m. _____her teachers report that she frequently asks for help outside of class.

A. In conclusion; Thus

B. First; Consequently

C. Although; In contrast

D. For instance; Furthermore

**42. The tone of a text is _____if the words say the opposite of what they really mean.**

A. ironic

B. earnest

C. confused

D. unambiguous

**43. The tone of a text is:**

A. a word or phrase that links ideas.

B. the reader's emotional response.

C. a structural pattern in a series of words.

D. the author's attitude toward the subject.

**Read the following passage and answer questions 44-47.**

When Dr. Kingston Hussein saw an announcement for a conference titled Ethics of Human Embryonic Research, he booked his tickets six months in advance.

"We need to stop and reflect on the ramifications of every new development in our research," said Dr. Hussein, the lead researcher in embryology at the Dampson Crockett Institute in Lewiston, Maine. "Every researcher in our field feels the weight of responsibility here. It's what we talk about when we go out for drinks after work."

Attitudes like Dr. Hussein's stand in stark contrast to common public perceptions of embryonic research. "These guys think they're gods," said Liz Goode, chairwoman of The Center for Ethical and Dignified Humanity, an organization that opposes all research on human embryos. "They want to get rich selling designer babies to billionaires. It's a nightmare."

An outside observer might expect a researcher like Dr. Hussein to avoid all contact with an activist like Goode. On the contrary, Dr. Hussein wrote to the organizers of the conference and requested that they invite Goode to host a panel. "We need dialogue," he said. "We need to hear what makes the public uncomfortable." He chuckled. "We also need to inform them about what we're actually doing."

And what *are* embryonic researchers doing? "Not building designer babies," he said. Dr. Hussein uses words like "run-of-the-mill medical" to describe his research goals. For instance, he is seeking causes and treatments for a variety of neurological disorders.

**44. Which adjective most accurately describes the author's tone?**

A. Scathing       B. Objective

C. Negative       D. Ironic

45. Reread the following quotation from the passage. Which adjective most accurately describes Dr. Hussein's tone?

"Every researcher in our field feels the weight of responsibility here. It's what we talk about when we go out for drinks after work."

A. Scathing     B. Apathetic

C. Earnest     D. Ironic

46. Reread the following quotation from the passage. Which adjective most accurately describes Liz Goode's tone?

"These guys think they're gods...They want to get rich selling designer babies to billionaires. It's a nightmare."

A. Harsh     B. Tolerant

C. Earnest     D. Ironic

47. Which phrase functions as a transition to juxtapose dissimilar ideas in the passage?

A. Attitudes like Dr. Hussein's

B. For instance

C. An outside observer

D. On the contrary

# SECTION III. VOCABULARY & GENERAL KNOWLEDGE

*You have 50 minutes to complete 50 questions*

1. Adding which of the following to prefixes to <u>cardium</u> would describe the membrane around the heart?

   A. Syn-    B. Epi-

   C. Peri-    D. Intra-

2. Select the meaning of the underlined word in the sentence. The critics claimed the ballerina gave a <u>superlative</u> performance.

   A. Dismal

   B. Acceptable

   C. Worthwhile

   D. Magnificent

3. <u>Monochromatic</u> most nearly means

   A. having one color

   B. having many parts

   C. having a lot of time

   D. having too much heat

4. In this sentence the root indicates that the doctor will surgically repair which body part? The surgeon was getting ready to perform a <u>rhinoplasty</u>.

   A. Ear    B. Nose

   C. Heart    D. Kidney

5. Select the meaning of the underlined word in the sentence. Jolie's has remained <u>intransigent</u> in her stance on the issue.

   A. Stubborn    B. Indefinite

   C. Passionate    D. Outspoken

6. Select the meaning of the underlined word in the sentence. The city's government is <u>infamous</u> for being corrupt and dishonest.

   A. Content    B. Regretful

   C. Notorious    D. Apologetic

7. Select the context clue from the following sentence that helps you define the multiple meaning word <u>refrain</u>. Shelby was going to tell a joke, but she decided to <u>refrain</u> because she did not want to offend anyone.

   A. "Shelby was going"

   B. "to tell a joke"

   C. "but she decided"

   D. "did not want to offend"

8. <u>Interject</u> most nearly means

   A. to debate an issue

   B. to introduce an idea

   C. to question a speaker

   D. to cut into a conversation

9. Based on your knowledge of roots, prefixes, and suffixes what does <u>encephalitis</u> mean?

   A. Around the spine

   B. Infection of the sinuses

   C. Inflammation of the brain

   D. Removal of the gallbladder

10. Select the context clue from the following sentence that helps you define the multiple meaning word <u>bind</u>. The mayonnaise is the key ingredient that will <u>bind</u> the egg salad together.

    A. "key"          B. "ingredient"

    C. "salad"        D. "together"

11. Select the context clue from the following sentence that helps you define the multiple meaning word <u>formula</u>. The mother gave her baby his <u>formula</u> after he woke up from his nap in the car.

    A. "mother"       B. "baby"

    C. "nap"          D. "car"

12. Based on your knowledge of roots, prefixes, and suffixes what is a <u>hypodermic</u> needle?

    A. A needle that goes under the skin

    B. A needle that goes inside the bone

    C. A needle that goes around the lungs

    D. A needle that goes between the ribs

13. Select the context clue from the following sentence that helps you define the word <u>laborious</u>. After cleaning out the garage for many hours, Sam was glad to be done with the <u>laborious</u> task.

    A. "cleaning out"   B. "garage"

    C. "many hours"     D. "task"

14. Adding which of the following prefixes to <u>glycemia</u> would show that a person has low blood sugar?

    A. Poly-          B. Hypo-

    C. Trans-         D. Hyper-

15. Which of the following suffixes means "to stop or control"?

    A. -osis          B. -tomy

    C. -stasis        D. -tropic

16. Which of the following root words means "bones"?

    A. Hidr           B. Tend

    C. Oste           D. Myel

17. Which of the following words means "inside the vein?"

    A. Advenous       B. Epivenous

    C. Ectovenous     D. Intravenous

18. Which of the following suffixes means "swelling of"?

    A. -oma           B. -osis

    C. -opsy          D. -orrhea

19. Which of the following root words means "veins"?

    A. Neur           B. Oste

    C. Myel           D. Phleb

20. Which of the following words means "pain of the kidneys"?

    A. Nephralgia     B. Nephrology

    C. Nephrotomy     D. Nephropathic

21. Which of the following suffixes means "hardening of"?

    A. -osis          B. -stasis

    C. -sepsis        D. -sclerosis

22. Which of the following root words means "small intestines"?

    A. Hidr           B. Enter

    C. Gastr          D. Myel

23. Which of the following words means "cancer-causing"?

    A. Malignant      B. Hematoxic

    C. Carcinogenic   D. Cardiovascular

24. Which prefix would you affix to the word "natal" to complete the following sentence? The nurses in the NICU provide _____natal care for premature babies.

   A. pre-
   B. peri-
   C. post-
   D. para-

25. Select the meaning of the underlined word in the sentence based on the context clues. If you wake up outside in your pajamas in the middle of the night, you may be a somnambulist.

   A. Explorer
   B. Magician
   C. Insomniac
   D. Sleepwalker

26. Select the word from the following sentence that has more than one meaning. Javier was overjoyed when he finally finished his application for college.

   A. Overjoyed
   B. Finally
   C. Application
   D. College

27. Select the meaning of the underlined word in the sentence based on the context clues. Since he was a novice at playing chess, he took lessons with a master to get more experience.

   A. Failure
   B. Natural
   C. Teacher
   D. Beginner

28. Select the meaning of the underlined word in the sentence based on the context clues. The cantankerous old man could usually be found screaming at all the kids for making too much noise.

   A. Irritable
   B. Talkative
   C. Concerned
   D. Meticulous

29. Which of the following suffixes means the study of?

   A. -less
   B. -able
   C. -ition
   D. -logy

30. Which of the following root words means to throw?

   A. ject
   B. dict
   C. rupt
   D. mort

31. Select the meaning of the underlined word in the sentence based on the context clues. Sheila has such an exuberant personality; she always has a smile on her face.

   A. Sincere
   B. Cheerful
   C. Appealing
   D. Interesting

32. Select the word from the following sentence that has more than one meaning. They need to prune the bushes every year or else they will lose their shape.

   A. Need
   B. Prune
   C. Lose
   D. Shape

33. Select the meaning of the underlined word in the sentence based on the context clues. You could spot her garish dress from a mile away with all its feathers and sequins.

   A. Glaring
   B. Dreadful
   C. Marvelous
   D. Impressive

34. Select the word from the following sentence that has more than one meaning. Only an animal with a strong constitution will be able to survive the Arctic's climate.

   A. Strong
   B. Constitution
   C. Survive
   D. Climate

35. Select the meaning of the underlined word in the sentence based on the context clues. When visiting the desert, the temperature tends to fluctuate, so you need to bring a variety of clothing.

   A. Rise
   B. Drop
   C. Change
   D. Stabilize

36. Which of the following prefixes means <u>after</u>?

    A.  post-            B.  auto-

    C.  trans-           D.  inter-

37. What is the best definition of the word <u>benevolent</u>?

    A.  Kind            B.  Selfish

    C.  Violent          D.  Mean

38. Select the word from the following sentence that has more than one meaning. The teacher was content with the quality of her students' work on their math exam.

    A.  Teacher         B.  Content

    C.  Quality          D.  Math

39. Which of the following root words means <u>far</u>?

    A.  tele            B.  trans

    C.  post            D.  ante

40. Which of the following root words means <u>foot</u>?

    A.  ped            B.  man

    C.  corp            D.  post

41. Which of the following suffixes means <u>belonging to</u>?

    A.  -er            B.  -ian

    C.  -ous            D.  -tion

42. Which of the following suffixes means <u>person who practices</u>?

    A.  -en            B.  -ist

    C.  -logy           D.  -able

43. Which of the following root words means <u>to say</u>?

    A.  vis            B.  vid

    C.  dict            D.  script

44. Which of the following suffixes means <u>made of</u>?

    A.  -er            B.  -en

    C.  -ful            D.  -ous

45. Which of the following root words means <u>to break</u>?

    A.  ject            B.  dict

    C.  rupt            D.  struct

46. Which of the following suffixes means <u>capable of</u>?

    A.  -ful            B.  -tion

    C.  -ous            D.  -ible

47. Which of the following suffixes means <u>having characteristics of</u>?

    A.  -ic            B.  -ed

    C.  -er            D.  -ist

48. Which of the following root words means <u>heat</u>?

    A.  terr            B.  therm

    C.  chrom           D.  fract

49. Which of the following prefixes means <u>too much</u>?

    A.  sub-           B.  non-

    C.  mis-           D.  over-

50. What is the best definition of the word <u>postscript</u>?

    A.  A summary       B.  A foreword

    C.  An introduction    D.  An afterword

# SECTION IV. GRAMMAR

*You have 50 minutes to complete 50 questions*

1. **People have ____arms and legs.**

   A. To
   B. Tu
   C. Too
   D. Two

2. **Choose the correct sentence.**

   A. My favorite day of the week is Tuesday. My favorite month is March, and Autumn is my favorite season.

   B. My favorite day of the week is Tuesday. My favorite month is March, and autumn is my favorite season.

   C. My favorite day of the week is tuesday. My favorite month is march, and Autumn is my favorite season.

   D. My favorite day of the week is tuesday. My favorite month is march, and autumn is my favorite season.

3. **Subjects ____to their king to show respect.**

   A. Bow
   B. Bou
   C. Baw
   D. Beau

4. **Choose the correct sentence.**

   A. The house of representatives has 435 members.

   B. The House of representatives has 435 members.

   C. The House Of Representatives has 435 members.

   D. The House of Representatives has 435 members.

5. **Choose the correct sentence.**

   A. Arnold Schwarzenegger was the governor of California.

   B. Arnold Schwarzenegger was the Governor of California.

   C. Arnold Schwarzenegger was the governor of california.

   D. arnold schwarzenegger was the governor of california.

6. **Since it is raining outside, I should ____a raincoat.**

   A. Wear
   B. Ware
   C. Where
   D. Whear

7. **What is the mistake in the following sentence?**

   He asked me, "What are you doing this weekend."

   A. The comma is misplaced.

   B. There should be a semicolon after *me*.

   C. There shouldn't be any quotation marks.

   D. There should be a question mark after *weekend*.

8. **What is the mistake in the following sentence?**

   Albert Einstein claimed "Imagination is more important than knowledge."

   A. *Albert Einstein*needs an apostrophe.

   B. There should be a colon after *claimed*.

   C. 'There should be a comma before *than*.

   D. There needs to be a comma after *claimed*.

9. **Fill in the blank with the correctly capitalized form.**

   Every week, they get together to watch _____.

   A. the bachelor
   B. The Bachelor
   C. The bachelor
   D. the Bachelor

10. **What is the correct use of a period in the following sentence?**

    A. She had a bad day
    B. She had a bad day.
    C. She had. a bad day.
    D. She. had. a. bad. day.

11. **On Earth, _____are seven continents.**

    A. Their
    B. There
    C. Theer
    D. They're

12. **What is the mistake in the following sentence?**

    Hospital's can be scary, because they are filled with sick people and needles.

    A. The comma is misplaced.
    B. There should be a colon after *with*.
    C. There should be a comma after *people*.
    D. *Hospital's* does not need an apostrophe.

13. **How many nouns are in the following sentence?**

    The team of scientists presented the results of their research at the conference.

    A. 2
    B. 3
    C. 4
    D. 5

14. **Identify the dangling or misplaced modifier, if there is one.**

    Having been repaired, we can drive the car again.

    A. Having been repaired
    B. we can drive
    C. the car again
    D. There is no dangling or misplaced modifier.

15. **Select the correct adverb to complete the following sentence.**

    Harry ran more _____than Olive.

    A. slow
    B. slowly
    C. slower
    D. slowest

16. **How many pronouns are in the following sentence?**

    We asked for his opinion, which he was happy to give.

    A. 1
    B. 2
    C. 3
    D. 4

17. **Select a verb that correctly completes the following sentence.**

    _____not worry about it.

    A. Is
    B. Do
    C. You
    D. Was

18. **Fill in the blank with the correct coordinating conjunction.**

    Would you like the soup _____would you like the salad?

    A. Or
    B. Yet
    C. But
    D. And

**19. How many verbs are in the following sentence?**

They toured the art museum and saw the conservatory.

A.  0          B.  1

C.  2          D.  3

**20. Which of the following is an example of a simple sentence?**

Which of the following options would give this sentence a parallel structure?

A.  Tamara's sporting goods store.

B.  Tamara has a sporting goods store in town.

C.  Tamara has a sporting goods store it is in town.

D.  Tamara's sporting goods store is in town, and she is the owner.

**21. The room was cleaned, painted and _____.**

Which of the following options would give this sentence a parallel structure?

A.  Tory redecorated it.

B.  redecorated by Tory.

C.  redecorating by Tory.

D.  Tory as redecorating it.

**22. Which of the following is an example of a complex sentence?**

A.  Roberto had a job through high school, he volunteered his time.

B.  Roberto had a job through high school, and he volunteered his time.

C.  Because Roberto had a job through high school he volunteered his time.

D.  Even though Roberto had a job through high school, he volunteered his time.

**23. Identify the conjunction in the following sentence.**

He is sick, yet he came to work.

A.  is          B.  yet

C.  came        D.  to

**24. Identify the direct object in the following sentence, if there is one.**

After hiking, the scouts cooked dinner over a campfire.

A.  scouts

B.  dinner

C.  campfire

D.  There is no direct object.

**25. Identify the dangling modifier in the following sentence.**

After reading the book, the movie that just came out must be pretty bad.

A.  After reading the book

B.  the movie

C.  that just came out

D.  must be really bad

**26. Timothy has a lot of goals in life like: getting his Masters in Education, volunteering his time to help others, and _____.**

Which of the following options would give this sentence a parallel structure?

A.  published his own book

B.  publishing his own book

C.  will publish his own book

D.  would publish his own book

**27. Select the correct word to complete the sentence.**

It's exciting to watch the nation rebuild ____ economy.

| A. its | B. it's |
| C. their | D. these |

**28. How many modifiers describe the underlined word in the following sentence?**

The royal <u>wedding</u> was beautiful and meaningful.

A. 0

B. 1

C. 2

D. 3

**29. Identify the dangling or misplaced modifier in the following sentence.**

When six years old, our family was transferred overseas by my father's company.

A. When six years old

B. our family

C. was transferred overseas

D. by my father's company

**30. How many nouns in the following sentence have incorrect capitalization?**

The Patel Family moved to the United States, and now they live in the Boston Area.

| A. 0 | B. 1 |
| C. 2 | D. 3 |

**31. Identify the direct object in the following sentence.**

Paulo accidentally locked his keys in his car.

| A. Paulo | B. accidentally |
| C. his keys | D. his car |

**32. How many nouns are in the following sentence?**

The team of scientists presented the results of their research at the conference.

| A. 2 | B. 3 |
| C. 4 | D. 5 |

**33. Identify the direct object in the following sentence, if there is one.**

Max tried so hard, but he did not succeed.

A. so

B. hard

C. not

D. There is no direct object.

**34. Identify the conjunction in the following sentence.**

I walked home even though my feet really hurt.

| A. home | B. even though |
| C. my | D. really hurt |

**35. How many plural nouns are in the following sentence?**

Marie's father's appendix was taken out.

| A. 0 | B. 1 |
| C. 2 | D. 3 |

**36. How many nouns are in the following sentence?**

I don't know her.

| A. 0 | B. 1 |
| C. 2 | D. 3 |

37. Select the correct word to complete the following sentence.

I don't think I did very ____ at the tryouts.

A. best                    B. well

C. good                   D. better

38. Identify the subordinating conjunction in the following sentence.

Don't leave until we get there.

A. until                   B. we

C. get                     D. there

39. Select the correct word to complete the following sentence.

It was a treacherous route, and they traveled more ____ when they had a guide.

A. safe                    B. safer

C. safest                  D. safely

40. Select the correct verb to complete the following sentence.

Neither Grandma nor Aunt Lucy ____ where the old photos are.

A. know                    B. knows

C. known                   D. knowing

41. Traveling gives people memorable experiences, exposes them to different cultures, and

_____.

Which of the following options would give this sentence a parallel structure?

A. broadens their perspective

B. to broaden their perspective

C. broadening their perspective

D. will broaden their perspective

42. Fill in the blank with the correct coordinating conjunction.

Julia wanted the new iPhone, ____ she could not afford it.

A. so                      B. or

C. but                     D. and

43. Identify the dangling or misplaced modifier, if there is one.

Hoping for sun, we went to the beach.

A. Hoping for sun

B. we went

C. to the beach

D. There is no dangling or misplaced modifier.

44. Identify the preposition in the following sentence.

It's really hot in that room.

A. It                      B. hot

C. in                      D. that

45. How many verbs are in the following sentence?

We read about World War I, World War II, and the Korean War in my history class.

A. 0                       B. 1

C. 2                       D. 3

46. Identify the direct object in the following sentence.

The doctor treated ten new patients last night.

A. doctor                  B. ten

C. patients                D. night

**47. Select the correct verb to complete the following sentence.**

Thanksgiving is my favorite holiday because the whole family ____together.

A. being
B. were
C. are
D. is

**48. Fill in the blank with the correct coordinating conjunction.**

My daughter is in the school play, ____I want to go to every performance.

A. so
B. or
C. but
D. and

**49. How many pronouns are in the following sentence?**

Suri and Marc asked about you.

A. 0
B. 1
C. 2
D. 3

**50. Select the correct verb to complete the following sentence.**

Our family ____staying home for the holidays this year.

A. is
B. be
C. am
D. are

# SECTION V. BIOLOGY

*You have 25 minutes to complete 25 questions*

1. In the taxonomic system, a class is grouped into which level?

   A. Order

   B. Family

   C. Species

   D. Phylum

2. A researcher characterizes a polymer that consists of glycerol molecules. What does she write in her notes about this polymer?

   A. These molecules will form lipid biomolecules.

   B. This polymer is capable of storing very little energy.

   C. The glycerol molecules are covalently bonded together.

   D. This polymer will help transmit genetic information in a cell.

3. A researcher characterizes the amino acid chain and structure of a novel substance. What type of substance is the researcher studying?

   A. Fat

   B. DNA

   C. Enzyme

   D. Sucrose

4. A study was performed to evaluate which type of road salt deiced a road most quickly. What is the independent variable?

   A. Deicing time period

   B. Road used for deicing

   C. Type of road salt used

   D. Amount of road salt used

5. A researcher predicts that a new drug will lower cholesterol in people. What is this statement called?

   A. Law

   B. Theory

   C. Variable

   D. Hypothesis

6. Which trait is used to distinguish living things from nonliving things?

   A. Size

   B. Genetics

   C. Homeostasis

   D. Environment

7. Why did it take many years for the cell theory to be developed?

   A. Advancements in microscopy took place slowly.

   B. Cells were difficult to isolate for experimental analysis.

   C. Researchers believed a cell formed from preexisting cells.

   D. Scientists already proved that cells were essential for life.

8. A researcher discovers a cell that is less than 0.5 millimeters in diameter. This cell has pili surrounding its cell wall. What does the researcher classify this cell as?

   A. Autotroph

   B. Eukaryote

   C. Heterotroph

   D. Prokaryote

9. Which structure do cells rely on for movement?

   A. Flagellum

   B. Microtubule

   C. Pili

   D. Vesicle

HESI

**10. What is a characteristic of eukaryotes?**

A. These organisms are all unicellular.

B. They lack a membrane-bound nucleus.

C. Many organelles are in their cytoplasm.

D. Bacteria and plants are examples of eukaryotes.

**11. What cellular process do autotrophs rely on to obtain energy?**

A. Carbon fixation

B. Cell respiration

C. Photosynthesis

D. Gluconeogenesis

**12. What is the most basic unit of structure in living things?**

A. Cell
B. Organelle

C. Oxygen
D. Pigment

**13. Glycolysis breaks down**

A. acetyl coA.
B. ATP.

C. glucose.
D. pyruvate

**14. During the $G_2$ phase, more copies of tubulin are made to separate**

A. histones.
B. chromosomes.

C. daughter cells.
D. sister chromatids.

**15. Which process involves crossing over?**

A. Mitosis
B. Meiosis

C. Calvin cycle
D. Cell respiration

**16. Chromosomes line up during**

A. anaphase.
B. interphase

C. prometaphase.
D. telophase.

**17. What is the correct order of the stages of the cell cycle?**

A. $G_1$, S, $G_2$, M
B. $G_2$, S, $G_1$, M

C. M, S, $G_2$, $G_1$
D. S, M, $G_1$, $G_2$

**18. What is made only during the light reaction phase of photosynthesis?**

A. ATP
B. $CO_2$

C. $H_2O$
D. $FADH_2$

**19. Which of the following is a segment of DNA that transmits information from parent to offspring?**

A. Centromere
B. Chromatid

C. Chromosome
D. Gene

**20. The replication of DNA ends with a twisted strand called a _____.**

A. base pair
B. nucleic acid

C. double helix
D. single strand

**21. Human cells have _____ sets of different chromosomes.**

A. 12
B. 23

C. 46
D. 50

**22. How can an organism have two alleles for each trait but only one of those alleles is expressed?**

A. One of the alleles is hidden in the chromosome.

B. One of the alleles is dominant over the other allele.

C. It depends on which allele is obtained from a parent first.

D. The allele closest to the top of the chromosomes is expressed.

362

23. An RNA copy of a gene used as a blueprint for a protein is called the ____.

    A. mRNA          B. pre-mRNA

    C. rRNA          D. tRNA

24. An offspring receives ____ allele(s) for a particular trait from each parent.

    A. 1             B. 2

    C. 3             D. 4

25. Crossing two heterozygous flowers, Bb x Bb, what is the chance of obtaining a homozygous, recessive trait?

    A. 25%           B. 50%

    C. 75%           D. 100%

# SECTION VI. CHEMISTRY

*You have 25 minutes to complete 25 questions*

1.  **Why must researchers consider the placebo effect?**

    A.  Monitor the outcome of the experiment

    B.  Ensure a proper independent variable is chosen

    C.  Account for the body's response to fake treatments

    D.  Create a baseline measure for experimental analysis

2.  **What step of the scientific method relies on logic reasoning to be formulated?**

    A.  Asking a question

    B.  Writing a conclusion

    C.  Researching information

    D.  Developing a hypothesis

3.  **Which term is used interchangeably with *negative variation*?**

    A.  Non-correlation

    B.  Direct correlation

    C.  Inverse correlation

    D.  Positive correlation

4.  **Look at the following image. What measuring tools are used?**

    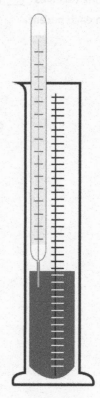

    A.  Ruler, barometer

    B.  Graduated cylinder, ruler

    C.  Barometer, thermometer

    D.  Thermometer, graduated cylinder

5.  **Light travels at a speed of almost $3 \times 10^5$ kilometers per second. How is this value written in standard notation?**

    A.  0.000003 km/s      B.  0.00003 km/s

    C.  30,000 km/s      D.  300,000 km/s

6. **Which of the following statements describes the mass of an electron?**

   A. The mass of an electron is less than the mass of a proton or neutron.

   B. The mass of an electron is about the same as the mass of a proton or neutron.

   C. The mass of an electron is greater than that of a neutron but less than that of a proton.

   D. The mass of an electron is greater than that of a proton but less than that of a neutron.

7. **Which of the following parts of an atom takes up the most space in terms of area?**

   A. Neutrons

   B. Electron cloud

   C. Individual electrons

   D. Protons and neutrons

8. **A neutral atom of aluminum has 13 electrons. How many electrons can be found in each shell in the electron cloud?**

   A. 6 in the first shell, 7 in the second shell

   B. 2 in the first shell, 11 in the second shell

   C. 2 in the first shell, 8 in the second shell, 3 in the third shell

   D. 3 in the first shell, 5 in the second shell, 5 in the third shell

9. **Which of the following is part of the metric system?**

   A. Celsius        B. Feet

   C. Ounces        D. Pound

10. **What is the Celsius value for 85 K?**

    A. −145        B. −188

    C. −205        D. −358

11. **A patient has a fever of 105°C. What is this value in Fahrenheit?**

    A. 137        B. 157

    C. 189        D. 221

12. **What is the temperature of 35°C in Kelvin?**

    A. 220        B. 238

    C. 308        D. 345

13. **Given the heating curve of iron, what are the approximate melting and boiling points?**

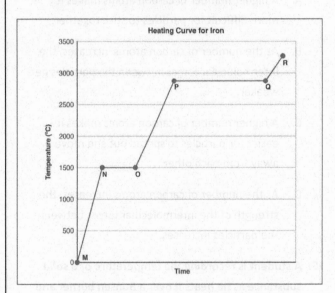

    A. 900°C, 2300°C    B. 1500°C, 2900°C

    C. 2300°C, 3100°C    D. 2900°C, 3400°C

14. Compare the boiling points of the alcohols in the table below. Molecules of these alcohols are similar, but they have different numbers of carbon atoms in a chain and, therefore, different masses. Based on the boiling point data in the table, what conclusion can be drawn about the relationship between the number of carbon atoms in a molecule and the interaction of the molecules?

| Alcohol | Formula | Mass (g/mol) | Boiling Point |
|---|---|---|---|
| Methanol | $CH_3OH$ | 32 | 65°C |
| Ethanol | $C_2H_5OH$ | 46 | 79°C |
| Propanol | $C_3H_7OH$ | 60 | 98°C |
| Butanol | $C_4H_9OH$ | 74 | 118°C |

A. A higher number of carbon atoms makes it more difficult for particles to stick together.

B. As the number of carbon atoms increases, the intermolecular forces between the particles get weaker.

C. A higher number of carbon atoms makes it easier for particles to spread out and move away from each other.

D. As the number of carbon atoms increases, the strength of the intermolecular forces between the particles increases.

15. A student is recording the temperature of a solid substance as he heats it over a Bunsen burner and notices that the temperature stays constant at 62°C for four minutes. How can the substance be described during these four minutes?

A. It is boiling.

B. It is melting.

C. It is entirely in the solid state.

D. It is entirely in the liquid state.

16. Flammability is an example of a _____.

A. polar substance

B. weak substance

C. physical property

D. chemical property

17. _____ is the diffusion of water molecules through a membrane in the direction of higher solute concentration.

A. Melting          B. Osmosis

C. Polarity          D. Sublimation

18. In the Lewis structure for carbon dioxide shown below, how many electrons is the carbon atom sharing with one oxygen atom?

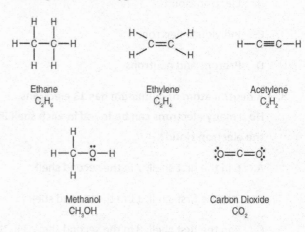

A. 2                      B. 4

C. 5                      D. 6

19. Consider the carbon-carbon bonds that exist in the molecules shown below. Which of the compounds below contains the strongest carbon-carbon bond?

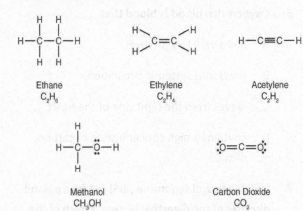

Ethane
$C_2H_6$

Ethylene
$C_2H_4$

Acetylene
$C_2H_2$

Methanol
$CH_3OH$

Carbon Dioxide
$CO_2$

A.  Acetylene

B.  Ethane

C.  Ethylene

D.  Methanol

20. According to the Lewis structure below, what is the formula for methanol?

Ethane
$C_2H_6$

Ethylene
$C_2H_4$

Acetylene
$C_2H_2$

Methanol
$CH_3OH$

Carbon Dioxide
$CO_2$

A.  CHO

B.  $CH_3O$

C.  $CH_4O$

D.  $C_3HO$

21. In which reaction are both the reactants and the products heterogeneous mixtures?

A.  $2H_2O(g) \rightarrow H_2(g) + O_2(g)$

B.  $2C_2H_2(g) + 5O_2(g) \rightarrow 4CO_2(g) + 2H_2O(g)$

C.  $2AgNO_3(aq) + Cu(s) \rightarrow 2Ag(s) + Cu(NO_3)_2(aq)$

D.  $CaCl_2(aq) + MgSO_4(aq) \rightarrow CaSO_4(s) + MgCl_2(aq)$

22. In the following single-replacement reaction, _____replaces _____.

$Cl_2 + 2NaI \rightarrow 2NaCl + I_2$

A.  sodium, iodine

B.  chlorine, iodine

C.  chlorine, sodium

D.  sodium, chlorine

23. What solution has a pH of 7?

A.  Aniline

B.  Pyridine

C.  Pure water

D.  Sodium hydroxide

24. An acid that dissociates into hydrogen ions is defined as a(n)

A.  weak acid.

B.  Arrhenuis acid.

C.  conjugate acid.

D.  Brønsted-Lowry acid.

25. What is the conjugate base of sulfuric acid?

A.  $HSO_4^-$

B.  $HSO_2^-$

C.  $HSO_3$

D.  $H_2SO_3$

# Section VII. Anatomy and Physiology

*You have 25 minutes to complete 25 questions*

1. **The knee is _____ to the foot.**

   A. distal

   B. inferior

   C. proximal

   D. superior

2. **The maintenance of normal blood sugar is what type of feedback mechanism?**

   A. Negative

   B. Neutral

   C. Positive

   D. Proximal

3. **Which wave is associated with a ventricle systole?**

   A. P wave

   B. T wave

   C. ST segment

   D. QRS complex

4. **What is the purpose of an electrocardiogram?**

   A. Indicate the rate of blood flow

   B. Display the heart's rate and rhythm

   C. Identify a person's blood group type

   D. Determine cell type in a blood sample

5. **Which statement is true regarding gas concentration of blood leaving the left side of the heart?**

   A. Oxygen levels are high.

   B. Carbon dioxide levels are high.

   C. Oxygen and carbon dioxide levels are low.

   D. Oxygen and carbon dioxide levels are high.

6. **Oxygen-rich blood is blood that**

   A. has a very low pH level.

   B. flows into systemic circulation.

   C. leaves from the right side of the heart.

   D. contains a high concentration of carbon dioxide.

7. **Irritable bowel syndrome (IBS) can be a painful disorder of the digestive system. Which of the following is a symptom of IBS?**

   A. Bloody stools

   B. Inflamed colon

   C. Abdominal pain

   D. Swollen abdomen

8. **The lining of the stomach is covered with rugae. What is a benefit of this?**

   A. Rugae increase the output of gastric juices.

   B. Rugae increase the surface area of the stomach.

   C. Rugae increase the permeability of the stomach walls.

   D. Rugae increase the types of nutrients that can diffuse.

9. **Sperm is combined with other components to form semen; these other components are formed mainly in the _____.**

   A. penis

   B. glans penis

   C. male accessory glands

   D. female accessory glands

10. The vulva is comprised of all of the following, except the _____.

    A. cervix

    B. clitoris

    C. labia majora

    D. vaginal opening

11. Why is glomerular filtrate important?

    A. Causes solutes to diffuse back into the renal artery

    B. Uses the forces of blood pressure to reabsorb urea

    C. Secretes nitrogenous wastes into the urine for excretion

    D. Increases the concentration of urine in the collecting duct

12. Roughly how many liters of blood flow through the kidneys each day?

    A. 75          B. 100

    C. 180         D. 425

13. Bones are primarily made of _____.

    A. chloride          B. magnesium

    C. sodium            D. phosphorus

14. Which organ does the vertebral column protect?

    A. Brain             B. Heart

    C. Spinal cord       D. Pelvic girdle

15. What does actin attach to?

    A. Z-line            B. I-band

    C. M-line            D. A-band

16. A study shows that decreased calcium content possibly contributes to poor skeletal muscle contractility. Which of the following structures was most likely observed to arrive at this conclusion?

    A. H-zone

    B. Actin myofilament

    C. Cardiac muscle fiber

    D. Sarcoplasmic reticulum

17. What substance is required to drive the slide filament process?

    A. ATP              B. Hormone

    C. Potassium        D. Water

18. A dermatologist explains to a patient that a bacterial infection has affected the sebaceous glands. Which layer does this form of acne directly affect?

    A. Stratum basale

    B. Stratum lucidum

    C. Stratum corneum

    D. Stratum granulosum

19. During basal cell carcinoma, the epidermal cells in the stratum basale

    A. invade the dermis.

    B. form a waterproof layer.

    C. undergo mitosis normally.

    D. fill with a large amount of keratin.

20. If a person smells something sweet, what form of information is this initially perceived as in the nervous system?

   A. Cognitive
   B. Integrative
   C. Motor
   D. Sensory

21. Which of the following most likely directly stimulates the excitation of a neuron?

   A. Astrocyte
   B. Muscle fiber
   C. Myelin sheath
   D. Neurotransmitter

22. What disease results when the pancreas cannot uptake the glucose in the bloodstream properly?

   A. Addison's
   B. Arthritis
   C. Diabetes
   D. Hyperthyroidism

23. In stressful situations, acetylcholine is produced. Which intercellular chemical signal is responsible for this action?

   A. Autocrine
   B. Neuromodulator
   C. Paracrine
   D. Pheromone

24. The B cells label invaders for later destruction by _____.

   A. antibodies
   B. macrophages
   C. proteins
   D. T cells

25. Antibodies attach to invading pathogens, marking them for _____.

   A. destruction
   B. penetration
   C. reproduction
   D. transformation

# VIII. PHYSICS

*You have 50 minutes to complete 25 questions*

1. **Which parameter is always a vector?**

   A. Acceleration      B. Mass

   C. Speed      D. Velocity

2. **Which statement about an object undergoing projectile motion is true? (Assume ideal conditions with no friction.)**

   A. The object's vertical velocity is constant.

   B. The object's vertical acceleration is zero.

   C. The object's horizontal velocity is constant.

   D. The object's horizontal acceleration is nonzero.

3. **Which statement about velocity and acceleration is correct?**

   A. Velocity is the magnitude of the speed.

   B. Speed is the magnitude of the velocity.

   C. Speed is the rate of change of the velocity.

   D. Velocity is the rate of change of the speed.

4. **A man applies a force to a wall by pushing on it. What does the wall do in response?**

   A. The wall applies a greater force in the same direction.

   B. The wall applies a smaller force in the opposite direction.

   C. The wall applies a force of equal magnitude in the same direction.

   D. The wall applies a force of equal magnitude in the opposite direction.

5. **Which situation best illustrates Newton's first law of motion?**

   A. A ball that is on a flat surface accelerates as a piston pushes it.

   B. A ball that is rolling on a flat surface maintains the same velocity.

   C. A ball that is on a sloped surface rolls down the slope because of gravity.

   D. A ball that is stationary on a flat surface does not fall despite the downward force of gravity.

6. **Which explanation best describes why individuals restrained on a spinning theme-park ride feel like they are being forced outward from the center of rotation?**

   A. They are undergoing linear motion.

   B. They are experiencing no acceleration.

   C. They are feeling the restraints pull them inward.

   D. They are accelerating outward from the center of rotation.

7. **A ball undergoing projectile motion loses horizontal velocity as it travels. Which factor best explains this deceleration?**

   A. Heat      B. Gravity

   C. Air resistance      D. Centrifugal force

8.  **Which of the following can be a result of friction on a moving object?**

    A.  Centripetal acceleration

    B.  An increase in the object's speed

    C.  Movement of a fluid surrounding the object

    D.  A net force in the direction of the object's velocity

9.  **Which of the following best explains why a block on a sloped surface remains stationary rather than sliding down the surface?**

    A.  The block undergoes centrifugal force.

    B.  The block experiences a net upward force.

    C.  The block is not subject to a gravitational force.

    D.  The block experiences a friction force that cancels other forces.

10. **Children on a turning bus feel a centrifugal force to the west. What is the direction of the centripetal force?**

    A.  East                  B.  North

    C.  South                 D.  West

11. **If a green laser hits a mirror at a 65° angle to the normal, at what angle will it reflect?**

    A.  25° to the normal

    B.  65° to the normal

    C.  90° to the normal

    D.  115° to the normal

12. **Which statement about a magnesium ion is correct?**

    A.  The number of protons differs from the number of neutrons.

    B.  The number of protons differs from the number of electrons.

    C.  The number of electrons differs from the number of neutrons.

    D.  The numbers of protons, electrons, and neutrons are all the same.

13. **Which of the following creates electromagnetic waves?**

    A.  An electron that is stationary

    B.  An electron that is approaching a proton

    C.  An electron that is moving at a constant velocity

    D.  An electron that is moving at a decreasing velocity

14. **Which type of wave is mechanical?**

    A.  Microwaves            B.  Radio waves

    C.  Seismic waves         D.  Infrared waves

15. **A reporter on the scene of an approaching hurricane notes that a pier has on one of its piles a large vertical ruler marked in feet. She uses it to measure ocean waves as they approach shore, finding that the waves are reaching as high as 12 feet and as low as 3 feet. What is the peak-to-peak amplitude of these waves?**

    A.  4.5 feet              B.  9 feet

    C.  12 feet               D.  15 feet

16. **What did Newton hypothesize when he watched the apple fall to the ground?**

    A. The force on the apple must be equal to its mass.

    B. The force on the apple must be unrelated to its mass.

    C. The force on the apple must be proportional to its mass.

    D. The force on the apple must be inversely proportional to its mass.

17. **How is an airbag useful in car accidents?**

    A. The airbag increases the force exerted by the driver.

    B. The airbag decreases the force exerted by the driver.

    C. The airbag increases the velocity exerted by the driver.

    D. The airbag decreases the velocity exerted by the driver.

18. **The impulse on an object is equal to the change in _____ that it causes.**

    A. energy          B. force

    C. momentum        D. velocity

19. **A volleyball of mass of 2.2 kg leaves the server's hand at 27 m/s. As the ball crosses above the 2.24 m high net, what kind(s) of energy does the ball possess?**

    A. Kinetic and potential

    B. Kinetic and electrical

    C. Potential and thermal

    D. Electrical and potential

20. **What characteristic of a force-time graph represents impulse?**

    A. The area under the curve

    B. The area above the curve

    C. The $y$-intercept of the curve

    D. The slope tangent to the curve

21. **Region X and region Y are approximately the same size, but the magnetic flux through region X is much higher. Which statement about these regions is correct?**

    A. The magnetic force in region X is less than in region Y.

    B. The magnetic force in region X is greater than in region Y.

    C. The magnetic force in region X and in region Y is about zero.

    D. The magnetic force in region X is about the same as in region Y.

22. **A physicist is accelerating ions in a vacuum chamber to examine their behavior. Considering only effects produced by the ions, which of the following will be absent?**

    A. Electric fields

    B. Magnetic fields

    C. Mechanical waves

    D. Electromagnetic waves

23. **Which term best describes a material that allows electric current to flow freely through it?**

    A. Conductor        B. Insulator

    C. Resistor         D. Voltage

24. **Which situation is impossible?**

    A.  An electric current in empty space

    B.  A north magnetic pole in empty space

    C.  A positive electric charge in empty space

    D.  An electromagnetic wave in empty space

25. **In a certain circuit, three wires connect at a node. If one of those wires carries 3 amps into the node and another carries 1 amp out of the node, what current does the third wire carry?**

    A.  2 amps into the node

    B.  2 amps out of the node

    C.  4 amps into the node

    D.  4 amps out of the node

# HESI Practice Exam 1 Answer Explanations

## Section I. Mathematics

**1. B.** The correct solution is 77. Use the subtraction algorithm. The process will involve borrowing from the tens place and then from the hundreds place. Alternatively, use a carefully drawn number line to estimate an answer or to check your results. **See Lesson: Basic Addition and Subtraction.**

**2. D.** To convert a ratio to a percent, divide the numbers in the ratio (noting that its equivalent fraction is $\frac{7}{3}$) to get approximately 2.33. Then, multiply by 100%. **See Lesson: Ratios, Proportions, and Percentages.**

**3. C.** The correct solution is $\frac{x^6 y^9}{z^3}$ because $(x^2 y^3 z^{-1})^3 = x^{2\times3} y^{3\times3} z^{-1\times3} = x^6 y^9 z^{-3} = \frac{x^6 y^2 z}{3z}$ . **See Lesson: Powers, Exponents, Roots, and Radicals.**

**4. B.** The correct solution is 1.7413 because 1.7413 contains the largest value in the tenths place. **See Lesson: Decimals and Fractions.**

**5. C.** The correct solution is 3 because $\frac{9}{4} \times \frac{4}{3} = \frac{36}{12} = 3$. **See Lesson: Multiplication and Division of Fractions.**

**6. D.** The correct solution is $1\frac{7}{8}$ because $\frac{5}{4} \times \frac{3}{2} = \frac{15}{8} = 1\frac{7}{8}$. **See Lesson: Multiplication and Division of Fractions.**

**7. D.** The correct solution is $3\frac{1}{2}$ because $\frac{3}{2} \times \frac{7}{3} = \frac{21}{6} = 3\frac{3}{6} = 3\frac{1}{2}$. **See Lesson: Multiplication and Division of Fractions.**

**8. B.** Answer B is correct. To convert 31% to a ratio, note that it is equal to $\frac{31}{100}$, which is 31:100 in colon ratio notation. **See Lesson: Ratios, Proportions, and Percentages.**

**9. B.** The correct solution is 7 because the cube root of 343 is 7. **See Lesson: Powers, Exponents, Roots, and Radicals.**

**10. D.** The correct solution is 6 because the landmass of the United States is about 4,000,000 square miles and the landmass of Alaska is about 700,000 square miles. So, the United States is about 6 times larger. **See Lesson: Powers, Exponents, Roots, and Radicals.**

**11. B.** The correct solution is 7. Since the biologist only has ringnecks and garters, any snake in her possession is a garter if it is not a ringneck. Because she has 13 snakes but 6 ringneck snakes, the number of garter snakes is the difference: 13 − 6 = 7. **See Lesson: Basic Addition and Subtraction.**

**12. B.** The correct answer is 20% because $\frac{1}{5}$ as a percent is 0.2 × 100 = 20%. **See Lesson: Decimals and Fractions.**

**13. D.** The correct solution is none of the above. Try some test cases. For example, −1 + 5 = 4, but −5 + 1 = −4. Also, −5 + 5 = 0. Counterexamples therefore show that statements A, B, and C are false. **See Lesson: Basic Addition and Subtraction.**

**14. D.** Division by 0 is undefined, and dividing a number by one yields that number. Also, 0 divided by any number is 0. **See Lesson: Basic Multiplication and Division.**

**15. D.** The correct answer is $\frac{29}{35}$ because $\frac{29}{10} \div \frac{7}{2} = \frac{29}{10} \times \frac{2}{7} = \frac{58}{70} = \frac{29}{35}$. **See Lesson: Multiplication and Division of Fractions.**

**16. B.** The correct answer is B. Ratios act just like fractions, so this product is the product of $\frac{8}{15}$ and 25% (which is equal to $\frac{1}{4}$). The answer is $\frac{8}{60} = \frac{2}{15}$. **See Lesson: Ratios, Proportions, and Percentages.**

**17. C.** The correct solutions are (2.2, 2.2) and (-2.2, -2.2).

| | |
|---|---|
| $x^2 + x^2 = 10$ | Substitute $x$ in for $y$ in the second equation. |
| $2x^2 = 10$ | Combine like terms on the left side of the equation. |
| $x^2 = 5$ | Divide both sides of the equation by 2. |
| $x = \pm 2.2$ | Apply the square root to both sides of the equation. |
| $y = 2.2$ | Substitute 2.2 in the first equation. |
| $y = -2.2$ | Substitute -2.2 in the first equation. |

**See Lesson: Equations with Two Variables.**

**18. B.** The correct solution is 3. The whole numbers include 0, 1, 2, 3,.... All whole numbers are greater than −3, but only 0, 1, and 2 are less than 3. **See Lesson: Basic Addition and Subtraction.**

**19. B.** Multiplication and division have equivalent priority in the order of operations. In this case, the expression must be evaluated from left to right. **See Lesson: Basic Multiplication and Division.**

**20. A.** The correct solution is −223. A negative number is always less than a positive number. Also, a negative number is less than another negative number if it is farther left on the number line: here,
−223 < −18. **See Lesson: Basic Addition and Subtraction.**

**21. C.** Because 462 is not evenly divisible by 53, remainder division is necessary. Use the division algorithm to obtain 8R38. **See Lesson: Basic Multiplication and Division.**

**22. B.** Because 26 is not evenly divisible by 9, the best answer in this case has a remainder. The division algorithm is used to obtain this result. **See Lesson: Basic Multiplication and Division.**

**23. A.** When multiplying signed numbers, remember that the product of a negative and a positive is negative. Other than the sign, the process is the same as multiplying whole numbers. **See Lesson: Basic Multiplication and Division.**

**24. D.** The correct answer is 21% because 0.21 as a percent is $0.21 \times 100 = 21\%$. **See Lesson: Decimals and Fractions.**

**25. C.** The correct answer is $11.\overline{1}\%$ because $0.\overline{1}$ as a percent is $0.\overline{1} \times 100 = 11.\overline{1}\%$. **See Lesson: Decimals and Fractions.**

**26. C.** The correct answer is 7.65 because $\frac{13}{20} = 13.00 \div 20 = 0.65$. **See Lesson: Decimals and Fractions.**

**27. D.** The correct answer is D. The fraction $\frac{36}{16}$ is 225%, meaning 36 is 225% of 16. **See Lesson: Ratios, Proportions, and Percentages.**

**28. B.** If 1 out of every 250 contract a disease, the fraction of people is $\frac{1}{250}$, which is equal to 0.004. Multiply by 100% to get 0.4%. **See Lesson: Ratios, Proportions, and Percentages.**

**29. C.** The correct solution is 8.48 quarts. $8L \times \frac{1.06 \, qt}{1 \, L} = 8.48 \, qt$. **See Lesson: Standards of Measure.**

**30. A.** The correct solution is 0.5 ton. 16,000 oz $\times \frac{1 \text{ lb}}{16 \text{ oz}} \times \frac{1 \text{T}}{2,000 \text{ lb}} = 16,\frac{000}{32},000 = 0.5\text{T}$. **See Lesson: Standards of Measure.**

**31. A.** The correct solution is 5.51 inches. 14 cm $\times \frac{1 \text{ in}}{2.54 \text{ cm}} = \frac{14}{2}.54 = 5.51$ in. **See Lesson: Standards of Measure.**

**32. C.** The correct solution is 8,000 pounds. 4T $\times \frac{2,000 \text{ lb}}{1 \text{ T}} = 8,000$ lb. **See Lesson: Standards of Measure.**

**33. B.** The correct solution is $x > -45$.

| | |
|---|---|
| $10x - 60 \leq 12x + 30$ | Multiply all terms by the least common denominator of 15 to eliminate the fractions. |
| $-2x - 60 \leq 30$ | Subtract 12x from both sides of the inequality. |
| $-2x \leq 90$ | Add 60 to both sides of the inequality. |
| $x \geq -45$ | Divide both sides of the inequality by –2. |

**See Lesson: Equations with One Variable.**

**34. A.** The correct solution is –20.

| | |
|---|---|
| $2x + 12 = x - 8$ | Multiply all terms by the least common denominator of 4 to eliminate the fractions. |
| $x + 12 = -8$ | Subtract x from both sides of the equation. |
| $x = -20$ | Subtract 12 from both sides of the equation. |

**See Lesson: Equations with One Variable.**

**35. D.** The correct solution is $\frac{9}{2}$.

| | |
|---|---|
| $5x - 3 = 3x + 6$ | Combine like terms on the left and right sides of the equation. |
| $2x - 3 = 6$ | Subtract 3x from both sides of the equation. |
| $2x = 9$ | Add 3 to both sides of the equation. |
| $x = \frac{9}{2}$ | Divide both sides of the equation by 2. |

**See Lesson: Equations with One Variable.**

**36. C.** The correct solution is $\frac{SA - 2\pi r^2}{2\pi r} = h$.

| | |
|---|---|
| $SA - 2\pi r^2 = 2\pi rh$ | Subtract $2\pi r^2$ from both sides of the equation. |
| $\frac{SA - 2\pi r^2}{2\pi r} = h$ | Divide both sides of the equation by $2\pi r$. |

**See Lesson: Equations with One Variable.**

**37. A.** The correct solution is $\frac{2ab}{1-2a} = c$.

| | |
|---|---|
| $2ab + 2ac = c$ | Apply the distributive property. |
| $2ab = c - 2ac$ | Subtract 2ac from both sides of the equation. |
| $2ab = c(1 - 2a)$ | Factor c from the right side of the equation. |
| $\frac{2ab}{1-2a} = c$ | Divide both sides of the equation by $1 - 2a$. |

**See Lesson: Equations with One Variable.**

**38. A.** The correct graph has the two lines intersect at (-3, 1). **See Lesson: Equations with Two Variables.**

**39. A.** The correct solution is (8, -1).

| | |
|---|---|
| $6x + 10y = 38$ | Multiply all terms in the first equation by 2. |
| $25x - 10y = 210$ | Multiply all terms in the second equation by 5. |
| $31x = 248$ | Add the equations. |
| $x = 8$ | Divide both sides of the equation by 31. |
| $3(8) + 5y = 19$ | Substitute 8 in the first equation for x. |
| $24 + 5y = 19$ | Simplify using order of operations. |
| $5y = -5$ | Subtract 24 from both sides of the equation. |
| $y = -1$ | Divide both sides of the equation by 5. |

**See Lesson: Equations with Two Variables.**

**40. C.** The correct solution is (2, 8).

| | |
|---|---|
| $4y = 32$ | Add the equations. |
| $y = 8$ | Divide both sides of the equation by 4. |
| $4x - 8 = 0$ | Substitute 8 in the second equation for y. |
| $4x = 8$ | Add 8 to both sides of the equation. |
| $x = 2$ | Divide both sides of the equation by 4. |

**See Lesson: Equations with Two Variables.**

**41. B.** The correct solution is $\frac{81y^6}{x^4}$ because $(9x^{-2}y^3)^2 = 9^2x^{-2\times2}y^{3\times2} = 9^2x^{-4}y^6 = 81x^{-4}y^6 = \frac{81y^6}{x^4}$. **See Lesson: Powers, Exponents, Roots, and Radicals.**

**42. D.** The correct solution is $3\frac{1}{2}$ because $\frac{3}{4}(3) + 2\frac{1}{2}\left(\frac{1}{2}\right) = \frac{3}{4}\left(\frac{3}{1}\right) + \frac{5}{2}\left(\frac{1}{2}\right) = \frac{9}{4} + \frac{5}{4} = \frac{14}{4} = \frac{7}{2} = 3\frac{1}{2}$ cups of sugar. **See Lesson: Solving Real World Mathematical Problems.**

**43. B.** The correct solution is $12.50 because she worked a total of $4.25(2) + 6.5(2) = 8.5 + 13 = 21.5$ hours. The hourly rate is $268.75 \div 21.50 = 12.50$. **See Lesson: Solving Real World Mathematical Problems.**

**44. B.** The correct solution is $4.50 because $21.25 - 7.75 = 13.50 \div 3 = 4.50$. **See Lesson: Solving Real World Mathematical Problems.**

**45. C.** The correct solution is $6\frac{1}{12}$ because $2\frac{3}{4} + 3\frac{1}{3} = 2\frac{9}{12} + 3\frac{4}{12} = 5\frac{13}{12} = 6\frac{1}{12}$ miles. **See Lesson: Solving Real World Mathematical Problems.**

**46. A.** The correct solution is $\frac{1}{10}$ because $1 - \left(\frac{1}{6} + \frac{2}{5} + \frac{1}{3}\right) = 1 - \left(\frac{5}{30} + \frac{12}{30} + \frac{10}{30}\right) = 1 - \frac{27}{30} = 1 = \frac{9}{10} = \frac{1}{10}$ of the yard remaining. **See Lesson: Solving Real World Mathematical Problems.**

**47. B.** The correct solution is $3x^3 - 9x^2 - 2x + 6$.

$(3x^2 - 2)(x - 3) = 3x^2(x - 3) - 2(x - 3) = 3x^3 - 9x^2 - 2x + 6$

**See Lesson: Polynomials.**

**48. D.** The correct solution is $2x^3 - 3x^2 - 17x - 12$.

$(2x + 3)(x^2 - 3x - 4) = (2x + 3)(x^2) + (2x + 3)(-3x) + (2x + 3)(-4) = 2x^3 + 3x^2 - 6x^2 - 9x - 8x - 12$
$= 2x^3 - 3x^2 - 17x - 12$

**See Lesson: Polynomials.**

**49. B.** The correct solution is $-20x^3y^5$. $-4x^2y^2(5xy^3) = -20x^3y^5$. **See Lesson: Polynomials.**

**50. B.** The correct solution is $(3x - 5)^2$. The expression $9x^2 - 30x + 25$ is rewritten as $(3x - 5)^2$ because the value of $a$ is 3x and the value of $b$ is 5. **See Lesson: Polynomials.**

# Section II. Reading Comprehension

**1. B.** If a book is describing information, its purpose is to inform. **See Lesson: Understanding the Author's Purpose, Point of View, and Rhetorical Strategies.**

**2. C.** This is an advertisement. Although it includes some information its primary purpose is to convince you to buy something. This makes it a persuasive text. **See Lesson: Understanding the Author's Purpose, Point of View, and Rhetorical Strategies.**

**3. D.** It is difficult to know much about the true feelings of advertising writers because it's their job to sell products, not say what they believe. However, it is a fair bet that advertising writers believe people will pay money for products presented the way they describe. **See Lesson: Understanding the Author's Purpose, Point of View, and Rhetorical Strategies.**

**4. D.** Celebrity endorsements in advertisements appeal to the emotions by associating a product for sale with a person who is widely admired. **See Lesson: Understanding the Author's Purpose, Point of View, and Rhetorical Strategies.**

**5. C.** Much of the information in this advertisement is not verifiable, but the fact that the clothing tracks the body's signals with sensors is a fact. **See Lesson: Understanding the Author's Purpose, Point of View, and Rhetorical Strategies.**

**6. C.** The advertisement highlights several aspects of WiseWear gear, such as the comfort and ease of use, that suggest the potential customer will feel good using the products. These details appeal to the emotions. **See Lesson: Understanding the Author's Purpose, Point of View, and Rhetorical Strategies.**

**7. B.** The first sentence of this paragraph expresses the main idea that people should be concerned by even a small amount of climate change. This makes it the topic sentence. **See Lesson: Main Ideas, Topic Sentences, and Supporting Details.**

**8. A.** The topic of a sentence is a word or phrase that describes what the text is about. **See Lesson: Main Ideas, Topic Sentences, and Supporting Details.**

**9. C.** This paragraph argues that a small change in global temperatures could have a major result. This idea is expressed in a topic sentence at the beginning of the paragraph. **See Lesson: Main Ideas, Topic Sentences, and Supporting Details.**

**10. D.** The information about temperature differences in the last ice age supports the main idea that people should be concerned by global climate change. This makes it a supporting detail. **See Lesson: Main Ideas, Topic Sentences, and Supporting Details.**

**11. B.** All of the above sentences relate to the topic of global climate change, but only the sentence about the Little Ice Age relates directly to the main idea that a small amount of climate fluctuation is cause for concern. **See Lesson: Main Ideas, Topic Sentences, and Supporting Details.**

**12. B.** The sentence above conveys factual information about Mars in an excited tone that suggests a positive interest in the subject. This makes it most likely to fit into an informational paragraph sharing facts about Mars. **See Lesson: Main Ideas, Topic Sentences, and Supporting Details.**

**13. D.** If the above sentence were a topic sentence, its supporting details would likely share information to develop the idea that Mars may have supported life in the past. **See Lesson: Main Ideas, Topic Sentences, and Supporting Details.**

**14. C.** The sentence above could act as an example to show how space discoveries teach us about Earth and ourselves. **See Lesson: Main Ideas, Topic Sentences, and Supporting Details.**

**15. B.** The argument that prison nursery programs can be beneficial is an opinion statement because it makes a judgment. **See Lesson: Facts Opinions and Evaluating an Argument.**

**16. B.** The statement makes a factual statement about how people said they felt. This makes it a fact even though it contains opinion information. **See Lesson: Facts Opinions and Evaluating an Argument.**

**17. C.** The main argument in this passage is that it may be beneficial to both mothers and babies if women who give birth in prison are allowed to keep their children with them. One assumption behind the passage is that society must promote the health and safety of children, but this is not the main argument. **See Lesson: Facts Opinions and Evaluating an Argument.**

**18. D.** The passage states explicitly that the idea of raising children in prison is controversial, so this is not an assumption. It does assume that our society should attempt to help children born to mothers in prison. **See Lesson: Facts Opinions and Evaluating an Argument.**

**19. B.** The sentence about putting babies in jail uses its own reason to defend its argument. It needs to provide evidence instead. **See Lesson: Facts Opinions and Evaluating an Argument.**

**20. A.** The paragraph about benefits to mothers shows that mothers who participate in the prison nursery program have better outcomes. It suggests but does not prove that their participation in the program is the cause of these outcomes. **See Lesson: Facts Opinions and Evaluating an Argument.**

**21. B.** The sentences above use a form of faulty reasoning called either/or reasoning. They suggest that there are only two possible ways for society to respond to the issue of babies being born in prison when in fact there are many. **See Lesson: Facts Opinions and Evaluating an Argument.**

**22. D.** An opinion statement includes feelings or beliefs that are not necessarily verifiably true, but it may be based on valid reasoning. **See Lesson: Facts Opinions and Evaluating an Argument.**

**23. C.** In the context of reading and writing, an argument is a statement meant to prove a point, not a heated disagreement. **See Lesson: Facts Opinions and Evaluating an Argument.**

**24. D.** Primary sources are written by people who witnessed the original creation or discovery of the information they present. This description does not apply to an encyclopedia entry. **See Lesson: Understanding Primary Sources Making Inferences and Drawing Conclusions.**

**25. D.** Readers must use judgment to determine how credible a source is in a particular circumstance. A researcher interested in modern farming technology would want an impartial recent article on the subject from a credible publisher. **See Lesson: Understanding Primary Sources Making Inferences and Drawing Conclusions.**

**26. D.** An online database of writings by a historical figure is primary, but a blog post reflecting on his contributions is secondary. **See Lesson: Understanding Primary Sources Making Inferences and Drawing Conclusions.**

**27. A.** The word *credible* means trustworthy. **See Lesson: Understanding Primary Sources Making Inferences and Drawing Conclusions.**

**28. C.** Emotional arguments may reasonably appear in a persuasive text, but not if they use manipulative strategies like scare tactics. **See Lesson: Understanding Primary Sources Making Inferences and Drawing Conclusions.**

**29. A.** A conference presentation reporting the results of scientific research is a primary source. Videos, photographs, and audio recordings of primary sources are also primary. **See Lesson: Understanding Primary Sources Making Inferences and Drawing Conclusions.**

**30. B.** Secondary sources add value to the discussion of a topic but are also removed from the original information. **See Lesson: Understanding Primary Sources Making Inferences and Drawing Conclusions.**

**31. A.** The authors of primary sources witnessed the original creation or discovery of the information they present. For this reason, they are considered the most trustworthy. **See Lesson: Understanding Primary Sources Making Inferences and Drawing Conclusions**

**32. D** The pie chart indicates the amount of time students of different genders contribute to discussions. The larger wedge for male speaking indicates that 70% of class discussion time is dominated by male speakers. **See Lesson: Summarizing Text and Using Text Features.**

**33. B.** If you read the labels carefully, you will see that the bar graph shows how many times students of each gender *are interrupted* during class discussions. The graph shows that students are interrupted more often than male students. **See Lesson: Summarizing Text and Using Text Features.**

**34. B.** The data in the chart and graph could help show that male students are receiving more chances to speak in class discussions, and that it would be a good idea to increase gender parity. **See Lesson: Summarizing Text and Using Text Features.**

**35. A.** A summary restates another author's ideas in different ways. **See Lesson: Summarizing Text and Using Text Features.**

**36. B.** This paragraph discusses the past and future in a way that shifts constantly between the two. Some events are vague and may overlap with others. However, coming to America is a clear event that happened before the escape from physical poverty and the entrance into the poverty of the soul. **See Lesson: Summarizing Text and Using Text Features.**

**37. C.** A bar graph shows relationships between numbers, so it could be used to illustrate how much of something a business has sold and which products have sold more than others. **See Lesson: Summarizing Text and Using Text Features.**

**38. B.** There is only one arrow leading from the start box, and it goes to the "look in the kitchen" box. **See Lesson: Summarizing Text and Using Text Features.**

**39. D.** The arrow that is labeled "No" directs readers to "Look in the kitchen." **See Lesson: Summarizing Text and Using Text Features.**

**40. A.** Transition words like "despite" express a contrast between ideas. **See Lesson: Tone and Mood, Transition Words.**

**41. D.** The sentences above would be best served with an example transition and an addition transition. **See Lesson: Tone and Mood, Transition Words.**

**42. A.** Words that say the opposite of what they really mean are ironic. Irony can be confusing to the reader at times, but it is not confused (which would imply that the writer does not know what he or she means). **See Lesson: Tone and Mood, Transition Words.**

**43. D.** Tone is the author's apparent attitude toward the subject of a text. It is distinguished from mood, which is the reader's emotional response. **See Lesson: Tone and Mood, Transition Words.**

**44. B.** The author of this passage is reporting on a controversial issue with an objective or impartial tone. **See Lesson: Tone and Mood, Transition Words.**

**45. C.** Dr. Hussein's words show that he cares deeply about the responsibility of his position. His tone could be described as earnest or concerned. **See Lesson: Tone and Mood, Transition Words.**

**46. A.** Liz Goode is highly critical of embryonic research. Her tone could be described as harsh, scathing, or critical. **See Lesson: Tone and Mood, Transition Words.**

**47. D.** The phrase "on the contrary" helps express a contrast. In other words, it introduces a juxtaposition of dissimilar ideas. **See Lesson: Tone and Mood, Transition Words.**

# Section III. Vocabulary and General Knowledge

**1. C.** Adding the prefix "peri" would make the word "pericardium," or the membrane around the heart. **See Lesson: Domain-Specific Words: Medical Terminology.**

**2. D.** The prefix *super* means "over or above," so a superlative performance would be a magnificent one. **See Lesson: Root Words, Prefixes, and Suffixes.**

**3. A.** The root *chrom* means "color" and the prefix *mono* means "one," so monochromatic means to having one color. **See Lesson: Root Words, Prefixes, and Suffixes.**

**4. B.** "Rhino" refers to the "nose," so the surgeon was going to operate on the patient's nose. **See Lesson: Domain-Specific Words: Medical Terminology.**

**5. A.** The prefix *in* means "not," and the root word "trans" means across. So an intransigent person is not willing to cross or bend, so this would be a stubborn person. **See Lesson: Root Words, Prefixes, and Suffixes.**

**6. C.** The prefix *in* means "not," so infamous means not known for being famous or for something good, so infamous means notorious. **See Lesson: Root Words, Prefixes, and Suffixes.**

**7. D.** The meaning of <u>refrain</u> in this context is "to stop from doing something." The phrase "did not want to offend" helps you figure out which meaning of <u>refrain</u> is being used. **See Lesson: Context Clues and Multiple Meaning Words.**

**8. D.** The root *ject* means "to throw" and the prefix *inter* means "between," so interject means to throw one's words between a conversation or cut into a conversation. **See Lesson: Root Words, Prefixes, and Suffixes.**

**9. C.** The word "encephalitis" means "inflammation of the brain." **See Lesson: Domain-Specific Words: Medical Terminology.**

**10. D.** The meaning of <u>bind</u> in this context is "to form a mass that stays connected." The word "together" helps you figure out which meaning of <u>bind</u> is being used. **See Lesson: Context Clues and Multiple Meaning Words.**

**11. B.** The meaning of <u>formula</u> in this context is "a liquid that is given to babies." The phrase "baby" helps you figure out which meaning of <u>formula</u> is being used. **See Lesson: Context Clues and Multiple Meaning Words.**

**12. A.** The word a "hypodermic" needle would go "under the skin." **See Lesson: Domain-Specific Words: Medical Terminology.**

**13. C.** The meaning of <u>laborious</u> in this context is "requiring a lot of time and effort." The phrase "many hours" helps you figure out the meaning of <u>unkempt</u>. **See Lesson: Context Clues and Multiple Meaning Words.**

**14. B.** Adding the prefix "hypo" would make the word "hypoglycemia," or low blood sugar. **See Lesson: Domain-Specific Words: Medical Terminology.**

**15. C.** The suffix –stasis means "to stop or control." **See Lesson: Domain-Specific Words: Medical Terminology.**

**16. C.** The root word that means "bones" is "oste." **See Lesson: Domain-Specific Words: Medical Terminology.**

**17. D.** "Intravenous" means "inside the vein." **See Lesson: Domain-Specific Words: Medical Terminology.**

**18. A.** The suffix –oma means "swelling of or tumor." **See Lesson: Domain-Specific Words: Medical Terminology.**

**19. D.** The root word that means "veins" is "phleb." **See Lesson: Domain-Specific Words: Medical Terminology.**

**20. A.** "Nephralgia" means "pain of the kidneys." **See Lesson: Domain-Specific Words: Medical Terminology.**

**21. D.** The suffix –sclerosis means "hardening of." **See Lesson: Domain-Specific Words: Medical Terminology.**

**22. B.** The root word that means "small intestines" is "enter." **See Lesson: Domain-Specific Words: Medical Industry.**

**23. C.** "Carcinogenic" means "cancer-causing." **See Lesson: Domain-Specific Words: Medical Terminology.**

**24. C.** The prefix "post" would make the word "postnatal" to complete the sentence. **See Lesson: Domain-Specific Words: Medical Terminology.**

**25. D.** The meaning of <u>somnambulist</u> in the context of this sentence is "sleepwalker." **See Lesson: Context Clues and Multiple Meaning Words.**

**26. C.** The word "application" has more than one meaning. **See Lesson: Context Clues and Multiple Meaning Words.**

**27. D.** The meaning of <u>novice</u> in the context of this sentence is "beginner." **See Lesson: Context Clues and Multiple Meaning Words.**

**28. A.** The meaning of <u>cantankerous</u> in the context of this sentence is "irritable." **See Lesson: Context Clues and Multiple Meaning Words.**

**29. D.** The suffix that means "the study of" is *logy*. **See Lesson: Root Words, Prefixes, and Suffixes.**

**30. A.** The root that means "to throw" is *ject*. **See Lesson: Root Words, Prefixes, and Suffixes.**

**31. B.** The meaning of <u>exuberant</u> in the context of this sentence is "cheerful." **See Lesson: Context Clues and Multiple Meaning Words.**

**32. B.** The word "prune" has more than one meaning. **See Lesson: Context Clues and Multiple Meaning Words.**

**33. A.** The meaning of <u>garish</u> in the context of this sentence is "glaring." **See Lesson: Context Clues and Multiple Meaning Words.**

**34. B.** The word "constitution" has more than one meaning. **See Lesson: Context Clues and Multiple Meaning Words.**

**35. C.** The meaning of <u>fluctuate</u> in the context of this sentence is "change." **See Lesson: Context Clues and Multiple Meaning Words.**

**36. A.** The prefix that means "after" is *post*. **See Lesson: Root Words, Prefixes, and Suffixes.**

**37. A.** The root *bene* means "good," so benevolent means kind. **See Lesson: Root Words, Prefixes, and Suffixes.**

**38. B.** The word "content" has more than one meaning. **See Lesson: Context Clues and Multiple Meaning Words.**

**39. A.** The root *tele* means "far." **See Lesson: Root Words, Prefixes, and Suffixes.**

**40. A.** The root that means "foot" is *ped*. **See Lesson: Root Words, Prefixes, and Suffixes.**

**41. B.** The suffix that means "belonging to" is *ian*. **See Lesson: Root Words, Prefixes, and Suffixes.**

**42. B.** The suffix that means "person who practices" is *ist*. **See Lesson: Root Words, Prefixes, and Suffixes.**

**43. C.** The root that means "to say" is *dict*. **See Lesson: Root Words, Prefixes, and Suffixes.**

**44. B.** The suffix that means "made of" is *en*. **See Lesson: Root Words, Prefixes, and Suffixes.**

**45. C.** The root that means "to break" is *rupt*. **See Lesson: Root Words, Prefixes, and Suffixes.**

**46. D.** The suffix that means "capable of" is *ible*. **See Lesson: Root Words, Prefixes, and Suffixes.**

**47. A.** The suffix that means "having characteristics of" is *ic*. **See Lesson: Root Words, Prefixes, and Suffixes.**

**48. B.** The root that means "heat" is *therm*. **See Lesson: Root Words, Prefixes, and Suffixes.**

**49. D.** The prefix that means "too much" is *over*. **See Lesson: Root Words, Prefixes, and Suffixes.**

**50. D.** The root *post* means "after," so postscript means something that was written after something else. **See Lesson: Root Words, Prefixes, and Suffixes.**

# Section IV. Grammar

**1. D.** *Two* is the correctly spelled form of the number. **See Lesson: Spelling.**

**2. B.** My favorite day of the week is Tuesday. My favorite month is March, and autumn is my favorite season. Days of the week and months of the year need to be capitalized, but seasons are not. **See Lesson: Capitalization.**

**3. A.** People *bow*, or bend down, to show respect. **See Lesson: Spelling.**

**4. D.** The House of Representatives had 435 members. National organizations need to be capitalized. Shorter prepositions, articles, and conjunctions in the names of organizations are not capitalized. **See Lesson: Capitalization.**

**5. A.** Arnold Schwarzenegger was the governor of California. Individual names and states are always capitalized. Professional titles are capitalized when they precede a name or are part of a direct address. **See Lesson: Capitalization.**

**6. A.** *Wear* is the only correctly spelled form of the word that fits with the sentence. **See Lesson: Spelling.**

**7. D.** *There should be a question mark after weekend*. What is a common question word. **See Lesson: Punctuation.**

**8. D.** *There needs to be a comma after claimed*. Commas are needed for introductory phrases and before the quoted material. **See Lesson: Punctuation.**

**9. B.** *The Bachelor*. The names of TV shows are capitalized. The is capitalized here because it is the first word in the name. **See Lesson: Capitalization.**

**10.** **B.** *She had a bad day*. A period is only used at the end of a sentence, and not anywhere in between. **See Lesson: Punctuation.**

**11.** **B.** *There* describes a place or position and is correctly spelled. **See Lesson: Spelling.**

**12.** **D.** *Hospital's does not need an apostrophe*. Hospitals is plural and is not possessive in this sentence. **See Lesson: Punctuation.**

**13.** **D.** The nouns are *team*, *scientists*, *results*, *research*, and *conference*. **See Lesson: Nouns.**

**14.** **A.** *Having been repaired* is placed where it references *we*, but it should reference *the car*. **See Lesson: Modifiers**

**15.** **B.** *Slowly* is an adverb that describes the verb *ran*. **See Lesson: Adjectives and Adverbs.**

**16.** **D.** *We, his, which*, and *he* are pronouns. **See Lesson: Pronouns.**

**17.** **B.** The helping verb *do* should be used to make a negative statement with the main verb *worry*. **See Lesson: Verbs and Verb Tenses.**

**18.** **A.** Or. It is the only conjunction that fits within the context of the sentence. **See Lesson: Types of Clauses.**

**19. C.** *Toured* and *saw* are verbs. **See Lesson: Verbs and Verb Tenses.**

**20. B.** This is a simple sentence since it contains one independent clause consisting of a simple subject and a predicate. **See Lesson: Types of Sentences.**

**21. B.** *Redecorated by Tory* would be parallel in structure since the list begins in passive voice and uses the past tense of the verbs. **See Lesson: Types of Sentences.**

**22. D.** This is a complex sentence because it has a dependent clause, an independent clause, and a subordinating conjunction, *even though*. **See Lesson: Types of Sentences.**

**23. B.** *Yet* is a conjunction. **See Lesson: Conjunctions and Prepositions.**

**24. B.** *Dinner* is the direct object of the verb *cooked*. **See Lesson: Direct Objects and Indirect Objects.**

**25. A.** *After reading the book* is a modifier that, by its placement, is incorrectly referenced to *the movie*. The modifier is dangling because there is no noun or pronoun that references the person who read the book. **See Lesson: Modifiers**

**26. B.** *Publishing his own book* would be parallel in structure to the other items since they are longer phrases and use the gerund form of the verb. **See Lesson: Types of Sentences.**

**27. A.** *Nation* is a singular noun, so the pronoun that refers to it should be a singular possessive pronoun. **See Lesson: Pronouns.**

**28. D.** *Royal, beautiful,* and *meaningful* describe *wedding*. **See Lesson: Modifiers**

**29. A.** *When six years old* is missing a reference. To add this reference, *I*, the sentence can be rewritten *When I was six years old, our family...* or *When six years old, I experienced our family's transfer.* **See Lesson: Modifiers**

**30. C.** *Family* and *area* are common nouns and should not be capitalized. **See Lesson: Nouns.**

**31. C.** *His keys* is the direct object of the verb *locked*. **See Lesson: Direct Objects and Indirect Objects.**

**32. D.** The nouns are *team, scientists, results, research,* and *conference*. **See Lesson: Nouns.**

**33. D.** Neither the verb tried nor the verb succeed has a direct object. *So* and *hard* are adverbs. **See Lesson: Direct Objects and Indirect Objects.**

**34. B.** *Even though* is a subordinating conjunction. It connects the clauses *I walked home* and *my feet really hurt*. **See Lesson: Conjunctions and Prepositions.**

**35. A.** *Marie's* and *father's* are possessive; neither is plural. *Appendix* is a singular noun. **See Lesson: Nouns.**

**36. A.** None of these words are nouns; *I* and *her* and pronouns. **See Lesson: Nouns.**

**37. B.** The adverb *well* describes the verb *did*. **See Lesson: Adjectives and Adverbs**

**38. A.** *Until* is a subordinating conjunction, connecting the main clause *don't leave* and the dependent clause *we get there*. **See Lesson: Conjunctions and Prepositions.**

**39. D.** *Safely* is an adverb that describes the verb *traveled*. **See Lesson: Adjectives and Adverbs**

**40. A.** With *neither/nor*, if both subjects are third person singular, the verb should take the third person singular form. **See Lesson: Subject and Verb Agreement.**

**41. A.** *Broadens their perspective* would be parallel in structure to the other items since they are longer phrases and use the same verb form. **See Lesson: Types of Sentences.**

**42. C.** But. It is the only conjunction that fits within the context of the sentence. **See Lesson: Types of Clauses.**

**43. D.** This sentence is correct. **See Lesson: Modifiers**

**44. C.** *In* is a preposition. **See Lesson: Conjunctions and Prepositions.**

**45. B.** *Read* is the only verb in the sentence. **See Lesson: Verbs and Verb Tenses.**

**46. C.** *Patients* is the direct object of the verb *treated*. **See Lesson: Direct Objects and Indirect Objects.**

**47. D.** This sentence has two predicates connected by *because*. In the second predicate, the verb *is* agrees with the subject *family*. **See Lesson: Subject and Verb Agreement.**

**48. A.** So. It is the only conjunction that fits within the context of the sentence. **See Lesson: Types of Clauses.**

**49. B.** *You* is the only pronoun listed. **See Lesson: Pronouns.**

**50. A.** The subject *family* is singular and takes the verb *is*. **See Lesson: Subject and Verb Agreement.**

# Section V. Biology

**1. D.** In a taxonomic system, each level is found in the level above it. Thus, the class level is found in the phylum and kingdom levels. **See Lesson: An Introduction to Biology.**

**2. C.** This polymer is a carbohydrate, so it must consist of several glycerol molecules that are covalently bonded together. **See Lesson: An Introduction to Biology.**

**3. C.** Amino acids are the monomers used to make proteins. An example of a protein is an enzyme. **See Lesson: An Introduction to Biology.**

**4. C.** The type of road salt used is the independent variable because it is the variable that is purposely changed during the study. It is the causative factor in the experiment. **See Lesson: An Introduction to Biology.**

**5. D.** The researcher is questioning whether taking a drug can lower cholesterol. The hypothesis is a predicted solution to this question: The drug will lower cholesterol. **See Lesson: An Introduction to Biology.**

**6. C.** Homeostasis is common to all living things, so this trait can be used to differentiate a living thing from a nonliving thing. **See Lesson: An Introduction to Biology.**

**7. A.** The cell theory is a theory because it is supported by a significant number of experimental findings. The cell theory took many years to be developed because microscopes were not powerful enough to make such observations. **See Lesson: Cell Structure, Function, and Type.**

**8. D.** Common characteristics of prokaryotic cells are that they are small and have hair-like structures called pili that surround their cell wall. **See Lesson: Cell Structure, Function, and Type.**

**9. A.** Flagella are tails attached to a cell that aid in locomotion, or movement throughout a cell's external environment. **See Lesson: Cell Structure, Function, and Type.**

**10. C.** Eukaryotic cells are unicellular or multicellular organisms that contain a membrane-bound nucleus. Eukaryotic cells contain several different organelles. **See Lesson: Cell Structure, Function, and Type.**

**11. C.** Plant cells are autotrophs that harness energy from the sun and use it to make food. This process of using energy to make food is done with the help of photosynthesis. **See Lesson: Cell Structure, Function, and Type.**

**12. A.** The most basic unit and building block of all living things is the cell. **See Lesson: Cell Structure, Function, and Type.**

**13. C.** Because *glycolysis* literally means "sugar breaking," this process involves the breakdown of glucose into pyruvate molecules to generate ATP. **See Lesson: Cellular Reproduction, Cellular Respiration, and Photosynthesis.**

**14. B.** The $G_2$ phase prepares for the M (mitotic) phase by making tubulin for microtubules. These microtubules, with the help of spindle fibers, separate chromosomes during mitosis. **See Lesson: Cellular Reproduction, Cellular Respiration, and Photosynthesis.**

**15. B.** Meiosis is a form of cell division that occurs when DNA from homologous chromosomes is exchanged. This exchange, or crossing over, increases genetic diversity in a population. **See Lesson: Cellular Reproduction, Cellular Respiration, and Photosynthesis.**

**16. C.** During prometaphase, the spindle fibers (that are attached to the centromere of the chromosome) pull the duplicated chromosome toward the poles of the cell. **See Lesson: Cellular Reproduction, Cellular Respiration, and Photosynthesis.**

**17. A.** During interphase, the cell undergoes an initial gap phase called $G_1$ before its DNA is copied in the S phase. After the DNA is copied, the cell undergoes a second gap phase called $G_2$. Then, the cell is ready to enter the mitotic phase, during which it divides into daughter cells. **See Lesson: Cellular Reproduction, Cellular Respiration, and Photosynthesis.**

**18. A.** ATP and NADH are produced are produced during the light reactions of photosynthesis. During the dark reactions, these organic molecules are used to create sugar molecules. **See Lesson: Cellular Reproduction, Cellular Respiration, and Photosynthesis.**

**19. D.** A gene is a segment of DNA that transmits information from the parent to the offspring.
**See Lesson: Genetics and DNA.**

**20. C.** The replication of DNA ends with a twisted strand called a double helix. **See Lesson: Genetics and DNA.**

**21. B.** Humans have 23 sets of chromosomes. **See Lesson: Genetics and DNA.**

**22. B.** One of the alleles is dominant, so it is expressed. **See Lesson: Genetics and DNA.**

**23. A.** A copy of a gene used as a blueprint for a protein is mRNA. **See Lesson: Genetics and DNA.**

**24. A.** Each offspring receives 1 allele for a particular trait from each parent. **See Lesson: Genetics and DNA.**

**25. A.** The probable outcome of this cross would be 1 homozygous dominant, 2 heterozygous dominants, and 1 homozygous recessive. **See Lesson: Genetics and DNA.**

# Section VI. Chemistry

**1. C.** The placebo is a false treatment given to a group to account for the body's psychological response to this type of treatment in a study. **See Lesson: Designing an Experiment.**

**2. D.** Researchers must use inductive and deductive reasoning to formulate a plausible hypothesis. **See Lesson: Designing an Experiment.**

**3. C.** Other terms for *negative variation* are indirect correlation, inverse correlation, and negative correlation. **See Lesson: Designing an Experiment.**

**4. D.** In the image, a thermometer is inserted into a graduated cylinder, which measures the volume of a solution. **See Lesson: Designing an Experiment.**

**5. D.** The exponent is positive 5, which means that the decimal point moves to the right five spaces when converting to standard notation. **See Lesson: Scientific Notation.**

**6. A.** The mass of a proton or neutron is 1.0 amu, and the mass of an electron is much less, 0.00054 amu. **See Lesson: Scientific Notation.**

**7. B.** The protons and neutrons are in the nucleus, which is very small and dense. The electron cloud makes up most of the atom in terms of area. **See Lesson: Scientific Notation.**

**8. C.** The electrons are found in the lowest possible shells. Only 2 can fit in the first shell, and only 8 can fit in the second shell. Filling those levels accommodates 10 electrons. The remaining 3 electrons will go into the third shell. **See Lesson: Scientific Notation.**

**9. A.** Celsius is part of metric system of measurement. It is a universally accepted way to record temperature values in science. **See Lesson: Temperature and the Metric System.**

**10. B.** Using the following formula, K = °C + 273: 85 − 273=−188. **See Lesson: Temperature and the Metric System.**

**11. D.** Use the following equation to convert Celsius to Fahrenheit: $F = \left(\frac{9}{5}\right)C + 32$

Where $F = \left(\frac{9}{5}\right) \times 105°C + 32 = 221$. **See Lesson: Temperature and the Metric System.**

**12. C.** To convert 35°C to Kelvin, 273 must be added to this value, which yields the value of 308K. **See Lesson: Temperature and the Metric System.**

**13. B.** The line between B and C is the melting point, around 1500°C, and the line between D and E is the boiling point, around 2900°C. **See Lesson: States of Matter.**

**14. D.** The number of carbon atoms in a molecule of each substance increases going down the chart, as do the boiling points. It takes more energy to separate molecules of alcohols that have a higher number of carbon atoms because the forces between the molecules are stronger. **See Lesson: States of Matter.**

**15. B.** When heating or cooling a substance, the temperature will not change while a substance is undergoing a phase change; it will only change when it is in a single state of matter before or after the phase change. The question indicates that the sample is a solid at the beginning of the experiment, and if the student is adding energy, the substance is melting. **See Lesson: States of Matter.**

**16. D.** Flammability is an indication of a chemical change. **See Lesson: Properties of Matter.**

**17. B.** Osmosis is the diffusion of water molecules through a membrane in the direction of higher solute concentration. **See Lesson: Properties of Matter.**

**18. B.** There is a double bond between carbon and oxygen. They share two pairs of electrons, which is a total of four electrons. **See Lesson: Chemical Bonds.**

**19. A.** The carbon-carbon bond in acetylene is a triple bond, which is stronger than the others because three pairs of electrons are being shared, rather than two or one pair. **See Lesson: Chemical Bonds.**

**20. C.** In a chemical formula, the subscript after each element symbol shows the number of atoms of that element in one molecule. In methanol, there is one carbon atom, four hydrogen atoms, and one oxygen atom. **See Lesson: Chemical Bonds.**

**21. C.** Both the reactants and products include one substance that is an aqueous solution and one solid substance. This means that there is a solution with a solid inside that does not dissolve, making it heterogeneous. **See Lesson: Chemical Solutions.**

**22. B.** In this reaction, chlorine ($Cl_2$) is an element in the reaction that replaces iodine in the compound sodium iodide (NaI). This allows chlorine to form a compound with sodium (NaCl) and leaves iodine ($I_2$) as an element. **See Lesson: Chemical Solutions.**

**23. C.** A pH of 7 is a neutral solution, which is how pure water is classified. **See Lesson: Acids and Bases.**

**24. B.** According to the Arrhenius theory for acids, these substances dissociate into hydrogen ions when dissolved in water. Arrhenius bases dissociate into hydroxide ions. **See Lesson: Acids and Bases.**

**25. A.** Hydrogen sulfate ($HSO_4^-$) is the conjugate base of sulfuric acid ($H_2SO_4$) because the acid donates a proton when it dissolves in an aqueous solution. **See Lesson: Acids and Bases.**

# Section VII. Anatomy and Physiology

**1. C.** The knee is closer to the point of attachment (where the thigh attaches to the trunk of the body) than the foot, so it is proximal to the foot. **See Lesson: Organization of the Human Body.**

**2. A.** The maintenance of normal blood pressure is a negative-feedback mechanism. **See Lesson: Organization of the Human Body.**

**3. D.** When a ventricular systole occurs, the ventricle is contracting. This is associated with the QRS complex on the electrocardiogram. **See Lesson: Cardiovascular System.**

**4. B.** An electrocardiogram records a person's heart rate and rhythm to evaluate how well the heart functions. **See Lesson: Cardiovascular System.**

**5. A.** Oxygen-rich blood, or blood with high oxygen levels, leaves the left side of the heart. **See Lesson: The Respiratory System.**

**6. B.** After deoxygenated blood is supplied with oxygen from the lungs within the pulmonary circuit, this oxygen-rich blood leaves the left side of the heart and is pumped out into systemic circulation.
**See Lesson: The Respiratory System.**

**7. C.** A hallmark symptom of irritable bowel syndrome is abdominal pain. **See Lesson: Gastrointestinal System.**

**8. B.** Rugae increase the surface area of the interior of the stomach. **See Lesson: Gastrointestinal System.**

**9. C.** Semen is formed in the male accessory glands (seminal vesicles, prostate gland, Cowper glands). These are all found within the male pelvis. **See Lesson: Reproductive System.**

**10. A.** The cervix is inside the pelvis; the vulva is comprised of external components. **See Lesson: Reproductive System.**

**11. D.** Filtration is important because it is the first of many steps along the nephrons during which necessary solutes and water are reabsorbed into the bloodstream, increasing the concentration of the urine that is formed. **See Lesson: The Urinary System.**

**12. C.** Roughly 180 liters of blood leave the renal artery on a daily basis, enter the glomerulus in the nephrons, and proceed through the renal tubules. The byproduct of this fluid, which is urine, empties into the bladder for storage. **See Lesson: The Urinary System.**

**13. D.** Bones make a mineral reservoir that contains roughly 9% of the body's calcium and 8% of the body's phosphorus. These minerals are used for various physiological functions performed in the body. **See Lesson: Skeletal System.**

**14. C.** The vertebral column is part of the axial skeleton. It protects the spinal cord from external damage. **See Lesson: Skeletal System.**

**15. A.** Actin is a thin band of myosin filament that attaches to a dark, striped band in the myofibril called the Z-line (or Z-disc). **See Lesson: Muscular System.**

**16. D.** The sarcoplasmic reticulum surrounds myofibrils in the skeletal muscle fiber and houses a certain concentration of calcium ion. Decreased levels of calcium in this structure can affect muscle contraction. **See Lesson: Muscular System.**

**17. A.** Molecules of ATP are used to energize and reenergize the protein molecules myosin according to the slide filament theory. The myosin myofilaments use ATP to attach their heads to thin actin filaments, pulling the thin filaments closer to the M-line during skeletal muscle contraction. **See Lesson: Muscular System.**

**18. C.** The outermost layer of the skin is the stratum corneum. The sebaceous glands are pores, or openings, in this layer. When acne forms due to a bacterial infection of the sebaceous glands, pimples forms on the stratum corneum. **See Lesson: Integumentary System.**

**19. A.** Basal cell carcinoma is a type of skin cancer that affects the epidermis. The stratum basale is the innermost layer of the epidermis. Within this layer, epidermal cells reproduce out of control and invade the dermis. **See Lesson: Integumentary System.**

**20. D.** Sensory nerves are responsible for receiving information from the external environment and sending that information to the CNS. Sensory nerves can collect this information using the senses like smelling. **See Lesson: The Nervous System.**

**21. D.** A neurotransmitter is a type of substance that is released from the presynaptic membrane of one neuron and binds to the receptor on the postsynaptic membrane of a different neuron. By binding, this substance stimulates excitation of the neuron causing a neural impulse to be transmitted. **See Lesson: The Nervous System.**

**22. C.** Diabetes results from improper uptake of glucose by insulin cells of the pancreas. **See Lesson: Endocrine System.**

**23. B.** Neuromodulators and neurotransmitters are secreted by nerve cells and aid the nervous system. As an example, acetylcholine is produced during stressful encounters. **See Lesson: Endocrine System.**

**24. B.** The B cells label invaders for later destruction by macrophages. **See Lesson: The Lymphatic System.**

**25. A.** Antibodies attach to any invading pathogens that might be present, marking them for destruction. **See Lesson: The Lymphatic System.**

# Section VIII. Physics

**1. D.** Mass and speed are always scalars. Acceleration can be a vector or a scalar, depending on the context. Velocity is always a vector; speed is the magnitude of the velocity. **See Lesson: Nature of Motion.**

**2. C.** An object undergoing projectile motion (in ideal conditions) has a constant horizontal velocity but a changing vertical velocity due to gravity. Thus, its horizontal acceleration is zero, but its vertical acceleration is nonzero. Only answer C is true. **See Lesson: Nature of Motion.**

**3. B.** Velocity is a vector, and its magnitude (or length) is the speed (a scalar). **See Lesson: Nature of Motion.**

**4. D.** According to Newton's third law, every action has an equal and opposite reaction—meaning the wall applies a force of equal magnitude but opposite in direction to the force that the man applies.
**See Lesson: Nature of Motion.**

**5. B.** Newton's first law is that an object's velocity remains fixed as long as no net force acts on that object. In this case, the ball on an ideal flat surface experiences no net forces, meaning its velocity will not change. **See Lesson: Nature of Motion.**

**6. D.** If the passengers were released at any point on the ride, they would move tangentially to the circle on which they were previously spinning. But because the ride holds onto them, it exerts a centripetal force constantly pulling them in. Thus, the passengers are experiencing the effects of inertia: their bodies tend to move linearly, so when they are pulled inward, inertia makes it feel like they are being thrown outward. **See Lesson: Friction.**

**7. C.** An object undergoing projectile motion maintains a constant horizontal velocity unless some force acts on it. The force in this case is friction due to air resistance. **See Lesson: Friction.**

**8. C.** Because friction is a force that generally acts in the direction opposite to an object's velocity, answers B and D are incorrect. Centripetal acceleration is a force perpendicular to velocity, eliminating answer A. Friction can cause movement of a fluid surrounding the object, such as in the case of a boat moving in the water. **See Lesson: Friction.**

**9. D.** Absent friction, the block would experience a net force due to gravity that would cause it to slide down the sloped surface. In this case, the friction force cancels any other forces, causing the block to remain stationary. **See Lesson: Friction.**

**10. A.** The centripetal force is equal in magnitude but opposite in direction to the centrifugal force, which is a ghost force. Thus, the children are experiencing a centripetal force to the east. **See Lesson: Friction.**

**11. B.** The angle of reflection of a wave is equal to the angle of incidence measured from the same line. In this case, the line is the normal or perpendicular line passing through the point at which the ray strikes the mirror. **See Lesson: Waves and Sounds.**

**12. B.** An ion is an atom with a net electric charge. Therefore, the number of protons must be different from the number of electrons. Neutrons have no electric charge and therefore have no bearing on the atom's net charge. **See Lesson: Waves and Sounds.**

**13. D.** Acceleration of a charge creates electromagnetic waves. Because the electrons in answers A and C are experiencing no acceleration, they do not create waves. In general, neither does an electron approaching a proton. An electron with a decreasing velocity is experiencing acceleration, creating electromagnetic waves. **See Lesson: Waves and Sounds.**

**14. C.** Mechanical waves involve oscillation of some material, such as water or air. Choices A, B, and D are electromagnetic waves—they can travel in the absence of a material. Seismic waves travel through solids and liquids as a result of geological events. **See Lesson: Waves and Sounds.**

**15. B.** The peak-to-peak amplitude is the distance between the crest and the trough. That distance is the difference between the measured heights of the crest and trough on the ruler: 12 feet – 3 feet = 9 feet.
**See Lesson: Waves and Sounds.**

**16. C.** He hypothesized that the force on the apple must be proportional to its mass. **See Lesson: Kinetic Energy.**

**17. B.** The airbag decreases the force exerted by the driver by extending the length of time over which the force is exerted. **See Lesson: Kinetic Energy.**

**18. C.** Impulse and momentum are directly proportional. **See Lesson: Kinetic Energy.**

**19. A.** The volleyball is moving, so it has kinetic energy. It is above ground level, so it also possesses potential energy. **See Lesson: Kinetic Energy.**

**20. A.** On a force-time graph, the impulse is the area under the curve. **See Lesson: Kinetic Energy.**

**21. B.** The greater the magnetic flux in a given region (alternatively, the denser the field lines in that region), the greater the magnetic force. Answer C is therefore correct. **See Lesson: Electricity and Magnetism.**

**22. C.** Ions are electrically charged particles, so they have electric fields associated with them. Also, since they are accelerating, they produce both magnetic fields and electromagnetic waves. Because they are moving in a vacuum, however, they have no medium in which to produce mechanical waves.
**See Lesson: Electricity and Magnetism.**

**23. A.** A material, such as many metals, that allows current to flow freely through it is called a conductor. **See Lesson: Electricity and Magnetism.**

**24. B.** Electric charges—positive or negative—can exist individually and separately from each other. Therefore, a positive electric charge and an electric current can both exist in empty space. Electromagnetic waves, which result from accelerated charge, can also exist in empty space. Magnetic poles, however, always come in pairs: a north pole and a south pole. **See Lesson: Electricity and Magnetism.**

**25. B.** The sum of currents going into a node must equal the sum of currents going out of the node. In this case, 3 amps are going in on one wire and 1 amp is going out on another. For the total in to equal the total out, the third wire must carry 2 amps out of the node. **See Lesson: Electricity and Magnetism.**